Biogenic Amines and Food Safety

Biogenic Amines and Food Safety

Editors

Maria Martuscelli
Dino Mastrocola

MDPI • Basel • Beijing • Wuhan • Barcelona • Belgrade • Manchester • Tokyo • Cluj • Tianjin

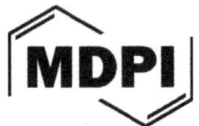

Editors
Maria Martuscelli
University of the Studies of
Teramo
Italy

Dino Mastrocola
University of the Studies of
Teramo
Italy

Editorial Office
MDPI
St. Alban-Anlage 66
4052 Basel, Switzerland

This is a reprint of articles from the Special Issue published online in the open access journal *Foods* (ISSN 2304-8158) (available at: https://www.mdpi.com/journal/foods/special_issues/biogenic_amines).

For citation purposes, cite each article independently as indicated on the article page online and as indicated below:

LastName, A.A.; LastName, B.B.; LastName, C.C. Article Title. *Journal Name* **Year**, *Volume Number*, Page Range.

ISBN 978-3-0365-0636-4 (Hbk)
ISBN 978-3-0365-0637-1 (PDF)

© 2021 by the authors. Articles in this book are Open Access and distributed under the Creative Commons Attribution (CC BY) license, which allows users to download, copy and build upon published articles, as long as the author and publisher are properly credited, which ensures maximum dissemination and a wider impact of our publications.

The book as a whole is distributed by MDPI under the terms and conditions of the Creative Commons license CC BY-NC-ND.

Contents

About the Editors . . . . **vii**

Maria Martuscelli, Luigi Esposito and Dino Mastrocola
Biogenic Amines' Content in Safe and Quality Food
Reprinted from: *Foods* 2021, *10*, 100, doi:10.3390/foods10010100 . . . . **1**

Martin Grootveld, Benita C. Percival and Jie Zhang
Extensive Chemometric Investigations of Distinctive Patterns and Levels of Biogenic Amines in
Fermented Foods: Human Health Implications
Reprinted from: *Foods* 2020, *9*, 1807, doi:10.3390/foods9121807 . . . . **3**

Young Kyoung Park, Jae Hoan Lee and Jae-Hyung Mah
Occurrence and Reduction of Biogenic Amines in Kimchi and Korean Fermented
Seafood Products
Reprinted from: *Foods* 2019, *8*, 547, doi:10.3390/foods8110547 . . . . **31**

**Chiu-Chu Hwang, Yi-Chen Lee, Chung-Yung Huang, Hsien-Feng Kung, Hung-Hui Cheng
and Yung-Hsiang Tsai**
Effect of Brine Concentrations on the Bacteriological and Chemical Quality and Histamine
Content of Brined and Dried Milkfish
Reprinted from: *Foods* 2020, *9*, 1597, doi:10.3390/foods9111597 . . . . **47**

Dalin Ly, Sigrid Mayrhofer, Julia-Maria Schmidt, Ulrike Zitz and Konrad J. Domig
Biogenic Amine Contents and Microbial Characteristics of Cambodian Fermented Foods
Reprinted from: *Foods* 2020, *9*, 198, doi:10.3390/foods9020198 . . . . **61**

Tianjiao Niu, Xing Li, Yongjie Guo and Ying Ma
Identification of a Lactic Acid Bacteria to Degrade Biogenic Amines in Chinese Rice Wine and
Its Enzymatic Mechanism
Reprinted from: *Foods* 2019, *8*, 312, doi:10.3390/foods8080312 . . . . **81**

**Young Kyoung Park, Young Hun Jin, Jun-Hee Lee, Bo Young Byun, Junsu Lee,
KwangCheol Casey Jeong and Jae-Hyung Mah**
The Role of *Enterococcus faecium* as a Key Producer and Fermentation Condition as an
Influencing Factor in Tyramine Accumulation in *Cheonggukjang*
Reprinted from: *Foods* 2020, *9*, 915, doi:10.3390/foods9070915 . . . . **95**

**Umile Gianfranco Spizzirri, Francesca Ieri, Margherita Campo, Donatella Paolino,
Donatella Restuccia and Annalisa Romani**
Biogenic Amines, Phenolic, and Aroma-Related Compounds of Unroasted and Roasted Cocoa
Beans with Different Origin
Reprinted from: *Foods* 2019, *8*, 306, doi:10.3390/foods8080306 . . . . **113**

**Johannes Delgado-Ospina, Carla Daniela Di Mattia, Antonello Paparella, Dino Mastrocola,
Maria Martuscelli and Clemencia Chaves-Lopez**
Effect of Fermentation, Drying and Roasting on Biogenic Amines and Other Biocompounds in
Colombian Criollo Cocoa Beans and Shells
Reprinted from: *Foods* 2020, *9*, 520, doi:10.3390/foods9040520 . . . . **133**

So Hee Yoon, Eunmi Koh, Bogyoung Choi and BoKyung Moon
Effects of Soaking and Fermentation Time on Biogenic Amines Content of *Maesil* (*Prunus Mume*) Extract
Reprinted from: *Foods* **2019**, *8*, 592, doi:10.3390/foods8110592 . . . . **153**

Annalisa Serio, Jessica Laika, Francesca Maggio, Giampiero Sacchetti, Flavio D'Alessandro, Chiara Rossi, Maria Martuscelli, Clemencia Chaves-López and Antonello Paparella
Casing Contribution to Proteolytic Changes and Biogenic Amines Content in the Production of an Artisanal Naturally Fermented Dry Sausage
Reprinted from: *Foods* **2020**, *9*, 1286, doi:10.3390/foods9091286 . . . . **167**

Hana Buchtova, Dani Dordevic, Iwona Duda, Alena Honzlova and Piotr Kulawik
Modeling Some Possible Handling Ways with Fish Raw Material in Home-Made Sushi Meal Preparation
Reprinted from: *Foods* **2019**, *8*, 459, doi:10.3390/foods8100459 . . . . **187**

About the Editors

Maria Martuscelli was born in Muro Lucano (PZ) in 1970. She is married and has two daughters. Maria Martuscelli is Associate Professor of Food Technology in the Faculty of Bioscience and Technology for Food, Agriculture, and Environment of University of the Studies of Teramo (Italy). She is a member of the Italian Society of Food Technology and entered in the Register of Experts in Industrial Research. Many outputs of her research are carried out in scientific projects which are supported by public institutions or private companies. Her research activity has seen her contribution in foreign institutions such as the 'Unite Mixte de Recherche et Flaveur Vision du consommateu comportment, of the' Institut National de la Recherche Agronomique, in Dijon (France); moreover, she was involved in data collection for the European Food Safety Autority, on "biogenic amines in food". She is the author of 96 scientific works, published in international and national journals, proceedings of national and international Congresses and chapters of books.

Dino Mastrocola was born in Guardiagrele (CH) in 1958. He is married and has a son. Dino Mastrocola is full professor of Food Technology in the Faculty of Bioscience and Technology for Food, Agriculture, and Environment of University of the Studies of Teramo (Italy) and Rector of the same institution since November 2018. He carries out research activities in the field of Food Science and Technology and is involved in national and international research projects. He participated in the Food Improvement Project in China, coordinated by prof. Antonino Zichichi at the International Centre for Scientific Culture - World Laboratory in Lausanne. He carried out a strict research activity in the R&D of Unilever Research in Colworth House (England) and at the Academy of Sciences in Beijing. From 1996 to 2003, he took part in the European food science dissemination project Flair Flow Europe. He is the author of 20 essays and over 180 scientific publications, and is also a founding member of the Italian Society of Food Sciences and Technologies.

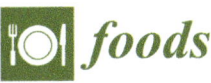

Editorial

Biogenic Amines' Content in Safe and Quality Food

Maria Martuscelli *, Luigi Esposito and Dino Mastrocola

Faculty of Bioscience and Technology for Food, Agriculture and Environment, University of Teramo, Via R. Balzarini 1, 64100 Teramo, Italy; lesposito2@unite.it (L.E.); dmastrocola@unite.it (D.M.)
* Correspondence: mmartuscelli@unite.it

Biogenic amines (BAs) are low-molecular-weight, nitrogenous compounds (mainly polar bases) coming from the decarboxylation of free amino acids or by amination or transamination of aldehydes and ketones. To our knowledge, BAs are essential for cellular development and growth, are important regulators of several processes such as brain activity, regulation of body temperature, stomach pH, gastric acid secretion, the immune response, and the synthesis of hormones and alkaloids, among others [1]. Decarboxylation of free amino acids represents the primary way of BAs' obtention. Microorganisms involved in this process are positive to the decarboxylase enzyme, with the pathways that seem to be strain dependent rather than species specific [2]. At any rate, the presence of proteins (amino acids), favorable growing and fermenting conditions, and the possibility of external contaminations during food processing are important factors in BAs' increase. An important contribution is also given by several pro-technological strains, in particular lactic acid bacteria (LAB) from the genera *Lactobacillus*, *Leuconostoc*, *Lactococcus*, *Enterococcus*, and *Streptococcus*, were recently deeply reviewed as they are high tyramine producers. Del Rio et al. [3] clarified the harmful effect of this amine in boosting histamine toxicity besides being responsible for the so-called "cheese reaction". Although starters are generally considered secure and good for both food safety and the general health status of the human body, there does not exist any regulation looking at the decarboxylase positivity of bacteria. As a matter of fact, it is challenging to use BAs' content in food as a unit of measure to establish food safety. Evidence of strict correlations between personal sensitivity and genetical predisposition for BAs' intoxication was found. In particular, the compromising of the detoxification system was enacted by mono and di-amine oxidase (MAO and DAO) enzymes in the intestinal epithelium that change for every individual. Great attention should be reserved not only to those subjects consuming mono and di-amino oxidase inhibitors (MAOI and DAOI) drugs, as they may become particularly sensitive to BAs' action, but should also include those experiencing any impairment in the functioning of the small intestine or kidneys and so, even coeliac subjects, people who suffered surgery, or those who are in treatment for cancer and other pathologies [4,5]. The scientific research is giving growing insights into BAs' presence in all food matrices including fresh fruit and vegetables, pulses, baby foods, alcoholic beverage [6–8], and halal foods [9]. This scenario forces scientists to turn their attention to the fact that all the population is at risk for experiencing BAs' accumulation by their choices in meal composition, food sources, and of course specific sensitivity. This editorial has collected papers giving an interesting outlook on the content of BAs' in food and a possible strategy to reduce their occurrence, BAs' role in the promotion of aroma, and the specific capacity of selected bacteria in promoting their accumulation and/or degradation. All these papers actively contribute to creating a more complete frame on the theme keeping constant the fact that the presence of BAs' in food represents an essential part of food quality and food safety.

Funding: This research received no external funding.

Conflicts of Interest: The authors declare no conflict of interest.

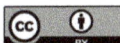

Citation: Martuscelli, M.; Esposito, L.; Mastrocola, D. Biogenic Amines' Content in Safe and Quality Food. *Foods* **2021**, *10*, 100. https://doi.org/10.3390/foods10010100

Received: 21 December 2020
Accepted: 2 January 2021
Published: 6 January 2021

Publisher's Note: MDPI stays neutral with regard to jurisdictional claims in published maps and institutional affiliations.

Copyright: © 2021 by the authors. Licensee MDPI, Basel, Switzerland. This article is an open access article distributed under the terms and conditions of the Creative Commons Attribution (CC BY) license (https://creativecommons.org/licenses/by/4.0/).

References

1. Wójcik, W.; Łukasiewicz, M.; Puppel, K. Biogenic amines—Formation, action and toxicity—A review. *J. Sci. Food Agric.* **2020**. [CrossRef] [PubMed]
2. Sudo, N. Biogenic Amines: Signals between Commensal Microbiota and Gut Physiology. *Front. Endocrinol.* **2019**, *10*, 504. [CrossRef] [PubMed]
3. Del Rio, B.; Redruello, B.; Linares, D.M.; Ladero, V.; Fernandez, M.; Martin, M.C.; Ruas-Madiedo, P.; Alvarez, M.A. The dietary biogenic amines tyramine and histamine show synergistic toxicity towards intestinal cells in culture. *Food Chem.* **2017**, *218*, 249–255. [CrossRef] [PubMed]
4. Del Rio, B.; Redruello, B.; Fernandez, M.; Cruz Martin, M.; Laderoa, V.; Alvarez, M.A. The biogenic amine tryptamine, unlike β-phenylethylamine, shows in vitro cytotoxicity at concentrations that have been found in foods. *Food Chem.* **2020**, *331*, 127303. [CrossRef] [PubMed]
5. Esposito, F.; Montuori, P.; Schettino, M.; Velotto, S.; Stasi, T.; Romano, R.; Cirillo, T. Level of Biogenic Amines in Red and White Wines, Dietary Exposure, and Histamine-Mediated Symptoms upon Wine Ingestion. *Molecules* **2019**, *24*, 3629. [CrossRef] [PubMed]
6. Dabadé, D.S.; Jacxsens, L.; Miclotte, L.; Abatih, E.; Devlieghere, F.; De Meulenaer, B. Survey of multiple biogenic amines and correlation to microbiological quality and free amino acids in foods. *Food Control* **2021**, *120*, 107497. [CrossRef]
7. Czajkowska-Mysłek, A.; Leszczynska, J. Risk assessment related to biogenic amines occurrence in ready-to-eat baby foods. *Food Chem. Toxicol.* **2017**, *107*, 82–92. [CrossRef] [PubMed]
8. Chaves-Lopez, C.; Serio, A.; Montalvo, C.; Ramirez, C.; Peréz Alvares, J.A.; Paparella, A.; Mastrocola, D.; Martuscelli, M. Effect of nisin on biogenic amines and shelf life of vacuum packaged rainbow trout (*Oncorhynchus mykiss*) fillets. *J. Food Sci. Technol.* **2017**, *54*, 3268–3277. [CrossRef] [PubMed]
9. Martuscelli, M.; Serio, A.; Capezio, O.; Mastrocola, D. Safety, Quality and Analytical Authentication of ḥalāl Meat Products, with Particular Emphasis on Salami: A Review. *Foods* **2020**, *9*, 1111. [CrossRef] [PubMed]

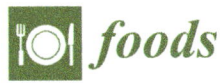

Article

Extensive Chemometric Investigations of Distinctive Patterns and Levels of Biogenic Amines in Fermented Foods: Human Health Implications

Martin Grootveld [1,*], Benita C. Percival [1] and Jie Zhang [2]

[1] Leicester School of Pharmacy, De Montfort University, The Gateway, Leicester LE1 9BH, UK; p11279990@alumni365.dmu.ac.uk
[2] Green Pasture Products, 416 E. Fremont Street, O'Neill, NE 68763, USA; gpplab@greenpasture.org
* Correspondence: mgrootveld@dmu.ac.uk; Tel.: +44-0-116-250-6443

Received: 19 October 2020; Accepted: 27 November 2020; Published: 5 December 2020

Abstract: Although biogenic amines (BAs) present in fermented foods exert important health-promoting and physiological function support roles, their excessive ingestion can give rise to deleterious toxicological effects. Therefore, here we have screened the BA contents and supporting food quality indices of a series of fermented food products using a multianalyte-chemometrics strategy. A liquid chromatographic triple quadrupole mass spectrometric (LC-MS/MS) technique was utilized for the simultaneous multicomponent analysis of 8 different BAs, and titratable acidity, pH, total lipid content, and thiobarbituric acid-reactive substances (TBARS) values were also determined. Rigorous univariate and multivariate (MV) chemometric data analysis strategies were employed to evaluate results acquired. Almost all foods analyzed had individual and total BA contents that were within recommended limits. The chemometrics methods applied were useful for recognizing characteristic patterns of BA analytes and food quality measures between some fermented food classes, and for assessing their inter-relationships and potential metabolic sources. MV analysis of constant sum-normalized BA profile data demonstrated characteristic signatures for cheese (cadaverine only), fermented cod liver oil (2-phenylethylamine, tyramine, and tryptamine), and wine/vinegar products (putrescine, spermidine, and spermine). In conclusion, this LC-MS/MS-linked chemometrics approach was valuable for (1) contrasting and distinguishing BA catabolite signatures between differing fermented foods, and (2) exploring and evaluating the health benefits and/or possible adverse public health risks of such products.

Keywords: biogenic amines (BAs); fermented foods; chemometrics; multivariate (MV) statistical analysis; liquid chromatographic triple quadrupole mass spectrometric (LC-MS/MS) analysis; public health; lipid peroxidation; antioxidants

1. Introduction

Biogenic amines (BAs) may be biosynthesized and degraded via normal metabolic activities in animals, plants, and micro-organisms. As such, these amines occur in a wide variety of foods, such as fish, meat, and cheese products, and especially in fermented foods such as wines, and yoghurts, etc. [1–3]. BA formation in foods usually occurs via the decarboxylation of amino acids [3], of which there are rich sources in these matrices; for example, amino acids are present at very high levels in grapes, and comprise ca. 30–40% of the total nitrogen content of wines [1–3].

Metabolic pathways available in lactic acid bacteria, which have the ability to grow and thrive in foods and beverages, generate significant levels of BAs. Routes available for this are the enzymatic production of putrescine from ornithine (catalyzed by ornithine decarboxylase) and/or from arginine via agmatine, a scheme involving prior conversion of the amino acid substrate to agmatine with arginine decarboxylase, followed by transformation of agmatine to N-carbamoylputrescine via the action of agmatine imino-hydroxylase, and then on to putrescine (a second route for its generation involves the conversion of arginine to ornithine and then to this product via the above ornithine decarboxylase-catalyzed route); putrescine to spermine, a process involving the enzyme spermine synthase, and then spermine to spermidine via the actions of spermidine synthase; cadaverine from lysine with lysine carboxylase and a pyridoxal phosphate co-factor; 2-phenylethylamine from phenylalanine catalyzed by aromatic amino acid carboxylases, including tyrosine decarboxylase; tyramine from tyrosine via tyrosine decarboxylase action; histamine from histidine with histidine decarboxylase; tryptamine from tryptophan with tryptophan decarboxylase, another pyridoxal phosphate-dependent enzyme; and trimethylamine from trimethylamine-N-oxide with a trimethylamine-N-oxide reductase (enzymes involved in the conversion of amino acids to BAs are classified as decarboxylase deaminases) [4,5]. BAs may also be biosynthesized from the amination and transamination of aldehydes and ketones [5], and this may be of some relevance to their detection in marine oil products which have been allowed to autoxidize. Indeed, a range of aldehyde species arise from the fragmentation of conjugated hydroperoxydienes, which are lipid oxidation products resulting from the peroxidation of polyunsaturated fatty acids (PUFAs) [6].

Overall, microbial sources of BAs include yeasts, as well as gram-positive and -negative bacteria [7]. The physiological activity of BA synthesis in prokaryotic cells predominantly appears to be associated with bacterial defense mechanisms employed to combat environmental acidity [8–10]. Hence, amino acid decarboxylation in this manner enhances survival under harsh acidic stress states [9] via proton consumption, and amine and CO_2 excretion required to facilitate restorations of internal pH values [11].

As with their biosynthesis, the catabolism of BAs is extensively outlined and reviewed in [5]. In view of their potentially toxic nature, fortunately humans have detoxification enzyme systems which catabolically oxidize BAs in vivo. These enzymes principally comprise monoamine and diamine oxidases (MAOs and DAOs respectively). MAOs are flavoproteins acting by the oxidative deamination of BAs to their corresponding aldehydes, along with hydrogen peroxide (H_2O_2) and ammonia. Two different forms of MAO have been identified in humans [5]. DAOs are responsible for histamine catabolism, as is histamine-N-methyltransferase, the latter catalyzing a ring methylation process [5].

Evidence available indicates that BAs may confer a series of human health benefits, which involve their interactions with a wide variety of intracellular macromolecules such as proteins, DNA, and RNA. Indeed, monoamines are typically precursors of neuromodulators and neurotransmitters [12]. Moreover, evidence is accumulating that the polyamines spermine and spermidine are important for sexual function and fertility [13], and polyamines in general are associated with cell growth and differentiation, including protein biosynthesis [14]. Indeed, the generation of BAs in eukaryotic cells is essential, since they are required for the critical biosynthesis of hormones, alkaloids, proteins, and nucleic acids [15]. One further plausible health benefit offered by both monoamine and polyamine forms of BAs is their antioxidant potential [16], and recent studies have shown that they function efficiently in this context, and protect against adverse unsaturated fatty acid peroxidation reactions when present in or supplemented to culinary oils, and other foods rich in PUFAs [6] (details regarding the nature and mechanisms of these antioxidant actions are provided in Section S1 of the Supplementary Materials).

Notwithstanding, the availability of these amines in the diet has not been without its problems. Indeed, adverse toxicological events may be stimulated by the ingestion of foods which are known to provide high concentrations of these agents, and one notable example is the provocation of deleterious hypertensive events in patients receiving therapies with monoamine oxidase inhibitor (MAOI) drug treatments [17]. A further problem is the depression of histamine oxidation, a process which arises from the ingestion of putrescine and agmatine, which serve as potentiators of this process; this promotes histamine toxicity episodes in humans [18]. Moreover, it has been reported that BAs such as putrescine and agmatine give rise to their corresponding carcinogenic nitrosoamines from reactions with nitrite anion, dietary or in vivo [19].

Human sensitivity to BAs is contingent on the availability and activities of detoxifying enzymes featured in BA metabolism, i.e., specific ones such as histamine methyltransferase, and those less specific such as mono- and diamine oxidases. However, since these enzymes are inhibited by different classes of drugs, including neuromuscular blocking agents such as alcuronium, antidepressants [20], and ethanol [21], the accumulation of BAs by the consumption of selected foods and beverages can, at least in principal, give rise to clinical disorders, including the extremely hazardous serotonin syndrome [22]. Further details regarding the adverse health effects associated with the excessive intake of BAs are delineated in Section S2 of the Supplementary Materials.

Current consumer demands for safer and healthier foods has prompted a high level of research investigations focused on BAs, although it should be noted that further studies are required to expand this area. High levels of BAs can build up in fermented foods, including fish, fish sauce, and cheese products. Their biosynthesis and accumulation therein are critically dependent on the availability of bacteria with decarboxylase-deaminase enzyme activities, environmental conditions that are unrestrictive towards their growth and propagation, and the efficient functioning of BA-generating enzymes, together with the presence of sufficient amounts of the relevant amino acid substrates required.

Hence, supporting analytical methodologies for the identification and measurement of BAs are of much importance to the food industry, and also from a public health perspective. Such methods should ideally offer high levels of reliability in order to monitor the potential health benefits offered by fermented food products, and also to circumvent any toxicological risks to consumers arising from their excessive production therein; realistic estimates of their human consumption are also major factors for consideration. To date, BA determinations in foods have represented a major challenge for analytical chemists in view of their non-chromophoric nature, their natural occurrence in complex multicomponent food and biological matrices, and high polarities, factors which are further complicated by a requirement for high analytical sensitivity, potential interferences, and, where relevant, chromatographic separation/resolution issues arising from the presence of many structurally-related agents in samples requiring such analysis [23]. Methods previously available for this purpose, and those for the screening of BA-producing bacteria, are outlined in Section S3 of the Supplementary Materials.

Notwithstanding, in principle, the simultaneous and direct multicomponent determination of BAs by the LC-MS/MS method described here, or a newly-developed strategy focused on largely non-invasive high-resolution proton (^{1}H) nuclear magnetic resonance (NMR) analysis [6], serve as valuable assets which, in combination with MV chemometrics strategies, may be employed for the recognition of patterns of these bacterial catabolites which are characteristic of differential bacterial sources of these agents.

Multivariate (MV) data analysis of multicomponent analytical datasets serves as an extremely powerful means of probing and tracking metabolic signatures that are characteristic of differential groups or classifications of samples, and when applied to explore the biochemical basis of human disease etiology, this technique is commonly known as metabolomics [24]. Indeed, to date this combination of multianalyte-MV analysis has been copiously utilized in many biomedical and clinical investigations, mainly for the identification of diagnostic or prognostic monitoring biomarkers for human diseases. However, when applied in a non-biomedical context, the technique can best be described as chemometrics, a technology which also commonly employs many of the MV data analysis strategies used in metabolomics experiments.

In view of the rich sources of BAs in fermented food products, in this study we determined the contents of a total of 8 different BAs in a series of commercially-available fermented fish, fish sauce/paste, vegetable sauce, cheese, wine/vinegar, and cod liver oil (FCLO) products. For this purpose, we employed both univariate and MV chemometrics analysis techniques in order to recognize differential patterns of these catabolites, which may be representative or characteristic of their food, bacterial, metabolic pathway, and/or food processing technology sources. Such analytical information also serves to furnish us with valuable information regarding the provision of these important nutrients in the human diet, and to evaluate the toxicological/adverse health risks presented by the ingestion of fermented foods containing portentously excessive levels of these agents. Currently, a total BA content of *ca.* 1000 ppm is linked to toxicity, and in recommended manufacturing practices, 100 ppm histamine, or a total BA content of 200 ppm, are considered acceptable levels which do not give rise to any associated adverse health effects [25].

These studies were supported by the consideration of further food quality determinations on these fermented food products, which consisted of pH values, titratable acidities (TAs), and total lipid contents, along with an adapted method for determining lipid peroxidation status (thiobarbituric acid-reactive substances (TBARS)).

With the exception of a small number of studies focused on BAs detectable in selected wine products, e.g., [26], to the best of our knowledge this is the first time that MV chemometrics techniques have been applied to explore potentially valuable "between-food classification: distinctions between the concentrations and patterns of BAs in a series of different food products, albeit fermented ones. Therefore, the aims of this investigation are to explore the abilities and reliabilities of LC-MS/MS-based chemometrics analysis techniques to: (1) evaluate the possible public health benefits and/or risks of BAs arising from the human consumption of fermented foods; and (2) effectively compare and distinguish between differing patterns of BA molecules in different classes of fermented food products.

2. Materials and Methods

2.1. Fermented Food Products

Fermented food products (cheese, fish, fish sauce/paste, vegetable sauce, and wine/vinegar classifications) were randomly selected and purchased from a variety of US retail outlets based in the state of Nebraska. These comprised $n = 4$ fish samples, $n = 9$ fish sauce/paste samples, $n = 4$ vegetable sauce samples, $n = 5$ cheeses, and $n = 4$ wine/vinegar samples (Table 1). Details of the fermentation processes employed by the manufacturers involved were unavailable. Prior to analysis, all samples were stored in a darkened freezer at a temperature of −20 °C for a maximal duration of 72 h.

Table 1. Details of fermented food products investigated for each classification.

Fermented Food Classification	Products Investigated
Cheeses	Full-fat pasteurized cow's milk soft cheese (washed with brandy); full-fat French cow's milk soft-ripened cheese; semi-soft washed rind Limberger cheese; full-fat pasteurized cow's milk soft cheese; French cow's milk soft cheese.
Fish	Pickled mud fish; pickled gourami fish; dried gourami fish; salted crab.
Fish Sauce/Paste	Loc fish sauce; scad fish sauce; anchovy fish sauce; Vietnamese fish sauce (×2); Thai fish sauce; standard U.S. fish sauce; shrimp paste (×2).
Vegetable Sauce	Bean curd; chili bean sauce; kimchi sauce; spicy tofu sauce.
Wine/Vinegar	Balsamic vinegar (×2); red wine vinegar; Casella wine.

Fermented cod liver oil (FCLO) was a natural product that was manufactured and kindly donated by Green Pastures LLC, 416 E. Fremont O'Neill, NE 68763, USA for this study. Separate batches ($n = 10$) of this FCLO product were randomly selected by independent visitors to its manufacturing site throughout a 6-month period, as noted in [6].

FCLO products were prepared from the fermentation of Pacific cod livers. Livers were frozen (−20 °C) within 40 min following their harvest from the Pacific Ocean, and then transported to a preparation facility whilst remaining in the frozen state. Fermented CLO was produced from these cod liver sources using a novel and proprietary fermentation technology. Briefly, cod livers were loaded into a fermentation tank, and both salt and the fermentation starter agent were added to induce the process. The tank was completely sealed during the fermentation and, following periods of 28–84 days, the raw FCLO product accumulated and was then isolated from the tank. Following fermentation, products were centrifuged, filtered to remove particulates, and then packed.

On arrival at the laboratory, FCLO product sample batches were de-identified through their transfer to coded but unlabeled universal storage containers. Each sample was subsequently stored in a darkened freezer at −80 °C until ready for analysis (predominantly within 24 h of their arrival).

2.2. Analysis of BAs in Fermented Food Product Samples

A liquid chromatographic triple quadrupole mass spectrometric (LC-MS/MS) technique was employed for the simultaneous analysis of up to 11 BAs in fermented food products using an adaption of the LC-MS/MS method reported in [27]. A Shimadzu 8045 LC-MS/MS facility was used for this purpose, the MS/MS detection system for the monitoring and molecular characterization of eluting BA analytes. Primarily, pre-set accurately weighed masses of food samples were shaken with a 20.0 mL volume of 70% (v/v) methanol/30% (v/v) water for 20 min, which were then centrifuged at 7000 rpm at 4 °C for another 20 min period. The clear supernatant was subsequently transferred to 1.7 mL volume amber auto-sampler vials for LC-MS/MS analysis. For wine/vinegar and FCLO samples, fixed aliquots were filtered using a 0.45 μm filter paper prior to the above methanol/water extraction stage.

The LC facility comprised a pump, vacuum degasser, auto-sampler, and column compartment, and finally a secondary variable wavelength spectrophotometric detection system was used for these analyses. This system could operate up to 800 bar. The internal standard (IS) utilized was tetra-deuterated histamine (histamine-$\alpha,\alpha,\beta,\beta-d_4$, (2HCl)), which was purchased from C/D/N Isotopes Inc. (Pointe-Claire, Quebec, Canada). IS m/z values employed for quantification purposes were 116.1 and 99.0 for precursor and product ions, respectively (112.1 and 95.1 respectively for undeuterated histamine).

A 3-μm 50 × 2.1 mm Pinnacle® DB pentaflurophenyl (PFP) base with propyl spacer column was employed for optimal BA analysis. Mobile phase 1 contained water solutions of the ion-pair reagent trifluoroacetic acid (TFA) (either 0.05 or 0.10% (w/v)), and mobile phase 2 was acetonitrile containing equivalent TFA concentrations. BA analytes were monitored in positive ion mode for the MS/MS detection system. Reporting limit values for fermented food samples were 1 ppm for all BAs determined.

Authentic BA calibration standards were purchased from Sigma-Aldrich Chemical Co. (St. Louis, MO, USA) (histamine, H7125; cadaverine, 33220; putrescine, D13208; 2-phenylethylamine, P6513; spermidine, 85578; tyramine, T2879; tryptamine, 193747), and Alfa Aesar Inc. (Heysham, UK) (spermine, J63060). BA contents were determined from calibration curves developed with standard solutions of concentrations 0.5, 1.0, 10.0, 50.00, 100.0, 200.0, and 400.0 ppb for each BA.

2.3. Total Lipid Analysis

Total lipid (fat) analysis was performed according to the AOAC 922.06 method. Briefly, homogenized samples were treated with HCl, and then washed at least two-fold with both petroleum ether and diethyl ether; solutions arising therefrom were then placed in pre-weighed beaker containers. Subsequently, the lipid-containing ether solutions were evaporated, and the (w/w) % content of lipid was determined directly from the weight gain of the container.

2.4. Determination of Thiobarbituric Acid-Reactive Substances (TBARS) Values

Primarily, accurately-weighed samples were digested with perchloric acid ($HClO_4$), and subsequently the resulting clear filtered supernatant solution was reacted with thiobarbituric acid (TBA) for a period of 15–18 h at 27.5 °C according to the method outlined in [28]. The absorbance value at a wavelength of 532 nm was then determined, and TBA-reactive substance (TBARS) values were reported as mg/kg (ppm) units following their quantification from a calibration curve developed with MDA standards.

2.5. Titratable Acidity (TA) and pH Value Determinations

Titratable acidity values were determined using the AOAC 947.05 method [29], and pH measurements were made using a modified FO PROC 31 protocol which is based on the USDA PHM method. The latter approach is based on the formation of a homogenized food/water slurry which was allowed to stand prior to pH determination with a probe.

2.6. Experimental Design and Statistical Analysis

2.6.1. Univariate Statistical Analysis

The experimental design for univariate analysis of the individual BA, TA, pH, and further variable dataset involved an analysis-of-variance (ANOVA) model, which incorporated 1 prime factor and 2 sources of variation: (1) that "between-fermented food classifications", a qualitative fixed effect (FF_i); and (2) experimental error (e_{ij}). The mathematical model for this experimental design is shown in equation 1, in which y_{ij} represents the (univariate) BA or alternative analyte dependent variable values observed, and μ their overall population mean values in the absence of any significant, influential sources of variation.

$$y_{ij} = μ + FF_i + e_{ij} \qquad (1)$$

ANOVA was conducted with *XLSTAT2016* and *2020* software. Datasets were autoscaled (i.e., the mean value of each parameter monitored was subtracted from each entry, and the residual then divided by food class standard deviation, which was computed with an $(n − 1)$ divisor) prior to analysis. In view of heterogeneities between the intra-sample variances of fermented food classifications, i.e., heteroscedasticities, the robust Welch test was employed to determine statistical significance of differences observed between the mean BA and other food quality variable values for each fermented food group. *post-hoc* ANOVA evaluations of the statistical significance of differences between the mean values of individual fermented food groups were performed using the Bonferroni test.

A similar ANOVA-based experimental design was applied to additional design models selected to determine the statistical significance and food class specificities of BA analytes only. For these purposes, the 8 BA dataset, which included those determined in the $n = 10$ batches of the FCLO product, was either constant sum (CS)-normalized or not, and then generalized logarithmically (glog)-transformed, and finally autoscaled prior to analysis. The CS normalization data preparation task was applied in order to evaluate the significance of fermented food classification-dependent BA profile patterns. The non-CS-normalized dataset also included total BA level as a further possible explanatory variable. *MetaboAnalyst 4.0* (University of Alberta and National Research Council, National Institute for Nanotechnology (NINT), Edmonton, AB, Canada) was utilized for the analysis of these data. Probability values obtained from *post-hoc* ANOVA comparisons of individual BA levels between fermented food classes were false discovery rate (FDR)-corrected.

Tests for the heteroscedasticity of ANOVA model residuals (Levene's test) were performed using *XLSTAT2020* (Addinsoft, Paris, France).

2.6.2. Multivariate Chemometrics and Algorithmic Computational Intelligence (CI) Analyses

Principal component analysis (PCA), partial least squares-discriminatory analysis (PLS-DA), correlation, and agglomerative hierarchical clustering (AHC) analyses of the combined BA dataset were performed using *XLSTAT2016* and *2020* and *MetaboAnalyst 4.0* [30] software module options. The dataset was generalized glog-transformed, and autoscaled prior *to MetaboAnalyst 4.0* analysis, but only autoscaled for *XLSTAT2016* and *2020* analyses. All these MV analysis strategies were primarily performed on non-CS-normalized data. For the PCA and PLS-DA analyses, limits for significant explanatory variable loadings vectors/coefficients were set at $≤−0.40$ or $≥0.40$. Validation of PLS-DA models was performed by determining component number-dependent Q^2 values (predominantly for two classification comparisons), and permutation testing with 2000 permutations. The significance of variable contributions to these models was determined by the computation of variable importance parameter (VIP) values (values >0.90 were considered significant).

Additional PCA analysis was performed in order to explore associations or independencies of individual BAs and other active variables considered, e.g., pH and TA values, total lipid contents, etc. For this purpose, a maximal 5 PC limit was applied, and PCA was then conducted on autoscaled data using varimax rotation and Kaiser normalization. The loadings of each analytical variable on successive orthogonal PCs was then sequentially evaluated. Similarly, this form of PCA was employed to investigate possible inter-relationships and orthogonalities between BA variables analyzed in FCLO batches sampled from the same manufacturing source specified above.

A further PCA model involved its application to the 8 BA dataset alone, which was either CS-normalized or not, glog-transformed, and autoscaled prior to analysis. As noted above, the CS-normalization data preparation step was utilized in order to evaluate the significance of any differential patterns or distributions of BA analytes which may be characteristic of fermented food classifications. This analysis was performed using *MetaboAnalyst 4.0*.

The random forest (RF) machine-learning algorithm approach was also utilized for classification and discriminatory variable selection purposes (*MetaboAnalyst 4.0* Random Forest module), with 1000 trees (*ntree*) and 4 predictors selected at each node (*mtry*) subsequent to tuning. The dataset was randomly split into training and test sets containing approximately two-thirds and one-third of entries respectively. The training set was employed to construct the RFs model, and an out-of-the-bag (OOB) error value was determined to evaluate the classification performance of this. Again, this analysis was performed on the glog-transformed and autoscaled dataset, either with or without prior CS-normalization as specified in the manuscript.

Missing data, specifically total lipid and (TBARS):(total lipid) ratios for 2 × fish sauce/paste, 1 × vegetable sauce, 1 × wine/vinegar, and 1 × cheese samples, were estimated by the support vector machine (SVM) impute technique [31] (*MetaboAnalyst 4.0*), or supplementation with the explanatory variable column mean values, along with a corresponding reduction in degrees of freedom available for parametric univariate statistical testing (*XLSTAT2016 or 2020*).

3. Results and Discussion

3.1. BA Levels and Food Quality Indices in Fermented Food Products, and Univariate Analysis of These Analytical Data

Mean ± SEM values for the individual and total BA contents of the FF products investigated are provided in Table 2. The major contributors towards the relatively high BA levels observed in fermented cheese samples were cadaverine (mean 60% of total) and tyramine (mean 21.5% of total). Although three of the cheese products analyzed had total BA concentrations of 30–63 ppm, two of them were found to be as high as 666 and 780 ppm, which were markedly above the recommended 200 ppm content limit. The ANOVA Welch test demonstrated that there were highly significant differences between these total BA values (Table 3), as expected ($p = 2.84 \times 10^{-4}$); such differences were largely explicable by those observed between the cheese and wine/vinegar product classifications investigated.

Hence, characteristic "markers" of fermented cheese samples appeared to be cadaverine and tyramine, which had contents markedly elevated over those of the other fermented food products evaluated, although there were very high intra-fermented food classification variances for these estimates.

Table 2. Biogenic amines (BA) contents and quality indices of fermented foods investigated. Mean ± SEM BA levels, and titratable acidity (TA), pH, total lipid, thiobarbituric acid-reactive substances (TBARS) and (TBARS):(total lipid) ratio values, for five classes of fermented food products (cheese, fish, fish sauce/paste, vegetable sauce, and wine/vinegar) purchased at a range of U.S. retail outlets (bracketed numbers represent the number of different products analyzed for each classification).

BA Variable/ppm	Cheese (5)	Fish (4)	Fish Sauce (9)	Vegetable Sauce (4)	Wine/Vinegar (4)
Cadaverine	191.6 ± 99.8	30.7 ± 5.6	45.2 ± 8.2	30.6 ± 14.0	0.7 ± 0.7
Histamine	5.7 ± 1.6	10.6 ± 2.9	20.0 ± 5.8	17.7 ± 9.5	1.9 ± 1.9
2-Phenylethylamine	11.1 ± 6.8	13.1 ± 8.0	8.3 ± 4.2	5.00 ± 5.00	nd
Putrescine	21.2 ± 14.9	14.9 ± 7.2	18.9 ± 5.1	18.4 ± 7.7	3.3 ± 0.15
Spermidine	9.6 ± 3.2	10.9 ± 2.5	15.0 ± 1.9	24.5 ± 10.1	4.4 ± 1.5
Spermine	3.5 ± 2.2	12.6 ± 4.5	18.7 ± 3.0	11.4 ± 4.3	1.5 ± 1.5
Tryptamine	7.0 ± 5.8	2.0 ± 0.7	5.6 ± 1.7	3.4 ± 1.0	nd
Tyramine	69.4 ± 42.5	8.9 ± 3.7	17.2 ± 4.0	36.4 ± 20.5	0.6 ± 0.4
Total BAs	322.2 ± 166.0	103.8 ± 12.7	155.9 ± 18.7	147.9 ± 56.2	12.4 ± 5.5
Titratable Acidity (g acid/100 g)	1.3 ± 1.1	0.6 ± 0.2	0.6 ± 0.1	0.7 ± 0.2	3.6 ± 1.2
pH	6.09 ± 1.38	6.33 ± 0.62	5.47 ± 0.28	5.18 ± 0.53	2.99 ± 0.20
Total Lipid (% w/w)	23.3 ± 2.0	6.9 ± 2.7	4.2 ± 1.4	5.1 ± 2.8	1.1 ± 0.2
TBARS Value (ppm)	0.07 ± 0.05	0.35 ± 0.14	0.47 ± 0.27	0.09 ± 0.03	0.83 ± 0.51
10^2.(TBARS):(Total Lipid) Ratio (ppm(% w/w)$^{-1}$)	0.5 ± 0.4	10.6 ± 6.85	33.1 ± 22.3	5.6 ± 3.55	98.3 ± 45.7

nd: not determined.

Table 3. Statistical significance and nature of differences between the mean BA contents and other food quality indices for fermented food products. Both robust Welch and Bonferroni-corrected *post-hoc* ANOVA test significance (p) values are provided. Abbreviations: ns, not statistically significant. * These values were close to statistical significance, but did not attain a p value of ≤0.05 with the robust Welch test.

BA/Index	Welch Test (WT) p Value	Post-hoc Significant Differences (All p < 0.05: Bonferroni Test)
Cadaverine (ppm)	0.0016	Cheese > Wine/Vinegar; Cheese > Fish Sauce/Paste; Cheese > Fish; Cheese > Vegetable Sauce
Histamine (ppm)	0.087 *	All ns
2-Phenylethylamine (ppm)	ns	All ns
Putrescine (ppm)	0.068 *	All ns
Spermidine (ppm)	0.029	Vegetable Sauce > Wine/Vinegar; Vegetable Sauce > Cheese; Vegetable Sauce > Fish
Spermine (ppm)	0.010	Fish Sauce/Paste > Wine/Vinegar; Fish Sauce/Paste > Cheese
Tryptamine (ppm)	ns	All ns
Tyramine (ppm)	0.021	Cheese > Wine/Vinegar
Total BAs	2.84×10^{-4}	Cheese >> Wine/Vinegar

Table 3. Cont.

BA/Index	Welch Test (WT) p Value	Post-hoc Significant Differences (All $p < 0.05$: Bonferroni Test)
Titratable acidity (g acid/100 g)	0.024	Wine/Vinegar > Fish; Wine/Vinegar > Fish Sauce/Paste; Wine/Vinegar > Vegetable Sauce; Wine/Vinegar > Cheese
pH	6.91×10^{-4}	Wine/Vinegar < Fish; Wine/Vinegar < Fish Sauce/Paste; Wine/Vinegar < Vegetable Sauce; Wine/Vinegar < Cheese
Total lipid (% w/w)	1.09×10^{-3}	Cheese > Wine/Vinegar; Cheese > Fish Sauce/Paste; Cheese > Fish; Cheese > Vegetable Sauce
TBARS value (ppm)	ns	ns
10^2.(TBARS):(Total Lipid) ratio (ppm(% w/w)$^{-1}$)	ns	Wine/Vinegar > Fish; Wine/Vinegar > Vegetable Sauce; Wine/Vinegar > Cheese

ns: not statistically significant.

Univariate statistical analysis performed by ANOVA (robust Welch test derivative), and also *post-hoc* Bonferroni test values, demonstrated that the mean values of each food classification examined were significantly or highly significantly different for 7 and 9 of the marker index variables respectively (p values ranging from <0.0003 to 0.04 for the former test, Table 3). Figure 1 shows a heatmap of the mean BA contents, and further variables included in this analysis; this clearly displays significantly higher tyramine, cadaverine, putrescine, and tryptamine levels in the fermented cheese products; higher histamine concentrations in the fish sauces/pastes explored, as expected (although vegetable sauces also had quite high levels of this BA); and also greater spermine contents in the fish paste/sauce products (*ca.* 1.5-fold greater than the mean value found for the fish classification, the next highest concentration). The vegetable sauce products had the highest mean spermidine levels, whereas the fermented fish group contained the largest amounts of 2-phenylethylamine detectable.

As expected, mean TA values were significantly greater for the wine/vinegar products than they were for all the other fermented food classes investigated, and correspondingly the mean pH value for the former group was significantly lower than those of all the other fermented foods. Of course, the mean total lipid content of the cheese group (23.3%) was significantly greater than all other food classifications tested (p *ca.* 10^{-3}), although no significant differences were found for the secondary lipid peroxidation TBARS marker. However, an examination of the mean ratio of TBARS index to total lipid content revealed that this value was markedly greater for the wine/vinegar group than that of all other food product types (Bonferroni-corrected *post-hoc* ANOVA tests), and significantly so over that of the cheese samples analyzed, as might be expected in view of the very low fat contents of fermented wine/vinegar samples (for example, it varies from 0.15–0.44% (w/v) in Zhenjiang aromatic vinegar samples [32]), and potentially substantially inflated TBARS levels resulting from quite high levels of TBA-reactive acetaldehyde and acrolein, amongst other aldehydes, present in such fermented products [33–36]. Indeed, many other aldehydes are reactive towards the TBA reagent, and also form chromophoric products on reaction with it [28]. Estimates for acetaldehyde in vinegar products can be as high as 1.0 g/kg respectively [33], but such levels are highly variable, with much lower levels being found, e.g., 2.6 mg/L (*ca.* 60 µmol/L) [37].

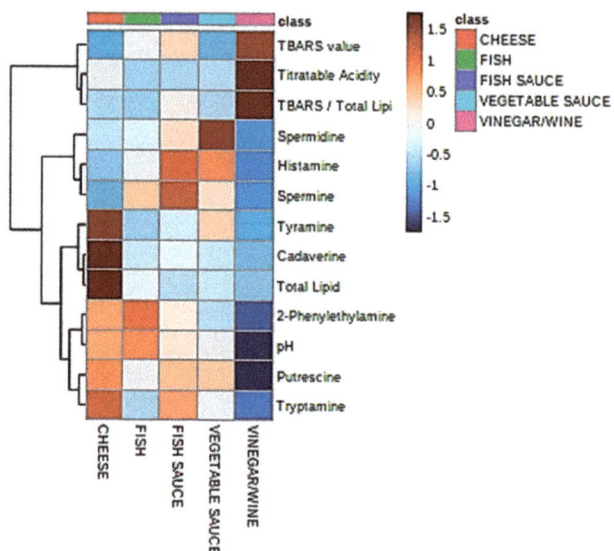

Figure 1. Heatmap diagram displaying the nature, extent and ANOVA-based significance of univariate differences between mean values of all 8 BA and further chemoanalytical food quality variables (near right-hand side *y*-axis) for the fermented cheese (red), fish (green), fish sauce/paste (dark blue), vegetable sauce (pale blue), and wine/vinegar (mauve) products. The complete dataset was glog-transformed and autoscaled prior to analysis, but not CS-normalized. Transformed analyte intensities are shown in the far right-hand side *y*-axis: deep blue and red colorations represent extremes of low and high contents respectively. The left-hand side of the plot shows results arising from an associated agglomerative hierarchical clustering (AHC) analysis of these variables, which reveals two major analyte clusterings, with three sub-clusterings for one of these. The top right-hand side major cluster comprises TBARS level, (TBARS):(total lipid) ratio and TA value, whereas the second contains all other analyte variables, including all BA contents. The first, second, and third sub-clusters within the bottom right-hand side major cluster feature spermine, spermidine, and histamine (the first two of these arising from the same putrescine and metabolically upstream ornithine and agmatine/arginine sources respectively); tyramine, cadaverine, and total lipid; and 2-phenylethylamine, putrescine, tryptamine, and pH respectively.

Acetaldehyde, a volatile flavor component of a variety of foods and beverages such as cheese, yoghurt, and wines [34], represents one of the most abundant carbonyl compounds detectable in wine, and typically accounts for *ca.* 90% of the total aldehydes present; its concentrations therein usually range from 10 to 200 mg/L (predominantly, it is generated as a yeast by-product during alcoholic fermentation processes [35], or from the chemical oxidation of ethanol [36]). However, very high levels of the unsaturated aldehyde acrolein are also present in red wine products [33]. Furthermore, a wide range of further aldehydes have been found to serve as major flavor constituents of traditional Chinese rose vinegar, and these include aliphatic *n*-alkanals such as heptanal, hexanal, nonanal, and dodecanal (ranging from 6–147 µg/kg), with larger amounts of benzaldehyde (851 µg/kg) [38].

Hence, overall these data clearly demonstrated that, in a univariate context, there were indeed significant differences between the mean contents of BAs and further parameters considered for the five classes of fermented food products studied.

Prior to the performance of MV statistical analysis of the dataset acquired, simple Pearson correlations were explored between all explanatory variables considered, and Figure 2 shows a correlation heatmap for these relationships. Clearly, there were moderate to strong positive correlations observed between all fermented food BAs present, the strongest observed between 2-phenylethylamine and tyramine (both aromatic BAs), tryptamine and spermine, and most notably, between cadaverine and histamine. Food pH values were found to have the strongest positive correlations with tyramine > putrescine > tryptamine, although spermidine was predominantly uncorrelated with this index. Moreover, as anticipated, TA was strongly negatively correlated with pH value > putrescine > tyramine ≈ histamine contents in that order. TBARS level, however, was largely independent of all BAs and their concentrations, with the exception of spermidine, which exhibited a weak positive relationship with this variable. Similarly, total lipid level was also mainly uncorrelated with all BA contents but was quite strongly anti-correlated with (TBARS):(total lipid) ratio and non-lipid-normalized TBARS value (both expected). The (TBARS):(total lipid) ratio was either strongly or moderately anti-correlated with all BA levels, and this may provide an indication of their potential antioxidant functions. In view of the complexity of these inter-relationships, the MV PCA and PLS-DA techniques were employed to explore them further.

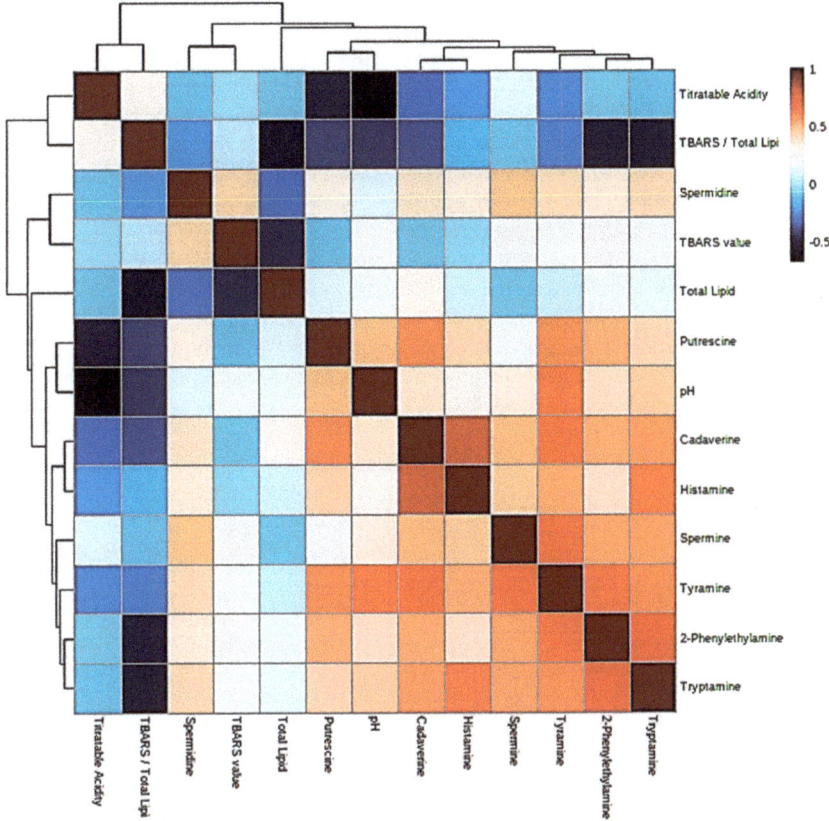

Figure 2. Correlation heatmap displaying positive and negative inter-relationships between BA concentrations, pH and TA values, total lipid contents, TBARS indices and (TBARS):(total lipid) ratios (TBARS/total lipid). The left-hand ordinate and top abscissa axes show AHC analysis based on these Pearson correlations (as a similarity criterion). From the top abscissa axis, of the two major clusterings revealed, that on the right-hand side contains all BA variable levels with the exception of spermidine, together with positively-correlated pH values, whereas the left-hand side one consists of all lipid- and lipid peroxidation-based variables, spermidine concentrations, and TA values.

3.2. Principal Component Analysis (PCA) of the Multivariate Fermented Food Dataset

PCA was primarily conducted in order to acquire an overview of the degree of distinctiveness between, i.e., clustering of, the fermented food classifications investigated, and also to identify any potential data outliers. An examination of two-dimensional (2D) scores plots from this analysis demonstrated that no significant outliers were detectable, and that PCs 1, 2, and 3 accounted for 41.5, 16.4, and 11.1% of the total variance respectively for the complete dataset which was glog-transformed and autoscaled. 2D and three-dimensional (3D) scores plots featuring these two most important PCs revealed that there was a reasonable level of distinction between the wine/vinegar and all other food product groups, and also between the cheese and fish classifications (Figure 3a); however, distinctions between the fish, fish sauce/paste, and vegetable sauce groups were not found, there being a significant degree of overlap between them. Notwithstanding, the sample sizes of the fermented fish and vegetable sauce groups involved were quite limited. A corresponding preliminary correlation circle diagram is shown in Figure 3b. Clear observations from this diagram are that (1) 2-phenylethylamine, tyramine, and cadaverine, and to a lesser extent, putrescine and tryptamine, are all correlated with PC1, and this observation indicates their communality in this model; (2) food pH values are also strongly correlated to PC1, and this indicates that higher values of this parameter may arise from the basicity of the above BAs (gas-phase primary amine basicity values increase with the length of its carbon chain substituents in view of their electron-donating positive charge-stabilizing effects—such values also increase with progression from primary to secondary to tertiary alkylamines [39]); (3) an at least partial correlation of histamine contents with PC2, which indicates distinction of this BA from those aligned with PC1; (4) an inverse correlation (anti-correlation) of total lipid level with the (TBARS):(total lipid) ratio index, as might be expected; and (5) a strong anti-correlation of TA value with BA levels, particularly tryptamine and putrescine, and this suggests that these amines serve to offer neutralization potential against acidic fermented food products. Also notable from this Figure are very strong correlations between the fermented food supplementary variable cheese and total lipid content, and between wine/vinegar and TA value, as indeed expected.

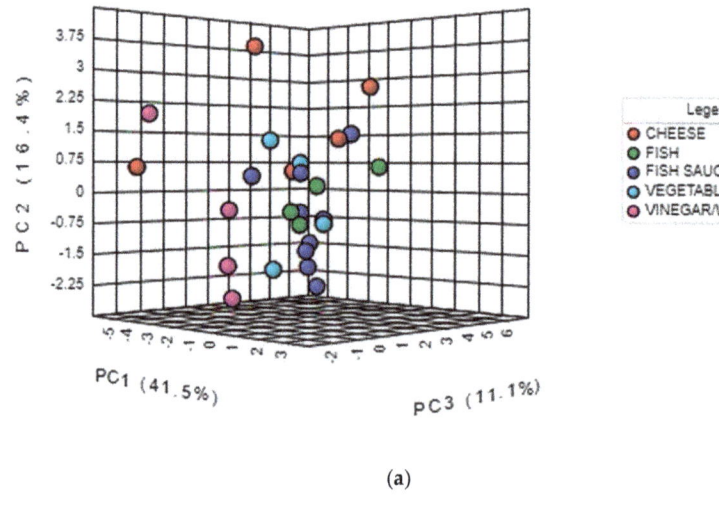

(a)

Figure 3. Cont.

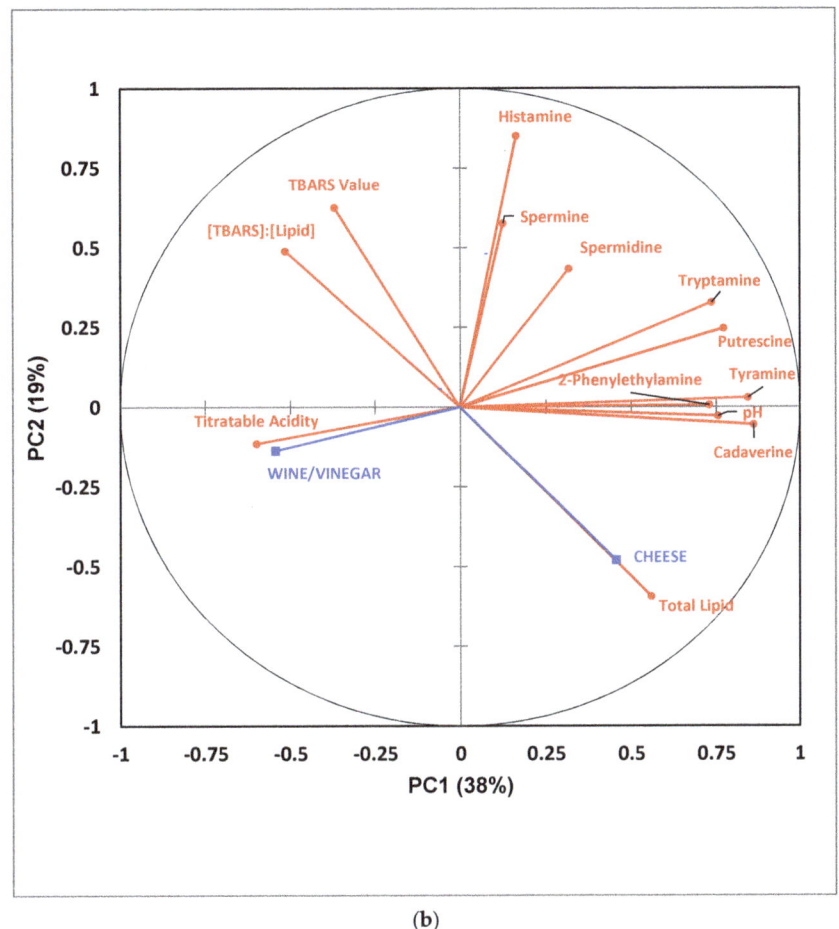

(b)

Figure 3. (a) 3D PCA scores plot of PC3 vs. PC2 vs. PC1, showing some degrees of distinction between different fermented food classes, i.e., those of cheese, fish, fish sauce/pastes, vegetable pastes, and wines/vinegars (particularly that between the wine/vinegar classification and all others). (b) Preliminary correlation circle diagram displaying correlations between all explanatory variables considered, and PCs 1 and 2 in a PCA model applied to the complete autoscaled (standardized) dataset. Active variables are depicted in red, whereas two of the supplementary variable classifications (cheese and wine/vinegar) are shown in blue. Variance contributions for PC1 and PC2 are indicated.

A more detailed analysis of these PCA loadings was made with the application of varimax rotation, Kaiser normalization, and a maximal number of 5 PCs considered. For this model, such variable loadings, and the percentage of total variance accounted for by each PC are available in Table 4. This analysis revealed that cadaverine, tryptamine, 2-phenylethylamine, and tyramine all strongly and positively loaded on PC1, spermidine and histamine strongly and positively loaded on PC3 (along with a more minor contribution from 2-phenylethylamine), and putrescine and spermidine loaded strongly and positively on PC5, albeit also with histamine to a much lesser extent. Interestingly, all aromatic BAs strongly loaded on PC1, as observed above (Figure 3b), whereas spermidine and its metabolic precursor putrescine both co-loaded onto the same PC (PC5).

Table 4. PCA loadings vectors for BAs and additional fermented food analyte parameters (including total lipid contents, and pH and TA values) for a 5 PC-limited model performed with varimax rotation and Kaiser normalization. Percentage variance contributions for PCs 1–5 and their (unrotated) analysis eigenvalues are also listed. Bold numbers are for a purpose specified in the Figure legends.

PC (Unrotated Eigenvalue):	PC1 (4.58)	PC2 (2.26)	PC3 (1.78)	PC4 (1.28)	PC5 (0.89)
% Variance Contribution	26.6	16.9	12.2	16.1	11.2
2-Phenylethylamine	**0.71**	−0.23	**0.43**	0.03	−0.06
Cadaverine	**0.90**	−0.07	−0.19	0.21	−0.04
Histamine	0.25	**0.45**	**0.63**	0.025	0.32
Putrescine	**0.57**	−0.04	−0.19	**0.42**	**0.50**
Spermidine	0.14	−0.19	0.20	0.06	**0.78**
Spermine	−0.08	−0.06	**0.85**	0.22	0.12
Tryptamine	**0.79**	0.07	0.11	0.13	0.30
Tyramine	**0.88**	−0.11	0.03	0.15	−0.03
Titratable acidity (TA)	−0.11	0.17	−0.30	**−0.86**	−0.09
pH	0.29	−0.10	0.04	**0.92**	−0.07
TBARS value	−0.08	**0.95**	0.08	−0.05	−0.05
Total lipid	**0.45**	−0.31	−0.21	0.37	**−0.61**
(TBARS):(Lipid) ratio	−0.14	**0.92**	−0.07	−0.23	−0.08

The TBARS secondary lipid oxidation index, along with its value normalized to total food lipid content, both loaded strongly and positively on PC2, as might be expected, although histamine also contributed somewhat towards this PC. Moreover, TA and pH values powerfully loaded on PC4 negatively and positively respectively, as would be expected from their anticipated negative correlation in fermented food products (putrescine also made a moderate positive contribution towards this component). Total lipid content was found to load significantly on PCs 1 and 5, positively and negatively so, respectively.

In a related study focused on PCA of both BAs and polyphenolics in Hungarian wines, Cosmos et al. [26] found that PC scores successfully clustered differential groups of these product classes, and that PC loadings vectors displayed significant patterns of BA and polyphenol levels. However, it should be noted that for this analysis, spermidine, and tyramine strongly loaded on PC1 (positively and negatively, respectively), agmatine and the sum total BA concentration loaded strongly and positively on PC2, spermine and cadaverine both strongly and negatively loaded on PC3, and that histamine loaded strongly and positively on PC4 alone. These associations between the BA analytes tested did not correspond to those found in the present study, although in the above MV analyses we elected not to include the total summed BA concentration value. Furthermore, our study also included the determinations of 2-phenylethylamine and putrescine, and not agmatine, but that reported in [26] monitored the latter BA but not 2-phenylethylamine and putrescine. However, as noted by the authors of [26], these PC loadings are only applicable to one region of Hungarian wine production, and their results will not be readily transferable to others, let alone other classes of fermented foods, especially in consideration of the often highly variable methods of fermentation, sources of fermentative micro-organisms, and conditions employed for these purposes. Notwithstanding, these researchers also concluded that in view of the loading patterns of BAs observed, it was unnecessary to measure all BA variables for quality assessments, and that only one per orthogonal PC was sufficient to provide acceptable levels of distinction between different sub-classes of such wines.

From this analysis, the unambiguously strong loadings vectors of the aromatic BAs 2-phenylethylamine and tyramine on PC1 provide evidence that they may indeed arise from the same biological and/or metabolic sources; however, this observation may also be rationalized by the natural production of tyrosine from phenylalanine, i.e., that involving the possible hydroxylation of the latter substrate to the former catalyzed by the enzyme phenylalanine hydroxylase (PAH) potentially available in fermentative lactobacilli employed for the production of fermented food products, followed by enzymatic transformation of the tyrosine product to tyramine by fermentative bacteria. To date, PAH is the only known aromatic amino acid hydroxylase found in bacteria [40].

The loadings of spermine and spermidine on different orthogonal PCs (PC3 and PC5, respectively) is not simply explicable, although the co-loading of spermidine's metabolic precursor putrescine on PC5 is consistent with them being featured in the same metabolic pathway. However, the co-loadings of BAs on differential PCs, particularly PC1, may reflect their engenderment from identical or related bacterial sources.

Notably, PC2 was dominated by powerful loading contributions from TBARS level and (TBARS):(total lipid) ratio (both positive), and PC4 by strong loadings from TA and pH values (negative and positive loadings vectors, respectively). These inter-relationships are, of course, expected, and are consistent with the data presented in Figure 3b. PC5 was retained in the model since it was the only one available which had a strong loading contribution from spermidine.

3.3. Distinction of Fermented Food Classifications Using PLS-DA

Similarly, PLS-DA of the dataset revealed an effective discrimination between the cheese and wine/vinegar classifications, although the fish, fish sauce/paste and vegetable sauce sample PC score datapoints were again unresolved; however, a visualized combination of these three fermented food classifications was at least partially resolved from the fermented cheese group (Figure 4). Permutation testing of the PLS-DA model confirmed its ability to distinguish between all the differing fermented food classifications evaluated ($p = 0.022$). For this model, key discriminatory variables were selected on the basis of their variable importance parameters (VIPs), and these were total lipid content (1.81) > cadaverine content (1.61) > (TBARS):(total lipid) ratio (1.36) > TA value (1.24) > histamine content (1.14) > 2-phenylethylamine content (0.78); data were glog-transformed and autoscaled prior to analysis. The top three discriminators largely arise from differential levels of lipids, cadaverine, and (TBARS):(total lipid) ratio between each of the fermented food groups, e.g., for the total lipids and cadaverine variables, the cheese content was significantly greater than that of all other fermented food groups, and for the above ratio, its value was significantly greater in the wine/vinegar group than it was in all other groups.

The quite strong distinctions observed between the cheese, wine/vinegar, and fish-fish sauce/paste-vegetable sauce composite products is readily explicable by significant or even substantial differences between the higher contents of cadaverine, tyramine, and, to a lesser extent, tryptamine in cheese, than those of the four other fermented food product classes. Further key discriminators are TA, pH, and total lipid contents, the latter of which is, of course, much higher in the cheese group.

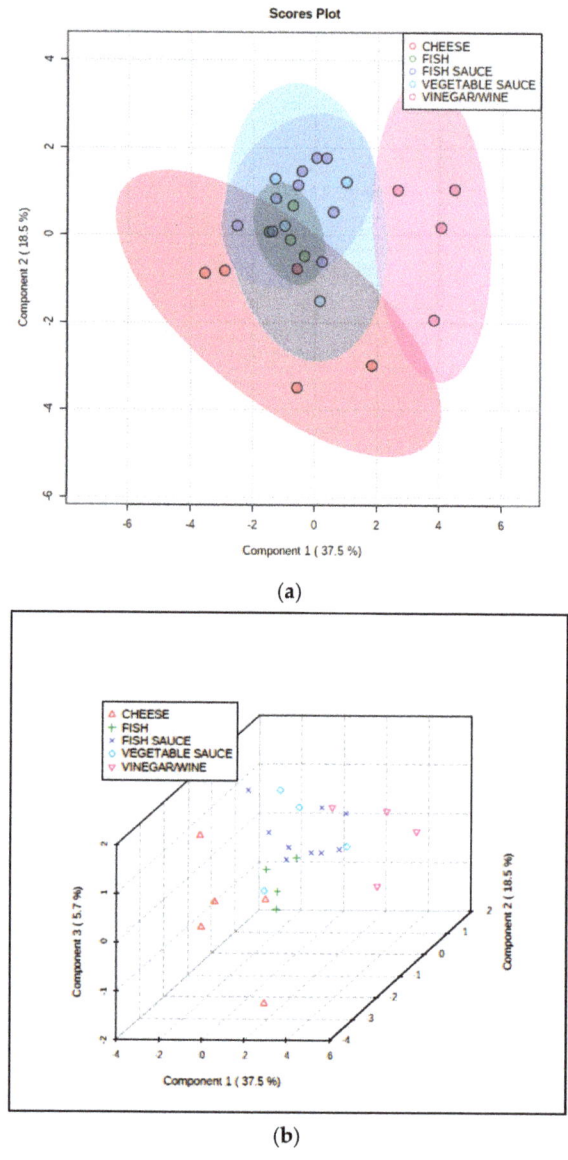

Figure 4. (**a**,**b**). 2D and 3D PLS-DA scores plots (PC2 vs. PC1, and PC3 vs. PC2 vs. PC1, respectively) revealing strong distinctions between the cheese, wine/vinegar, and a considered combination of fish, fish sauce/paste and vegetable sauce fermented food groups ((**a**) also shows 95% confidence ellipses for each fermented food classification). Little or no distinction between the latter three fermented food groups were discernable using this MV analysis approach.

3.4. RF Modelling of Fermented Food Classifications

Application of the RF CI classification technique was found to be only partially successful for the classification of the different fermented food groups investigated. Using the models described in Section 2.6.2, this approach correctly classified 4/4 wine vinegar, 6/9 fish sauce/paste, and 3/5 cheeses, but 0/4 for both fish and vegetable sauce products.

3.5. PCA of FCLO BAs

The FCLO product considered was primarily investigated separately since only BA contents, and not parameters such as pH and TA were available for it. Moreover, its total lipid content is, of course, not far removed from a value of 100%, and therefore it would be inappropriate to test this index in the above MV analysis models (similarly, total lipid level-normalized TBARS values would also be inappropriate to test in these systems). However, it was possible to explore inter-relationships between FCLO BA concentrations and/or their orthogonality status using a rigorous PCA approach featuring varimax rotation and Kaiser normaliszation in order to maximize success with the assignment of individual BA variables to PCs.

Table 5 lists the BA contents of $n = 10$ FCLO product batches. The total concentrations of BAs in these samples was higher than the recommended "limit" of 200 ppm in only two out of ten batches of the samples tested, albeit marginally so (only 14 and 20% higher). Similarly, bioactive histamine was completely undetectable in this product. As noted in [6], all BAs monitored were completely undetectable in three other natural, albeit unfermented, CLO products included for comparative purposes. All BAs tested were found to be reasonably soluble in FCLO lipidic matrices, and also in 1/3 (v/v) diluted solutions of this product in deuterochloroform (C^2HCl_3), presumably as the uncharged species with their amine functions deprotonated (solubility in these media is expected to increase with increasing amine function substituent chain length and hydrophobicity).

Table 5. (BA concentrations (ppm) of $n = 10$ separate batches of a FCLO product. Total BA and corresponding mean ± SEM values are also provided. Histamine and spermine were undetectable in all samples analyzed.

Biogenic Amine (ppm)	FCLO Batch										Mean ± SEM
	1	2	3	4	5	6	7	8	9	10	
2-PE	86	103	50	17	76	0	1.4	0	1.9	1.3	33.7 ± 13.0
Tyramine	70	88	43	8	32	0	1.8	0	1.1	0	24.4 ± 10.3
Tryptamine	35	24	26	3	8	0	0	0	1.7	1.5	9.9 ± 4.2
Cadaverine	23	11	25	0	7	0	0	0	0	0	6.6 ± 3.1
Putrescine	14	10	14	0	0	0	0	0	0	0	3.8 ± 2.0
Spermidine	0	4	0	0	0	0	0	0	0	0	0.4 ± 0.4
Total	228	240	158	28	123	0	3.2	0	4.7	2.8	78.8 ± 31.3

PCA performed on the FCLO BA dataset revealed that cadaverine, putrescine, and tryptamine all loaded strongly and positively on the first of two automatically-selected PCs (PC1), whereas the aromatic BAs 2-phenylethylamine and tyramine loaded strongly and positively on the second (PC2), along with spermidine (Table 6). These data displayed some consistency with PC loading values obtained on the full fermented food dataset (Table 4), which had 2-phenylethylamine and tyramine both strongly loading on one PC (PC1). However, such levels will, of course, be critically dependent on the microbial fermentation sources, parameters employed for fermented food production, and production conditions for these processes.

Table 6. PCA loadings vectors for FCLO BAs in a two PC-limited PCA model performed with varimax rotation and Kaiser normalization. Percentage variance contributions for these PCs and their (unrotated) analysis eigenvalues are also listed. Bold numbers are for a purpose specified in the Figure legends.

PC (unrotated Eigenvalue)	PC1 (4.03)	PC2 (1.58)
% Variance Contribution	52.8	40.6
2-PE	0.35	**0.84**
Tyramine	**0.54**	**0.84**
Tryptamine	**0.93**	0.33
Cadaverine	**0.99**	−0.01
Putrescine	**0.95**	0.23
Spermidine	−0.11	**0.93**

3.6. MV Chemometric Analysis of BA Data Only: Recognition of Fermented Food Class-Distinctive BA Patterns Using CS-Normalization

Additionally, we conducted univariate and MV analyses of datasets which were restricted to the BA profiles only, but also included the $n = 10$ FCLO samples reported above. Additionally, these analyses were performed with and without application of constant sum (CS) normalization. The CS-normalized data format was employed in order to facilitate the recognition of fermented food class-specific BA patterns. For the non-CS-normalized format, the total BA content value was also included as an explanatory variable, as indeed it was in [26].

Firstly, ANOVA performed on the CS-normalized, glog-transformed, and autoscaled dataset found very highly significant, albeit FDR-corrected p values for three of the sum-proportionate mean BA concentration differences observed between the fermented food classifications explored in this manner. Notably, these differences were observed for cadaverine, 2-phenylethylamine, and tryptamine (Table 7), and *post-hoc* testing revealed that for cadaverine, the cheese products had significantly greater proportionate levels than three others, and for both 2-phenylethylamine and tryptamine, FCLO had significantly higher ones than all other products examined. These differences in CS-normalized values are readily visualizable in the form of an ANOVA-based heatmap (Figure 5a), which revealed characteristic BA signatures for three of the fermented food product classifications. Clearly, the cheese, FCLO, and wine/vinegar sampling groups have high proportionate levels of cadaverine, 2-phenylethylamine/tyramine/tryptamine (all aromatic BAs), and metabolic pathway-associated putrescine/spermidine/spermine, respectively. However, when evaluated in this univariate system, "between-fermented food class" mean differences observed for putrescine, spermine, spermidine, histamine, and tyramine were not found to be statistically significant.

Secondly, both PCA and PLS-DA models were employed, and these approaches were successful in providing evidence for the MV distinctiveness of the FCLO, cheese, and wine/vinegar groups; however, as noted for the analyses conducted on the combined BA/further food quality parameter dataset, unfortunately no distinctions were observed between the fermented fish, fish sauce/paste, and vegetable sauce products (Figure 5b,c).

For the CS-normalized dataset (without total BA concentrations as an additional variable), PLS-DA variable importance parameter (VIP) values were in the order spermidine (1.48) > putrescine (1.34) > spermine (1.20) > histamine (1.06) > 2-phenylethylamine (0.94), whereas those for the non-CS-normalized dataset were spermidine (1.56) > spermine (1.35) > 2-phenylethylamine (1.32) > putrescine (0.84) (total BA level was a very poor predictor variable for the latter). As expected, there were significant differences between the sequential orders of these values when prior CS-normalization was implemented.

Table 7. Univariate statistical significance and nature of differences observed between the mean CS-normalized, glog-transformed, and autoscaled BA contents of fermented food samples (cheese, FCLO, fish, fish sauce/paste, vegetable sauce, and wine/vinegar products) in a completely randomized, one-way ANOVA model. The significance of FDR-corrected *post-hoc* ANOVA tests are also provided (significant differences are ranked in order of their decreasing statistical significance, i.e., increasing p value). The "between-fermented food class" source of variation was not statistically significant for putrescine, spermidine, spermine, histamine, or tyramine when tested in this model.

BA	FDR-Corrected p Value	Significant post-hoc *ANOVA* Differences
Cadaverine	1.49×10^{-5}	Cheese > FCLO; Cheese > Vegetable Sauce; Cheese > Wine/Vinegar; Fish > FCLO; Fish Sauce > FCLO; Vegetable Sauce > FCLO; Fish > Wine/Vinegar; Fish Sauce > Wine/Vinegar; Vegetable Sauce > Wine/Vinegar.
2-Phenylethylamine	8.25×10^{-4}	FCLO > Cheese; FCLO > Fish; FCLO > Fish Sauce; FCLO > Vegetable Sauce; FCLO > Wine/Vinegar; Fish > Vegetable Sauce.
Tryptamine	2.93×10^{-2}	FCLO > Cheese; FCLO > Fish; FCLO > Fish Sauce; FCLO > Vegetable Sauce; FCLO > Wine/Vinegar.

Moreover, for the PLS-DA model adopted without CS-normalization, histamine, spermidine, and spermine contents all loaded significantly on component 1 (loading vector coefficients 0.48, 0.57, and 0.47 respectively); 2-phenylethylamine, cadaverine, tyramine, and total BA levels on component 2 (loadings vector coefficients 0.42, −0.61, −0.57, and −0.61 respectively); 2-phenylethylamine and tryptamine levels on PC3 (loadings vector coefficients 0.50 and 0.57 respectively); and putrescine and spermine on PC4 (loadings vector coefficients 0.75 and −0.73 respectively). For this dataset, a four-component model was found to be most effective (permutation p value 0.0055).

Importantly, it should be noted that one now common issue in chemometrics/metabolomics experiments is the occurrence of a univariately-insignificant variable which remains multivariately-significant. Such observations are readily rationalized, firstly by the complementation (i.e., correlation) between explanatory variables, i.e., separately they do not, but when combined together as a MV composite (e.g., as a sufficiently-loading PC variable), they do serve to explain "between-classification" differences detected; secondly, consistency effects arising from the "masking" of potential univariately-significant differences by high levels of biological source sampling and/or measurement variation may be responsible (such variation may be averaged out via the conversion of datapoints to orthogonal component scores as in the PCA and PLS-DA models applied here); and thirdly, relatively small sample sizes for each classification involved (fermented foods in this case)—unfortunately, strategies applied to correct for FDRs promote the risk of statistical type II errors (i.e., false negatives) [24].

The PLS-DA evaluation was then extended and performed for pairwise comparisons of the differing fermented food classifications (CS-normalized dataset only). Firstly, as expected, Q^2 values for the fish vs. fish sauce/paste, fish sauce/paste vs. vegetable sauce, and fish vs. vegetable sauce comparisons were all moderately negative, and p values for associated permutation tests were all >0.10. However, these values for the wine/vinegar vs. FCLO, and FCLO vs. cheese two classification model comparisons revealed that Q^2 (permutation p values) indices for these comparisons were 0.71 (0.059) and 0.72 (0.090), but only 0.38 (0.16) for the wine/vinegar vs. cheese one (values were based on models containing two, five, and one components respectively). Hence, these results provide some evidence for the success of this strategy in distinguishing between the FCLO product, and both the cheese and wine/vinegar ones, although permutation test p values obtained for these models were a little higher than the 0.05 significance level, i.e., they were close to statistical significance.

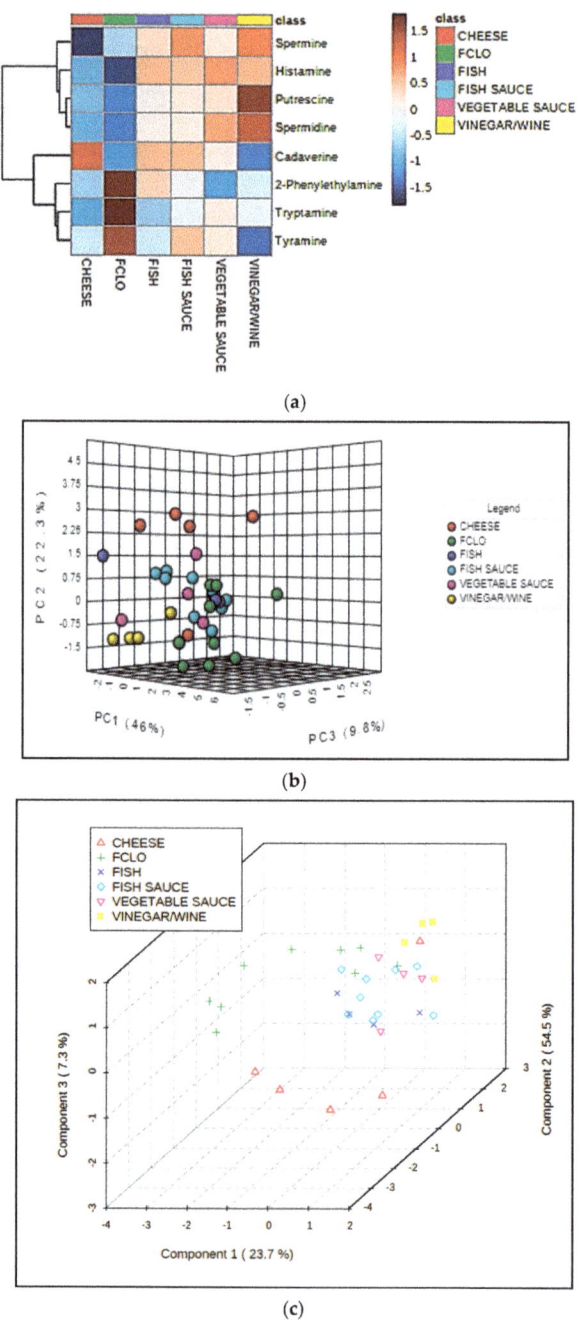

Figure 5. (a) Heatmap diagram displaying the most univariately-significant differences between mean values of eight BA explanatory variables (near right-hand side y-axis) for the fermented cheese (red), FCLO (green), fish (dark blue), fish sauce/paste (pale blue), vegetable sauce (purple), and wine/vinegar (yellow) products. The complete BA dataset was CS-normalized, glog-transformed, and autoscaled

prior to analysis. AHC analysis shown on the left-hand side ordinate axis demonstrated two major analyte clusterings, the upper one consisting of putrescine, spermidine, and spermine pathway biomolecules (and histamine), whereas the lower one features all aromatic BAs, along with cadaverine. (**b**) 3D PCA PC3 vs. PC2 vs. PC1 scores plot for the same CS-normalized dataset shown in (**a**), showing reasonable or strong distinctions between the cheese, wine/vinegar and FCLO fermented food classes. (**c**) 3D PLS-DA PC3 vs. PC2 vs. PC1 scores plot for the corresponding non-CS-normalized dataset, which also incorporated total BA content as a potential explanatory variable (again, effective distinctions between the cheese, FCLO, and wine/vinegar classes were notable).

We then elected to statistically combine the fish, fish sauce/paste, and vegetable sauce groups, and repeated the PLS-DA modelling in order to compare the sauce/fish composite, cheese, FCLO, and wine/vinegar groups using the CS-normalized dataset. This analysis exhibited a quite high level of classification success (Figure 6a); Q^2 for this comparative four-classification analysis was 0.44, and a PLS-DA permutation test confirmed its significance ($p = 0.031$). The loadings of each BA variable on PLS-DA components 1 and 2 is shown in Figure 6b, and this demonstrates three groups of these predictors: the first with highly positive component 1 and highly negative component 2 loadings (all aromatic BAs, i.e., 2-phenylethylamine, tyramine, and tryptamine); the second with low to intermediate positive component 1 but highly positive component 2 loadings (metabolically-related putrescine, spermidine, and spermine, together with histamine); and the third with highly negative loadings on component 1, but negligible loadings on component 2 (cadaverine only). These grouped BA loadings vectors were very consistent with other observations made from the MV analysis of these data as a full six fermented food classification dataset. Specifically, they are completely reflective of the patterns of BA "markers" found in fermented FCLO, wine/vinegar, and cheese products respectively (Figure 5a).

Finally, RF analysis of this revised dataset showed that this approach had an at least reasonable level of classification success, with all (10/10) FCLO and 88% (15/17) of the fish/sauce combination samples being correctly classified; notwithstanding, only 60 and 50% of the cheese and wine/vinegar fermented food products, respectively, were.

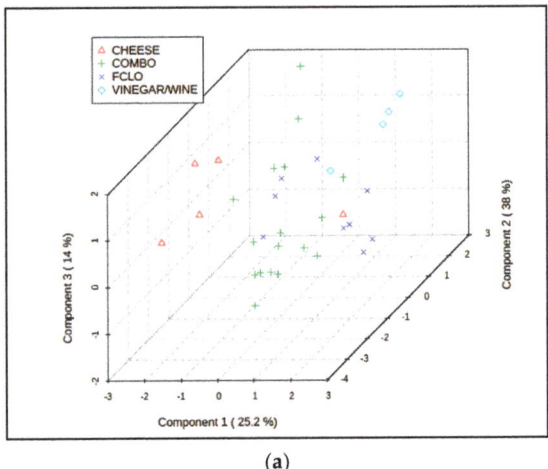

(**a**)

Figure 6. *Cont.*

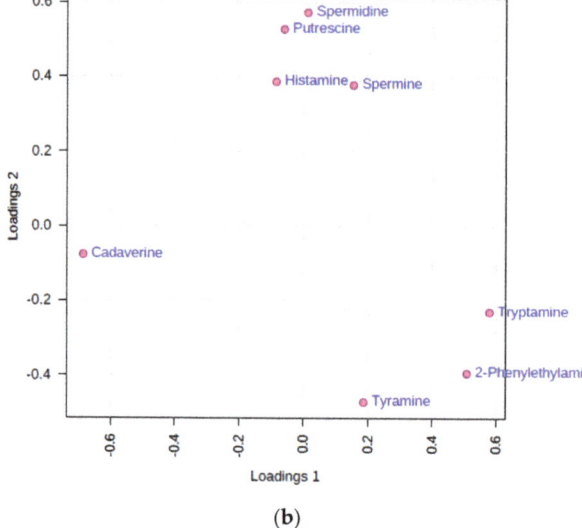

Figure 6. PLS-DA evaluation of revised dataset with combined fish, fish sauce/paste, and vegetable sauce classifications (abbreviated COMBO); CS-normalization was applied to the dataset prior to analysis. (**a**) 3D PLS-DA component 3 vs. component 2 vs. component 1 scores plot revealing some clustering of the fermented food classifications (i.e., cheese, wine/vinegar, FCLO, and COMBO). (**b**) Corresponding component 2 vs. component 1 loadings plot for this PLS-DA analysis.

3.7. Scientific Significance and Human Health Implications of Results Acquired

Results acquired from the combined applications of univariate and MV chemometrics techniques in this study clearly demonstrated that the latter strategy was valuable for distinguishing between fermented wine/vinegar products and cheeses, and the discrimination between both of these food classes from either fish, fish sauce/paste, or vegetable sauce products (or a statistical combination of them) was possible on the basis of their BA, total lipid, pH, and TA values; nevertheless, such techniques were not readily able to distinguish between the latter three fermented food classes. However, a rigorously-constrained univariate analysis method selected to overcome complications arising from intra-food classification heteroscedasticities and FDRs was able to successfully distinguish between the vegetable sauce and fish groups through significantly higher and lower levels of spermidine and 2-phenylethylamine, respectively, present in the former class. Moreover, experimental results indicated that cadaverine, tyramine, putrescine, and tryptamine concentrations may all contribute significantly towards food pH values in view of their strong positive correlations with this parameter found, together with corresponding negative ones with TA values (Figure 3b).

Moreover, BA-targeted univariate and multivariate analyses of CS-normalized data was found to be valuable for providing useful discriminatory information, which highlighted the characteristic patterns of BA biomolecules, which may be valuable for further investigations of the particular nature and/or geographic origins of fermented foods, and the mechanisms involved in their formation. Indeed, the present study found that such patterns comprised cadaverine only for cheese samples, three aromatic BAs (2-phenylethylamine, tyramine, and tryptamine), for FCLOs (sourced from fermented cod livers), and those from the sequential metabolic pathway which transforms the amino acid substrates ornithine or arginine to spermine (i.e., putrescine, spermidine, and spermine itself) for wine/vinegar products. Such idiosyncratic, fermented food product-dependent signatures for CS-normalized fermented food BA concentrations may serve to provide valuable information regarding the fermentative bacterial sources, routes involved in fermentation, and product manufacturing conditions employed for them.

For the putrescine → spermidine → spermine metabolic pathway, which was identified as representing a wine/vinegar-specific one from analysis of the CS-normalized dataset, and which accounted for >70% of total BAs in this fermented food class (Table 2), both positive or negative correlations could arise between a BA catabolite and its immediate upstream precursor, but not necessarily between the terminal spermine metabolite and that upstream of its spermidine substrate (i.e., putrescine).

With regard to toxic concentrations and health risk recommendations available in [25], it should be noted that all mean histamine levels determined in the fermented food samples tested here lie markedly below the recommended 100 ppm limit for it (with no single product exceeding this value—the highest level observed was 57 ppm in one of the fish sauce products assessed). Furthermore, with the exception of the cheese products evaluated, the mean total BA values all food groups were <200 ppm, the wine/vinegar classification substantially so (Table 2). However, although three of the cheese products tested had total BA contents of <200 ppm, two of them had levels ranging from 600–800 ppm, and therefore their dietary consumption may present a health risk for susceptible individuals.

Mean BA concentrations for the FCLO product examined ranged from 0 (histamine) to only 34 ppm (2-phenylethylamine), with the highest levels observed for the most predominant species, 2-phenylethylamine and tyramine, being 103 and 88 ppm. Since the United States of America's recommended dietary intake of health-friendly, highly unsaturated omega-3 (O-3) fatty acids (FAs) is a maximum of 1.0 g/day [41], and the oil explored here contains a mean of 29% (w/w) total O-3 FAs (predominantly the sum of eicosapentaenoic and docosahexaenoic acids) [6], then daily consumption of $100/29\% \times 1.0$ g = 3.45 g of this FCLO product would provide estimated absolute maximal daily intake levels of 3.45×103 µg = 355 µg, and 3.45×88 µg = 304 µg of 2-phenylethylamine and tyramine, respectively. Based on the 10 samples of this product analyzed, estimated mean daily intakes of these BAs will be 111 and 95 µg only. Therefore, it appears that daily consumption of this product at the recommended U.S.-recommended dosage levels will certainly not provide any health risks to consumers, even if they are susceptible to the adverse effects experienced by their excessive intake (e.g., migraines induced by 2-phenylethylamine).

As noted above, one potentially important health benefit offered by the ingestion of dietary BAs is their novel antioxidant properties, both for the prevention of food spoilage during storage or transport episodes, but also in vivo following their ingestion. Indeed, our laboratory recently explored the powerful antioxidant capacities of BA-containing natural FCLO products, and their resistivities to thermally-mediated oxidative damage to unsaturated FAs therein, particularly O-3 PUFAs [6]. These marine oil products, which arise from the pre-fermentation of cod livers (Section 2), were indeed found to display a very high level of antioxidant activity, and PUFAs therein were also more resistant towards thermally-mediated peroxidation than other natural cod liver oil products evaluated. Resonances assignable to aromatic BAs, specifically those arising from 2-phenylethylamine and tyramine, were directly observable in the ^{1}H NMR profiles of ca. 1/3 (v/v) diluted solutions of these products with C^2HCl_3. Additionally, corresponding spectra acquired on both ^2H_2O and $C^2H_3O^2H$ extracts of these oils confirmed the presence of both these BAs, together with a series of others, both aromatic and aliphatic. In the present study, mean concentrations of 2-phenylethylamine and tyramine detectable in these products were found to be 34 and 24 ppm, respectively. Antioxidant actions of the phenolic BA antioxidant tyramine found in this FCLO product may be explicable by its chain-breaking antioxidant effects, and this may offer contributions towards the potent resistance of PUFAs, particularly O-3 FAs, present therein. However, in view of the absence of a phenolic function in 2-phenylethylamine, its antioxidant potential is likely to involve an alternative radical-scavenging mechanism, presumably that involving O_2-consuming carbon-centered pentadienyl radical species, as found in [22,23].

The TBARS method employed here to determine the lipid peroxidation status of fermented foods, which involved an extended low temperature equilibration process [28], successfully avoids the artefactual generation of TBA-reactive aldehydes, including malondialdehyde (MDA), during commonly-employed alternative protocols for this assay system, which generally involve a short (ca. 10–15 min) heating stage at 95–98 °C in order to develop the monitored pink/red chromophore rapidly. However, from an analysis of TBARS and (TBARS):(total lipid) ratios determined on the preliminary FCLO-excluded fermented food samples, there appears to be only little evidence for the ability of BAs to offer any protection against lipid peroxidation in such products. Although Table 3 shows that the above ratio is significantly greater in the wine/vinegar group, this observation is perceived to be derived from their very low lipid contents, and the presence of a range of non-MDA TBA-reactive aldehydes present therein, including acetaldehyde and acrolein, for example, although these are also lipid oxidation products. Moreover, despite taking steps to avoid the artefact-generating heating stage of this assay, this test still remains poorly specific in view of the reactions of a variety of non-aldehydic substrates to react with it to form interfering chromophores, which also absorb at a monitoring wavelength of 532 nm. Nevertheless, TBARS level appeared to be positively correlated with fermented food spermidine concentration (Figure 2), and both this lipid peroxidation index and its lipid-normalized value appeared to be positively correlated with fermented food histamine content (loading on PC2, Table 4). However, in view of the many complications associated with this TBARS lipid peroxidation index, which offers only a very limited and still often erroneous viewpoint on the highly complex lipid peroxidation process [42], such observations cannot be rationally considered at this stage. As expected, the lipid-normalized TBARS value was negatively correlated with total lipid content (Figure 3b). The latter variable also appeared to be negatively correlated with histamine and putrescine levels (loading on PC5, Table 4). Unfortunately, results from unspecific TBARS assays are still widely employed as important quality indices throughout the food industry.

One quite surprising observation made in the current study was the detection of lipids, albeit at low levels, in wine and vinegar samples. Notwithstanding, as noted above, FAs have been detected in Zhenjiang aromatic vinegar products at similar contents to those found here [32]. Furthermore, Yunoki et al. [43] explored the FA constituents of some commercially-available red wine products, and found that lipid constituent concentrations varied from 27 to 96 mg/100 mL for $n = 6$ domestic (Japanese) wines, and 31 to 56 mg/100 mL for $n = 6$ foreign products, and that a total of 12 different FAs were detectable, mainly saturated ones. Although the extraction method described in the latter report was a 2:1 chloroform:methanol (Folch) one that targets non-polar triacylglycerols (TAGs) and more polar phospholipids, it is likely that the FAs detectable in the wine/vinegar products explored here, and also those present in Zhenjiang aromatic vinegars [32], are present as free non-glycerol-esterified species and their corresponding anions, and this would account for their higher levels detectable in these studies than those reported in [43]. Indeed, fermentation processes readily induce the hydrolysis of TAGs to free FAs, together with mono- and diacylglycerol adducts, and free glycerol [44]; such FAs will be expected to contribute towards the food pH values determined here. Similarly, Phan et al. [45] found a broad spectrum of lipidic species, specifically TAGs, polar lipids, free FAs, sterols, and cholesterol esters present in pinot noir wines.

The official AOAC gravimetric method for lipid determination employed in the current study involves an acid hydrolysis step involving HCl in any case, followed by extraction with mixed ethers, i.e., both diethyl and petroleum ethers. Hence, the HCl added will be sufficient to hydrolyze any residual TAGs present to free FAs and glycerol, and also fully protonate the former so that they are extractable as such into ether solvents. Indeed, it has been demonstrated that such free FAs are readily soluble and extractable into these ether solvent systems [46,47]. Hence, the passage of lipidic species from grapes and/or micro-organisms to finalized bottled wine and vinegar products has been confirmed in further investigations.

Interestingly, ^{1}H NMR analysis of ^{2}H$_2$O extracts of the FCLO product investigated found proportionately high concentrations of free FAs and free glycerol therein (data not shown). These FAs were mainly present as PUFAs, as would be expected from the overall lipid composition of this product which contains high levels of omega-3 FAs as TAG species prior to fermentation induction. This observation is fully consistent with the ability of lactobacilli-mediated fermentation processes to partially hydrolyze TAGs in such a product. High levels of the short-chain organic acids propionic and acetic acids (as their propionate and acetate anions in neutral solution media), both lactobacilli fermentation catabolites, the former arising from the metabolic reduction of lactate [48], were also detectable in these extracts. These results will be reported in detail elsewhere.

4. Limitations of the Study

One important limitation of this study is the limited sample sizes of some of the fermented food sampling classes incorporated into our primary experimental design. This was largely a consequence of only small numbers of differing fermented food products being available for purchase locally, for example vegetable sauce and fish products. However, it should be noted that the cheese and wine/vinegar classifications had BA contents and patterns which markedly contrasted with those of the other fermented food groups evaluated. These differences, along with those for other food quality markers observed (Table 3, Figures 1 and 3–5), were found to be very highly statistically significant, even with these limited sample sizes. Hence, this did not present a major constraining issue. Moreover, the performance of additional MV analyses on a revised model including a combined fish, fish sauce/paste, and vegetable sauce classification (on the basis of only a limited level of significant differences between them) with $n = 17$ overall served to overcome this problem (Figure 6), and this incentive did not distract from the main objectives and focus of the investigation in view of their predominant MV similarities in BA contents. However, univariate analysis found that the mean spermidine concentration was significantly higher in fermented vegetable sauces than it was in corresponding fish products (Table 3), and vice-versa for mean 2-phenylethylamine levels (Table 7). Further evidentiary support was provided by data analysis strategies applied, which were highly rigorous, and included the preliminary tracking of sample outliers. Furthermore, rigorous Welch tests were implemented for the ANOVA models employed, and either Bonferroni or FDR corrections were applied for *post-hoc* "between-fermented food classification" tests in order to circumvent potential problems with false positives (type I errors).

Another limitation of the current study was the unavailability of differing manufacturing sources of FCLO products, and therefore unlike other fermented food products assessed here, statistical evaluations involved an investigation of 10 separate, randomly-selected batches of a single product, both separately (Table 5) and jointly with all other classes involved in the primary statistical analysis conducted (Table 7, and Figures 5 and 6). However, the very wide between-batch variance of all FCLO samples explored facilitated this approach.

Finally, one further limitation is the poor specificity and interpretability of the TBARS method employed for the quality assessment of fermented food products here, specifically for assessments of their degrees of lipid peroxidation. However, one major precautionary step was taken in this study to minimize problems and potential interferences in this assay system, and this involved the avoidance of an aldehydic artefact-forming heating stage. Future investigations of the lipid oxidation status of fermented foods should therefore employ more reliable and specific methodologies such as those involving high-resolution ^{1}H NMR analysis for the direct, simultaneous, multicomponent analysis of a series of both primary and secondary lipid oxidation products, e.g., conjugated hydroperoxydienes and their aldehydic fragmentation products, respectively. This protocol may be applied directly to solution-state products, or indirectly to either aqueous or lipid/deuterochloroform extracts of fermented food products.

5. Conclusions

This study demonstrated that almost all fermented foods tested had total BA levels which lay below the maximum recommended values for them. A composite application of univariate and MV chemometrics techniques clearly demonstrated that the MV approach applied was valuable for discriminating between fermented wine/vinegar products and cheeses, and the distinction between these two fermented food classes and a combination of fish, fish sauce/paste, and vegetable sauce products. Further MV analysis performed on CS-normalized BA profiles revealed distinctive patterns for cheese (cadaverine only), FCLOs (the aromatic BAs 2-phenylethylamine, tyramine, and tryptamine), and wine/vinegar products (pathway-associated putrescine, spermidine, and spermine). Such distinctive signatures for fermented food BA contents may offer useful information regarding the nature of, and regulatory conditions employed for, fermentation processes utilized during their commercial production.

The simultaneous untargeted analysis of eight or more BAs using the LC-MS/MS analysis strategy employed here offers major advantages which are unachievable by alternative, more targeted techniques with the ability to determine only single or very small numbers of chemometrically-important analytes. Notably, the diagnostic potential of a series of n (for example, five or more) BA content analyte variables in a MV chemometrics investigation offers major advantages over the analytical acquisition of only a single possible marker. Indeed, food sample patterns of BAs and related food quality indices, which are characteristic of a particular fermented food product classification, will be expected to provide a much higher level of statistical power, reliability, and confidence concerning the accurate distinction between these classifications, and their accurate and selective assignment to one of them, than that discernable from a single BA analyte level only. Secondly, the patterns of BAs and associated food quality criteria determined, together with their correlations to particular factors or components (predominantly linear, but occasionally quadratic or higher combinations of predictor BA and supporting variables), may potentially serve to supply extensive information regarding the sources of such BAs, bacterial, commercial, or otherwise.

Supplementary Materials: The following are available online at http://www.mdpi.com/2304-8158/9/12/1807/s1, S1: Summary of Antioxidant Activities of BAs, S2: Potential Adverse Health Effects of Dietary Bas, S3: Outline of Analytical Techniques Available for BA Determinations and the Screening of BA-Generating Bacteria in Foods.

Author Contributions: J.Z. was responsible for the manufacture of FCLO samples and the random distribution of these samples from different batches for analysis; he was also responsible for surveys of the availabilities, and purchases of all fermented food products from US retail outlets, together with their distribution for analysis. M.G. and B.C.P. monitored and validated all chemical analysis methods for fermented food products, involving those for BAs, TA and pH values, total lipid contents, and TBARS levels. M.G. was responsible for study experimental design, and also performed the univariate and MV chemometrics analyses of analytical datasets acquired, with assistance from B.C.P. M.G. also prepared, drafted, and finalized the manuscript for submission purposes. J.Z., B.C.P., and M.G. reviewed and edited manuscript drafts, and also contributed towards the interpretation of experimental results obtained. M.G. also fully supervised the complete study. All authors have read and agreed to the published version of the manuscript.

Funding: This research was part-funded by The Weston-Price Foundation, grant number WP1-MG3.

Acknowledgments: All authors are very grateful to the Weston A. Price Foundation (DC, USA) for part-funding the study, and to Midwest Laboratories (13611 B Street, Omaha, NE 68144-3693, USA) for performing the laboratory analysis of BAs. We are also grateful to Dave Wetzel of Green Pastures Products Inc. (NE, USA) for valuable discussions.

Conflicts of Interest: J.Z. is an employee of Green Pasture Products, 416 E. Fremont Street, O'Neill, NE 68763, USA. None of the other authors declare any conflicts of interest. The sponsoring body had no role in the design, execution, interpretation, or writing of the study.

References

1. Vidal-Carou, M.C.; Ambatle-Espunyes, A.; Ulla-Ulla, M.C.; Marine Â-Font, A. Histamine and tyramine in Spanish wines: Their formation during the winemaking process. *Am. J. Enolog. Viticul.* **1990**, *41*, 160–167.
2. Izquierdo-Pulido, M.; Marine Â-Font, A.; Vidal-Carou, M.C. Biogenic amine formation during malting and brewing. *J. Food Sci.* **1994**, *59*, 1104–1107. [CrossRef]
3. Perpetuini, G.; Tittarelli, F.; Battistelli, N.; Arfelli, G.; Suzzi, G.; Tofalo, R. Biogenic amines in global beverages. In *Biogenic Amines in Food: Analysis, Occurrence and Toxicity*; Saad, B., Tofalo, R., Eds.; The Royal Society of Chemistry: Cambridge, UK, 2020; pp. 133–156.
4. Halaasz, A.; Barath, A.; Simon-Sakardi, L.; Holzapel, W. Biogenic amines and their production by microorganisms in food. *Trends Food Sci. Technol.* **1994**, *5*, 42–49. [CrossRef]
5. Tittarelli, F.; Perpetuini, G.D.; Gianvito, P.; Tofalo, R. Biogenic amines producing and degrading bacteria: A snapshot from raw ewes' cheese. *LWT Food Sci. Technol.* **2019**, *101*, 1–9. [CrossRef]

6. Percival, B.C.; Wann, A.; Zbasnik, R.; Schlegel, V.; Edgar, M.; Zhang, J.; Ampem, G.; Wilson, P.; Le-Gresley, A.; Naughton, D.; et al. Evaluations of the peroxidative susceptibilities of cod liver oils by a ^{1}H NMR analysis strategy: Peroxidative resistivity of a natural collagenous and biogenic amine-rich fermented product. *Nutrients* **2020**, *12*, 3075. [CrossRef]
7. Alvarez, M.A.; Moreno-Arribas, M.V. The problem of biogenic amines in fermented foods and the use of potential biogenic amine-degrading microorganisms as a solution. *Trends Food Sci. Technol.* **2014**, *39*, 146–155. [CrossRef]
8. Vandekerckove, P. Amines in dry fermented sausage: A research note. *J. Food Sci.* **1977**, *42*, 283–285. [CrossRef]
9. Rhee, J.E.; Rhee, J.H.; Ryu, P.Y.; Choi, S.H. Identification of the cadBA operon from *Vibrio vulnificus* and its influence on survival to acid stress. *FEMS Microbiol. Lett.* **2002**, *208*, 245–251. [CrossRef] [PubMed]
10. Lee, Y.H.; Kim, B.H.; Kim, J.H.; Yoon, W.S.; Bang, S.H.; Park, Y.K. CadC has a global translational effect during acid adaptation in Salmonella enterica serovar typhimurium. *J. Bacteriol.* **2007**, *189*, 2417–2425. [CrossRef]
11. Van de Guchte, M.; Serror, P.; Chervaux, C.; Smokvina, T.; Ehrlich, S.D.; Maguin, E. Stress responses in lactic acid bacteria. *Antonie van Leeuwenhoek* **2002**, *82*, 187–216. [CrossRef]
12. D'Aniello, E.; Periklis, P.; Evgeniya, A.; Salvatore, D.A.; Arnone, M.I. Comparative neurobiology of biogenic amines in animal models in deuterostomes. *Front. Ecol. Evolut.* **2020**, *8*, 322.
13. Bendera, R.; Wilson, L.S. The regulatory effect of biogenic polyamines spermine and spermidine in men and women. *Open J. Endocrin. Metab. Dis.* **2019**, *9*, 35–48. [CrossRef]
14. Tabor, C.; Tabor, H. Polyamines. *Ann. Rev. Biochem.* **1984**, *53*, 749–790. [CrossRef] [PubMed]
15. Premont, R.T.; Gainetdinov, R.R.; Caron, M.G. Following the trace of elusive amines. *Proc. Natl. Acad. Sci. USA* **2001**, *98*, 9474–9475. [CrossRef]
16. Santos, M.H.S. Biogenic amines: Their importance in foods. *Int. J. Food Microbiol.* **1996**, *29*, 213–231. [CrossRef]
17. Arena, M.E.; de Nadra, M.C.M. Biogenic amine production by Lactobacillus. *J. Appl. Microbiol.* **2001**, *90*, 158–162. [CrossRef]
18. Taylor, S.L. Histamine food poisoning: Toxicology and clinical aspects. *Crit. Rev. Toxicol.* **1986**, *17*, 91–128. [CrossRef]
19. Hotchkiss, J.H.; Scanlan, R.A.; Libbey, L.M. Formation of bis (hydroxyalkyl)-N-nitrosamines as products of the nitrosation of spermidine. *J. Agric. Food Chem.* **1977**, *25*, 1183–1189. [CrossRef]
20. Livingston, M.G.; Livingston, H.M. Monoamine oxidase inhibitors. An update on drug interactions. *Drug Saf.* **1996**, *14*, 219–227. [CrossRef]
21. Prell, G.D.; Mazurkiewicz-Kwilecki, I.M. The effects of ethanol, acetaldehyde, morphine and naloxone on histamine methyltransferase activity. *Prog. Neuro-Psychopharmacol.* **1981**, *5*, 581–584. [CrossRef]
22. Lonvaud-Funel, A. BAs in wines: Role of lactic acid bacteria. *FEMS Microbiol. Lett.* **2001**, *199*, 9–13. [CrossRef] [PubMed]
23. Jastrzębska, A.; Piasta, A.; Kowalska, S.; Krzemiński, M.; Szłyk, E. A new derivatization reagent for determination of biogenic amines in wines. *J. Food Comp. Anal.* **2016**, *48*, 111–119. [CrossRef]
24. Grootveld, M. *Metabolic Profiling: Disease and Xenobiotics*; Issues in Toxicology Series; Royal Society of Chemistry: Cambridge, UK, 2014; ISBN 1849731632.
25. Nout, M.J.R. Food Technologies: Fermentation. *Encycl. Food Saf.* **2014**, *3*, 168–177. [CrossRef]
26. Cosmos, E.; Heberger, K.; Simon-Sarkadi, L. Principal component analysis of biogenic amines and polyphenols in Hungarian wines. *J. Agric. Food Chem.* **2002**, *50*, 3768–3774.
27. Quilliam, M.A.; Blay, P.; Hardstaff, W.; Wittrig, R.E.; Bartlett, V.; Bazavan, D.; Schreiber, A.; Ellis, R.; Fernandes, D.; Khalaf, F.; et al. LC-MS/MS analysis of biogenic amines in foods and beverages. In Proceedings of the 123rd AOAC Annual Meeting and Exposition, Philadelphia, PA, USA, 13–16 September 2009.
28. Witte, V.C.; Krause, G.F.; Bailey, M.E. A new extraction method for determining 2-thiobarbituric acid value of pork and beef during storage. *J. Food Sci.* **1970**, *35*, 582–585. [CrossRef]
29. FAO. Appendix XXV, Replies of the 6th Session of the CCMMP to Questions Referred by the 23rd Session of the CCMAS. Available online: http://www.fao.org/3/j2366e/j2366e25.htm (accessed on 27 September 2020).
30. Chong, J.; Soufan, O.; Li, C.; Caraus, I.; Li, S.; Bourque, G.; Wishart, D.S.; Xia, J. MetaboAnalyst 4.0: Towards more transparent and integrative metabolomics analysis. *Nucleic Acids Res.* **2018**, *46*, W486–W494. [CrossRef]

31. Pelckmans, K.; De Brabanter, J.; Suykens, J.A.K.; De Moor, B. Handling missing values in support vector machine classifiers. *Neural Netw.* **2005**, *18*, 684–692. [CrossRef]
32. Zhao, C.; Xia, T.; Du, P.; Duan, W.; Zhang, B.; Zhang, J.; Zhu, S.; Zheng, Y.; Wang, M.; Yu, Y. Chemical composition and antioxidant characteristic of traditional and industrial Zhenjiang aromatic vinegars during the aging process. *Molecules* **2018**, *23*, 2949. [CrossRef]
33. Grootveld, M.; Percival, B.C.; Leenders, J.; Wilson, P. Potential adverse public health effects afforded by the ingestion of dietary lipid oxidation product toxins: Significance of fried food sources. *Nutrients* **2020**, *12*, 974. [CrossRef]
34. Fugelsang, K.C. *Wine Microbiology*; Chapman & Hall: New York, NY, USA, 1997.
35. Romano, P.; Suzzi, G.; Turbanti, L.; Polsinelli, M. Acetaldehyde production in *Saccharomyces cerevisiae* wine yeasts. *FEMS Microbiol. Lett.* **1994**, *118*, 213–218. [CrossRef]
36. Liu, S.-Q.; Pilone, G.J. An overwiew of formation and roles of acetaldehyde in winemaking with emphasis on microbiological implications. *Int. J. Food Sci. Technol.* **2000**, *35*, 49–61. [CrossRef]
37. Uebelacker, M.; Lachenmeier, D.W. Quantitative determination of acetaldehyde in foods using automated digestion with simulated gastric fluid followed by headspace gas chromatography. *J. Anal. Meth. Chem.* **2011**. [CrossRef] [PubMed]
38. Zhao, G.; Kuang, G.; Li, J.; Hadiatullah, H.; Chen, H.; Wang, X.; Yao, Y.; Pan, Z.-H.; Wang, Y. Characterization of aldehydes and hydroxy acids as the main contribution to the traditional Chinese rose vinegar by flavor and taste analyses. *Food Res. Int.* **2020**, *129*, 108879. [CrossRef] [PubMed]
39. Vijisha, K.R.; Muraleedharan, K. The pKa values of amine based solvents for CO_2 capture and its temperature dependence—An analysis by density functional theory. *Int. J. Greenh. Gas. Cont.* **2017**, *58*, 62–70. [CrossRef]
40. Flydal, M.I.; Martinez, A. Phenylalanine hydroxylase: Function, structure, and regulation. *IUBMB Life* **2013**, *65*, 341–349. [CrossRef] [PubMed]
41. Harris, W.S. Fish oil supplementation: Evidence for health benefits. *Cleveland Clin. J. Med.* **2004**, *71*, 208–221. [CrossRef]
42. Janero, D.R. Malondialdehyde and thiobarbituric acid-reactivity as diagnostic indices of lipid peroxidation and peroxidative tissue injury. *Free Rad. Biol. Med.* **1990**, *9*, 515–540. [CrossRef]
43. Yunoki, K.; Tanji, M.; Murakami, Y.; Yasui, Y.; Hirose, S.; Ohnishi, M. Fatty acid compositions of commercial red wines. *Biosci. Biotechnol. Biochem.* **2004**, *68*, 2623–2626. [CrossRef]
44. Anihouvi, V.B.; Kindossi, J.M.; Hounhouigan, J.D. Processing and quality characteristics of some major fermented fish products from Africa: A critical review. *Int. Res. J. Biol. Sci.* **2012**, *1*, 72–84.
45. Phan, Q.; Tomasino, E.; Osborne, J. Influences of yeast product addition and fermentation temperature on changes in lipid compositions of pinot noir wines (abstract). In Proceedings of the 3rd Edition of International Conference on Agriculture and Food Chemistry, Rome, Italy, 23–24 July 2018.
46. Markley, K.S.; Sando, C.E.; Hendricks, S.B. Petroleum ether-soluble and ether-soluble constituents of grape pomace. *J. Biol. Chem.* **1938**, *123*, 641–654.
47. Sun, R.C.; Tomkinson, J. Comparative study of organic solvent and water-soluble lipophilic extractives from wheat straw I: Yield and chemical composition. *J. Wood Sci.* **2003**, *49*, 47–52. [CrossRef]
48. Zhang, C.; Brandt, M.J.; Schwab, C.; Gänzle, M.G. Propionic acid production by cofermentation of *Lactobacillus buchneri* and *Lactobacillus diolivorans* in sourdough. *Food Microbiol.* **2010**, *27*, 390–395. [CrossRef] [PubMed]

Publisher's Note: MDPI stays neutral with regard to jurisdictional claims in published maps and institutional affiliations.

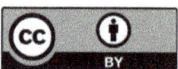

© 2020 by the authors. Licensee MDPI, Basel, Switzerland. This article is an open access article distributed under the terms and conditions of the Creative Commons Attribution (CC BY) license (http://creativecommons.org/licenses/by/4.0/).

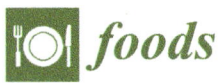

Review

Occurrence and Reduction of Biogenic Amines in Kimchi and Korean Fermented Seafood Products

Young Kyoung Park, Jae Hoan Lee and Jae-Hyung Mah *

Department of Food and Biotechnology, Korea University, 2511 Sejong-ro, Sejong 30019, Korea; eskimo@korea.ac.kr (Y.K.P.); jae-lee@korea.ac.kr (J.H.L.)
* Correspondence: nextbio@korea.ac.kr; Tel.: +82-44-860-1431

Received: 4 October 2019; Accepted: 24 October 2019; Published: 4 November 2019

Abstract: Biogenic amines produced during fermentation may be harmful when ingested in high concentrations. As current regulations remain insufficient to ensure the safety of fermented vegetable products, the current study determined the risks associated with the consumption of kimchi by evaluating the biogenic amine concentrations reported by various studies. Upon evaluation, some kimchi products were found to contain histamine and tyramine at potentially hazardous concentrations exceeding the recommended limit of 100 mg/kg for both histamine and tyramine. The biogenic amines may have originated primarily from metabolic activity by microorganisms during fermentation, as well as from *Jeotgal* (Korean fermented seafood) and *Aekjeot* (Korean fermented fish sauce) products commonly used as ingredients for kimchi production. Many studies have suggested that *Jeotgal* and *Aekjeot* may contribute to the histamine and tyramine content in kimchi. Microorganisms isolated from kimchi and *Jeotgal* have been reported to produce both histamine and tyramine. Despite the potential toxicological risks, limited research has been conducted on reducing the biogenic amine content of kimchi and *Jeotgal* products. The regulation and active monitoring of biogenic amine content during kimchi production appear to be necessary to ensure the safety of the fermented vegetable products.

Keywords: kimchi; *Jeotgal*; *Aekjeot*; *Myeolchi-jeot*; *Myeolchi-aekjeot*; biogenic amines; recommended limits; occurrence; reduction; starter cultures

1. Introduction

Kimchi refers to a group of traditional Korean fermented vegetable products consumed worldwide [1]. Dating back to the 12th century during the Three Kingdoms period of ancient Korea, salted and fermented vegetable products represent the earliest form of kimchi, however, the addition of several ingredients such as the introduction of red peppers in the 16th century was eventually adopted for kimchi production [2]. The availability of local ingredients across different provinces in Korea led to the development of many regional kimchi varieties [3] (Figure 1). Currently, there are over 200 varieties of kimchi with over 100 different ingredients used for kimchi production [4]. Each kimchi variety is categorized according to the ingredients selected for production [5]. Kimchi in its current form has been recognized globally through international standardization as well [6]. Kimchi is prepared by trimming Napa cabbage, followed by salting, rinsing, and then draining excess water. The seasoning ingredients include red pepper powder, garlic, ginger, radish, glutinous rice paste, sugar, *Jeotgal*, and *Aekjeot*. The salted Napa cabbage is then mixed with the seasoning and stored at low temperatures (typically 0–10 °C in Korea [5]) to ferment until ripened [6]. While the production method described by the Codex only describes *Baechu* kimchi (Napa cabbage kimchi), slight variations are used to produce other kimchi varieties.

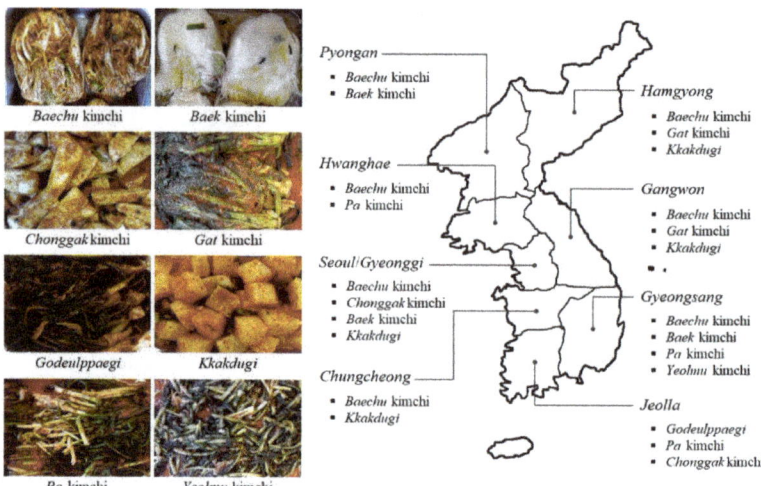

Figure 1. Kimchi varieties available across different provinces in Korea. *Baechu* kimchi: Napa cabbage kimchi; *Baek* kimchi: Napa cabbage kimchi prepared without red pepper powder; *Chonggak* kimchi: ponytail radish kimchi; *Gat* kimchi: mustard leaf kimchi; *Godeulppaegi*: Korean lettuce kimchi; *Kkakdugi*: diced radish kimchi; *Pa* kimchi: green onion kimchi; *Yeolmu* kimchi: young radish kimchi.

Nonetheless, nearly every kimchi variety benefits from preliminary brining, which inhibits the growth of pathogenic bacteria while selecting for lactic acid bacteria (LAB) known for promoting beneficial effects such as gastrointestinal regulation and prevention of colon cancer [7,8]. The LAB such as *Leuconostoc*, *Lactobacillus*, and *Weissella* species as well as the enzymes present in the ingredients are responsible for kimchi fermentation [9,10]. Consumption of kimchi is reported to provide numerous health benefits such as anti-oxidative, anti-carcinogenic, anti-mutagenic, and anti-aging effects [8,11,12].

Despite the numerous beneficial functional qualities, fermented foods such as kimchi may contain potentially harmful substances known as biogenic amines (BA). The nitrogenous compounds are mostly produced by microorganisms during fermentation through enzymatic decarboxylation of amino acids, as well as transamination of ketones and aldehydes [13]. BA are often categorized as aliphatic: putrescine, cadaverine, spermidine, spermine; aromatic: β-phenylethylamine, tyramine; heterocyclic: tryptamine, histamine [14,15]. The intake of BA at high concentrations as well as amine oxidase inhibition and deficiency may lead to toxic effects [16]. Recently, histamine, tyramine, putrescine, cadaverine, spermidine, and spermine were found to be cytotoxic toward human intestinal cells [17–19]. Furthermore, BA may also be converted to potentially carcinogenic N-nitrosamines in the presence of nitrites [20,21]. Excessive intake of foods containing high concentrations of histamine may potentially induce "scombroid poisoning" with symptoms such as headaches, hives, diarrhea, dyspnea, and hypotension [22]. Similarly, ingestion of foods with excessive tyramine content may cause a "cheese crisis" with symptoms that include severe headaches, hemorrhages, hypertensive effects or even heart failure [23]. As a result, many countries have implemented regulations on the production of histamine-rich seafood products, however many other food products are not currently regulated [24]. Several studies have suggested limits for BA content in food products of 100 mg/kg for histamine, 100–800 mg/kg for tyramine, 30 mg/kg for β-phenylethylamine, and 1000 mg/kg for total BA content [14,15]. The concentrations of BA in many fermented food products such as fermented meats and cheese have been widely reported to exceed limits for safe consumption. Similarly, BA have been detected in kimchi products, the most widely consumed traditional Korean food. High concentrations of BA have also been detected in kimchi ingredients *Jeotgal* (Korean fermented seafood) and *Aekjeot* (Korean fermented fish sauce), which contribute to the overall BA content in kimchi [25]. In addition, microorganisms isolated from kimchi as well as the fermented seafood products *Jeotgal* and *Aekjeot* have been reported to produce BA. Current regulations remain insufficient to address the potential health risks associated with the consumption of kimchi with high concentrations of BA. Therefore, the current article evaluated the risks associated with the BA content of kimchi products according to intake limits for β-phenylethylamine (30 mg/kg), histamine (100 mg/kg), and tyramine (100 mg/kg) as recommended by Ten Brink et al. [15], and reviewed potential sources of BA, and methods for reducing BA content.

2. Biogenic Amine Content in Kimchi Products

Table 1 displays the BA content of kimchi products as reported by various studies. The BA content of *Baechu* kimchi (Napa cabbage kimchi), the most popular kimchi variety consumed worldwide, has been reported by several studies. Cho et al. [25] reported histamine and tyramine concentrations in *Baechu* kimchi that exceeded recommended limits. Another study also showed that tyramine content in *Baechu* kimchi exceeded the recommended limit [26]. Tsai et al. [27] notably reported the highest histamine content which exceeded the recommended limit by a factor of 53. Tsai et al. [27] suggested that the high concentration of histamine in kimchi might be due to ingredients such as fish sauce or shrimp paste used in the kimchi production process. Shin et al. [28] reported β-phenylethylamine, histamine, and tyramine content at safe concentrations below 30 mg/kg. Similarly, Mah et al. [29] reported both histamine and tyramine content at safe concentrations below 30 mg/kg. In ripened *Baechu* kimchi, Kang et al. [26] reported tyramine content at concentrations that nearly reached the recommended limit.

Aside from *Baechu* kimchi, several studies have also reported the BA content of other kimchi varieties as well. *Chonggak* kimchi (ponytail radish kimchi) as reported by Jin et al. [30] contained histamine concentrations that exceeded the recommended limit. Tyramine content in *Chonggak* kimchi as reported by Kang et al. [26] were at safe concentrations, while Mah et al. [29] reported safe concentrations of both histamine and tyramine below recommended limits. As for *Gat* kimchi (mustard leaf kimchi), Lee et al. [31] reported histamine concentrations which exceeded the recommended limit by a factor of 2, while tyramine content slightly exceeded the limit. In contrast, Mah et al. [29] reported that *Gat* kimchi did not contain histamine and tyramine at detectable levels. *Kkakdugi* (diced radish kimchi) as reported by Jin et al. [30] contained tyramine at safe concentrations below the recommended limit, however, histamine concentrations exceeded the recommended limit. In contrast, Mah et al. [29] reported that histamine was not detected in *Kkakdugi*, and tyramine content was at safe concentrations below recommended limits. Similarly, Kang et al. [26] also reported tyramine concentrations in *Kkakdugi* below the recommended limit. As for *Pa* kimchi (green onion kimchi), Lee et al. [31] reported histamine and tyramine concentrations exceeded recommended limits by a factor of 4 and 2, respectively. In contrast, Mah et al. [29] reported histamine and tyramine in *Pa* kimchi at safe concentrations as tyramine content was not detected while histamine content remained below 30 mg/kg. Other kimchi varieties such as *Baek* kimchi (Napa cabbage kimchi prepared without red pepper powder), *Godeulppaegi* (Korean lettuce kimchi), and *Yeolmu* kimchi (young radish kimchi) were reported to contain histamine and tyramine at safe concentrations below 100 mg/kg [29].

Nonetheless, as the vast majority of studies are primarily focused upon *Baechu* kimchi, further research on the BA content of other kimchi varieties remains necessary. Currently, the severity of the risks associated with the BA content of kimchi remains difficult to thoroughly assess as limited research has been conducted. Though various BA have been detected in kimchi products, several studies have reported histamine and tyramine content at concentrations that exceeded the recommended intake limits of 100 mg/kg. Furthermore, the risk of nitrosamine formation entails the need for continuous monitoring of BA content during fermentation, especially as putrescine and cadaverine were detected at particularly high concentrations. Due to the toxicological risks associated with the consumption of BA, the content in kimchi necessitates regulation and control to ensure its safety.

Table 1. Biogenic amine content of Korean fermented vegetable products.

Korean Fermented Vegetable Products	N [1]	Biogenic Amines (mg/kg) [2]								Ref.
		TRP [3]	PHE	PUT	CAD	HIS	TYR	SPD	SPM	
	3	NT [3]	NT	11.2–89.0 [4]	ND [5]–151.8	ND-5.1	ND-28.2	ND	ND	[29]
Baechu kimchi (Napa cabbage kimchi)	20	2.3–22.6	ND-6.8	15.1–240.4	3.6–44.9	0.6–142.3	9.7–118.2	7.7–16.5	ND-3.7	[25]
	37	ND-114	ND	ND-73	ND-1550	ND-5350	ND-42	ND-88	ND-121	[27]
	18	ND-43.9	NT	ND-245.9	ND-63.3	NT	ND-103.6	ND-74.8	NT	[26]
	20	ND-74.8	ND-2.0	2.3–148.6	0.9–39.8	ND-21.8	1.1–27.9	ND-6.7	ND-5.1	[28]
Baek kimchi (Napa cabbage kimchi prepared without red pepper powder)	3	NT	NT	ND-54.7	ND-94.8	ND	ND	ND	ND	[29]
	3	tr [6]	NT	1.9–39.6	11.5–25.6	NT	7.8–64.9	ND-1.7	NT	[26]
Chonggak kimchi (ponytail radish kimchi)	3	NT	NT	ND-11.2	ND-70.7	ND	ND	ND	ND	[29]
	3	2.3–15.2	NT	ND-20.3	ND-85.7	NT	20.2–58.1	ND	NT	[26]
	5	ND-23.70	ND-2.80	3.89–853.70	2.00–148.50	8.24–131.20	0.79–18.70	6.10–14.00	ND-20.74	[30]
Gat kimchi (mustard leaf kimchi)	3	NT	NT	ND-10.4	ND-11.6	ND	ND	ND	ND	[29]
	13	ND-26.74	ND-15.75	1.89–720.82	2.12–52.43	3.30–232.10	1.28–149.77	12.26–32.62	ND-61.94	[31]
Godeulppaegi (Korean lettuce kimchi)	3	NT	NT	ND-6.4	ND-26.7	ND	ND	ND	ND	[29]
Kkakdugi (diced radish kimchi)	3	NT	NT	ND-15.4	ND-55.1	ND	ND-9.0	ND	ND	[29]
	5	5.5–18.6	NT	ND-51.6	ND-56.2	NT	ND-10.8	ND-21.8	NT	[26]
	5	ND	ND-15.24	10.85–982.32	ND-124.60	18.75–127.78	2.97–76.95	ND-16.76	ND-3.10	[30]
Pa kimchi (green onion kimchi)	3	NT	NT	ND-7.8	ND-15.9	ND-21.7	ND	ND	ND	[29]
	13	ND-15.95	ND-5.97	ND-254.47	ND-123.29	8.67–386.03	ND-181.10	2.32–18.74	ND-33.84	[31]
Yeolmu kimchi (young radish kimchi)	3	NT	NT	ND	ND	ND	ND	ND	ND	[29]

[1] N: Number of samples examined; [2] TRP: tryptamine, PHE: β-phenylethylamine, PUT: putrescine, CAD: cadaverine, HIS: histamine, TYR: tyramine, SPD: spermidine, SPM: spermine; [3] NT: not tested; [4] Values are the minimum and maximum concentrations reported. The same number of digits is used after the decimal point in the values, as was presented in the corresponding references; [5] ND: not detected; [6] tr: trace.

3. Biogenic Amine Content of Other Vegetable Products

Research has also been conducted on the BA content of vegetable products originating from other countries (Table S1). The popular fermented food sauerkraut is produced through lactic acid fermentation of white cabbage [32,33]. Among European fermented food products, sauerkraut most closely resembles Korean kimchi [34]. Despite its popularity, Taylor et al. [35] reported that sauerkraut contained histamine concentrations that exceeded recommended limits. Ten Brink et al. [15] also reported that histamine and tyramine in sauerkraut exceeded recommended limits by a factor of 1 and 2, respectively. Many varieties of Japanese *Tsukemono* are preserved vegetables produced utilizing methods such as fermentation, salting, and pickling [36]. *Tsukemono* are differentiated based on ingredients, pickling method, and microorganisms responsible for fermentation [5]. Handa et al. [37] reported that histamine and tyramine in *Tsukemono* exceeded recommended limits by a factor of 3 and 4, respectively. As an important part of the Taiwanese diet, mustard pickle is prepared using mustard greens submerged in 14% NaCl brine for 4 months [38]. Kung et al. [38] reported that mustard pickles contained histamine and tyramine at safe concentrations below 100 mg/kg. Though fermented vegetable products are consumed worldwide, limited research has been conducted on the BA content of vegetable-based fermented foods. The few studies available had reported a wide range of BA content, including concentrations that exceeded recommended limits. Therefore, as the risks associated with the consumption of fermented vegetables remains largely undetermined, additional research is necessary to ensure the safe consumption of fermented foods.

4. Determinants for Biogenic Amine Content in Kimchi

4.1. Biogenic Amine Content of Kimchi Ingredients: Jeotgal and Aekjeot

Kimchi production involves the use of many ingredients including the fermented seafood products *Jeotgal* and *Aekjeot*. Used as seasoning ingredients during the production of kimchi [39], *Jeotgal* and *Aekjeot* contain flavor compounds that contribute greatly to the ripening process during kimchi fermentation [40]. Reports of the fermented seafood products as kimchi ingredients date back to the 16th century during the age of the *Chosun* dynasty of Korea [41]. Though *Jeotgal* and *Aekjeot* used during modern kimchi production vary by region, the most commonly used varieties include *Myeolchi-jeot* (salted and fermented anchovy), *Myeolchi-aekjeot* (salted and fermented anchovy sauce), *Saeu-jeot* (salted and fermented shrimp), and *Kkanari-aekjeot* (salted and fermented sand lance sauce) [42]. *Jeotgal* production typically involves submersion of seafood in brine with 20% salinity for 2–3 months at room temperature, and results in the final product resembling the initial seafood ingredient [43]. Some *Jeotgal* products undergo additional seasoning for consumption as side dishes rather than as ingredients during kimchi production [44,45]. Similarly, *Aekjeot* production involves the submersion of seafood in brine with salinity ranging from 20 to 30% for 1–2 years, however solid particles are removed through filtration for the final product [46]. In both *Jeotgal* and *Aekjeot*, the salt content inhibits putrefactive bacteria, and the enzymatic activity partially breaks down the proteins to develop a rich flavor [41]. Also, the addition of *Jeotgal* contributes to the protein, amino acid, and mineral content of kimchi, further reinforcing the nutritional value of kimchi products [5].

Despite the benefits described above, *Jeotgal* and *Aekjeot* have been reported to contain high concentrations of potentially hazardous BA such as histamine and tyramine [29]. Table 2 displays the BA content of the fermented seafood products. The reported BA content of *Aekjeot* and *Jeotgal* were evaluated according to recommended limits for intake. *Myeolchi-jeot* was reported to contain histamine and tyramine concentrations which exceeded recommended limits by a factor of approximately 6 and 2, respectively [47]. *Myeolchi-aekjeot* reportedly contained histamine and tyramine at concentrations that exceeded recommended limits by a factor of approximately 12 and 4, respectively [29]. The BA content of *Myeolchi-aekjeot* as studied by Cho et al. [25] showed β-phenylethylamine, histamine, and tyramine content at concentrations that exceeded recommended limits by a factor of about 2, 11, and 6, respectively. Moon et al. [48] also studied the BA content of *Myeolchi-aekjeot* by reporting β-phenylethylamine, histamine, and tyramine content at concentrations that exceeded recommended limits by a factor of approximately 3, 12, and 4, respectively. Similarly, Shin et al. [28] reported that *Myeolchi-aekjeot* contained β-phenylethylamine, histamine, and tyramine at concentrations that exceeded recommended limits by a factor of approximately 1, 4, and 4, respectively. Cho et al. [49] and Joung and Min [50] reported histamine concentrations in *Myeolchi-aekjeot* which greatly exceeded recommended limits by a factor of about 21 and 11, respectively.

As for *Kkanari-aekjeot*, histamine and tyramine content were reported at concentrations that exceeded recommended limits by a factor of approximately 10 and 2, respectively [29]. Cho et al. [25] also reported the β-phenylethylamine, histamine, and tyramine content in *Kkanari-aekjeot* at concentrations which exceeded recommended limits by a factor of 2, 11, and 6, respectively. Moon et al. [48] reported histamine and tyramine content at concentrations that exceeded recommended limits by a factor of about 7 and 3, respectively. Similarly, Shin et al. [28] reported that *Kkanari-aekjeot* contained β-phenylethylamine, histamine, and tyramine at concentrations that exceeded recommended limits by a factor of approximately 1, 10, and 3, respectively. Notably, the highest histamine content in *Kkanari-aekjeot* was reported by Cho et al. [49] as concentrations greatly exceeded the recommended limit by a factor of approximately 18.

As for *Saeu-jeot*, Mah et al. [47], Cho et al. [25], Moon et al. [48], and Shin et al. [28] reported BA content at safe concentrations below recommended limits for β-phenylethylamine, histamine, and tyramine, respectively.

Overall, the considerably high BA concentrations, especially histamine, reported for both retail *Jeotgal* and *Aekjeot* products may be potentially hazardous. All *Kkanari-aekjeot* and *Myeolchi-aekjeot* products contained histamine concentrations which exceeded 100 mg/kg indicating that safety regulations are necessary. According to Mah et al. [29], the high BA content may be due to the considerably long fermentation duration for the production of the fermented seafood. Furthermore, the results of the research conducted by Moon et al. [48] suggested that total BA content increased alongside crude protein concentrations for both *Jeotgal* and *Aekjeot*. After all, the high concentrations of BA reported for kimchi appears to originate partly from fish sauce such as *Myeolchi-aekjeot* and *Kkanari-aekjeot* [25]. Given the high concentrations of BA detected in kimchi and fermented seafood products, safety regulation and standardization of the manufacturing process appears to be necessary.

High BA concentrations were not limited to *Jeotgal* and *Aekjeot* products as the similar observations were reported for fermented seafood products originating from other countries (Table S1). Saaid et al. [51] studied the BA content of Malaysian seafood. The study showed that *Cincalok* (salted and fermented shrimp) contained histamine and tyramine at high concentrations that exceeded the recommended limits by a factor of approximately 3 and 7, respectively. *Budu* (salted and fermented anchovy) also contained high histamine and tyramine concentrations that exceeded recommended limits by a factor of 4 and 9, respectively. Similarly, research conducted by Rosma et al. [52] revealed histamine concentrations in *Budu* exceeding the recommended limit by a factor of 11.

The reported results indicated that fermented seafood products tended to contain high concentrations of BA, especially histamine. As the BA content exceeded well beyond recommended limits, consumption of the fermented seafood products may lead to adverse effects on human health. Due to the potential toxicological risks, expansion of current regulations regarding the BA content of seafood appears to be necessary to cover the aforementioned fermented seafood products as well as to include other amines such as tyramine and β-phenylethylamine.

Table 2. Biogenic amine content of Korean fermented seafood products.

Korean Fermented Seafood Products	N [1]	Biogenic Amines (mg/kg) [2]								Ref.
		TRP [3]	PHE	PUT	CAD	HIS	TYR	SPD	SPM	
Myeolchi-jeot (salted and fermented anchovy)	3	NT [3]	NT	92–241 [4]	ND [5]–665	155–579	63–244	ND–43	ND–77	[47]
Myeolchi-aekjeot (salted and fermented anchovy sauce)	4	NT	NT	86.1–178.9	ND	684.6–1154.7	222.6–383.1	ND–358.6	ND	[29]
	8	60.1–296.8	9.3–54.1	33.8–182.1	81.6–263.6	352.5–1127.6	93.9–611.3	4.7–27.1	1.9–12.2	[25]
	15	ND–382.2	ND–85.3	ND–680.0	ND–126.1	684.5–1205.0	77.5–381.1	ND	ND	[48]
	10	NT	NT	NT	NT	584.59–2070.58	NT	NT	NT	[49]
	12	NT	NT	NT	NT	150–1112	NT	NT	NT	[50]
	5	35.0–193.5	20.0–36.9	41.8–173.3	100.0–253.0	196.0–393.2	211.4–446.0	0.8–6.7	1.4–4.1	[28]
Kkanari-aekjeot (salted and fermented sand lance sauce)	4	NT	NT	55.5–136.4	ND–2.8	308.2–959.7	131.0–203.1	ND–30.9	ND	[29]
	8	62.0–187.2	10.4–51.7	1.6–311.6	52.1–314.8	215.4–1124.1	142.7–583.0	4.0–23.4	2.2–12.8	[25]
	16	ND–410.0	ND–17.9	ND–674.3	ND–96.9	308–732.2	112.3–328.0	ND	ND	[48]
	10	NT	NT	NT	NT	194.01–1839.68	NT	NT	NT	[49]
	5	122.5–242.5	18.3–32.5	30.8–43.8	52.5–168.3	183.4–1038.9	155.7–252.4	3.4–6.4	1.2–5.6	[28]
Saeu-jeot (salted and fermented shrimp)	2	NT	NT	ND	ND	ND	ND	ND	33–62	[47]
	5	5.3–10.6	ND–1.9	2.0–5.2	6.7–8.5	28.6–33.0	11.2–15.2	1.6–2.9	ND–0.7	[25]
	8	11.8–14.5	5.3–10.6	5.2–12.4	6.7–8.5	28.6–32.0	ND–45.5	ND	ND	[48]
	5	3.3–8.1	ND–4.2	2.8–5.4	ND–1.5	2.3–12.7	1.4–7.4	ND–0.8	0.4–9.6	[28]

[1] N: Number of samples examined; [2] TRP: tryptamine, PHE: β-phenylethylamine, PUT: putrescine, CAD: cadaverine, HIS: histamine, TYR: tyramine, SPD: spermidine, SPM: spermine; [3] NT: not tested; [4] Values are the minimum and maximum concentrations reported. The same number of digits is used after the decimal point in the values, as was presented in the corresponding references; [5] ND: not detected.

4.2. Biogenic Amine Production by Bacterial Strains from Kimchi and Fermented Seafood Products

Microorganisms play a major role in the production of BA during fermentation through the decarboxylation of free amino acids. LAB responsible for fermentation have been reported to produce putrescine, cadaverine, histamine, and tyramine [15]. Table 3 displays the BA production by bacterial strains isolated from various kimchi and fermented seafood products. Tsai et al. [27] reported that LAB strains isolated from kimchi products purchased from Taiwanese markets were capable of producing histamine and other BA. The isolated strains identified as *Lactobacillus paracasei* subsp. *paracasei*, *Lb. brevis*, and *Brevibacillus brevis* were tested for β-phenylethylamine, putrescine, cadaverine, histamine, and spermine production in assay media. The reported results showed that *Lb. paracasei* subsp. *paracasei*, *Lb. brevis*, and *Bb. brevis* produced histamine at concentrations of 15.1, 13.6, and 16.3–43.1 µg/mL, respectively. Other BA were detected at concentrations lower than 15 µg/mL. Kim and Kim [53] isolated LAB strains from kimchi identified as *Lb. brevis*, *Lb. curvatus*, *Leuconostoc mesenteroides*, and *Staphylococcus hominis* that demonstrated tyramine production capabilities at over 200 µg/mL in assay media. Jeong and Lee [54] reported on putrescine, cadaverine, histamine, and tyramine production in assay media by LAB isolated from kimchi including *Leu. citreum*, *Leu. lactis*, *Leu. mesenteroides*, *Weissella cibaria*, *W. confusa*, and *W. paramesenteroides*. The results revealed that *Leuconostoc* spp. did not produce histamine and tyramine, however, putrescine and cadaverine were produced at concentrations lower than 20 µg/mL. *Weissella* spp. also produced putrescine and cadaverine at concentrations lower than 20 µg/mL, however, some strains produced histamine and tyramine at concentrations higher than 50 µg/mL. Compared to *Leuconostoc* spp., *Weissella* spp. produced a wider variety of BA at higher concentrations, prompting recommendations for stricter safety guidelines for screening starter *Weissella* strains suitable for kimchi fermentation [54].

Other varieties of kimchi were also reported to contain microorganisms capable of BA production. While the majority of the LAB strains isolated from *Chonggak* kimchi and *Kkakdugi* did not produce BA at detectable levels, some isolated LAB strains reportedly produced tyramine in the ranges of 260.93–339.56 µg/mL and 287.23–386.17 µg/mL, respectively, in BA production assay media [30]. Aside from tyramine, other BA were not detected in the same assay media. Although the study did not specify the bacterial species capable of producing BA, *Lb. brevis* was suggested as a strong producer of BA. Lee et al. [31] reported the BA production in assay media by LAB strains isolated from *Gat* kimchi and *Pa* kimchi. From *Gat* kimchi, *Enterococcus faecium*, *Lb. brevis*, and *Leu. mesenteroides* produced the highest concentrations of tyramine in the ranges of 259.10–269.57 µg/mL, ND–365.96 µg/mL, and 145.14–301.67 µg/mL, respectively. *Lb. brevis* strains also produced putrescine ranging from ND to 320.42 µg/mL. From *Pa* kimchi, the isolated LAB strains identified as *Lb. brevis* and *Lb. sakei* produced the highest concentration of BA such as tyramine in the ranges of ND–301.52 µg/mL and 113.98–131.36 µg/mL, respectively. Also, a *Lb. brevis* strain produced putrescine at 362.44 µg/mL. Aside from putrescine and tyramine, other BA produced by LAB strains were reported at concentrations lower than 60 µg/mL. Based on the reported BA production capabilities of isolated strains, LAB appear to contribute to the BA content in kimchi, especially tyramine which were produced at the highest concentrations.

Aside from LAB, other bacterial species isolated from *Jeotgal* products were reported to have BA production capabilities. *S. equorum* strains isolated from *Saeu-jeot* and *Myeolchi-jeot* were reported to be capable of producing putrescine, cadaverine, histamine, and tyramine in assay media [55,56]. The reported results showed that all BA were detected at concentrations below 50 µg/mL. Lim [57] isolated bacterial strains from *Myeolchi-jeot* which were identified as *Bacillus licheniformis*, *Serratia marcescens*, *S. xylosus*, *Aeromonas hydrophila*, and *Morganella morganii*, and the strains were capable of producing high concentrations of histamine in assay media at 1699.3 ± 35.6 µg/mL, 1987.2 ± 27.8 µg/mL, 2257 ± 30.7 µg/mL, 1655.5 ± 41.2 µg/mL, and 2869.4 ± 49.0 µg/mL, respectively. Mah et al. [58] suggested that *Bacillus* species, especially *B. licheniformis*, contributed towards BA content as the isolated strains isolated from *Myeolchi-aekjeot* were capable of producing putrescine, cadaverine, histamine, and tyramine. Thus, the isolated bacterial strains appear to contribute to the high histamine content of fermented seafood products, which in turn contribute to the BA content of kimchi.

Table 3. Biogenic amine production by bacterial strains isolated from Korean fermented vegetable and seafood products.

Korean Fermented Vegetable and Seafood Products	Strains	N[1]	Biogenic Amines (µg/mL)[2]								Ref.
			TRP[3]	PHE	PUT	CAD	HIS	TYR	SPD	SPM	
	Lactobacillus paracasei subsp. *paracasei*	1	NT[3]	ND[4]	ND	0.3	15.1	NT	NT	4.5	[27]
	Lactobacillus brevis	1	NT	4.3	0.2	0.8	13.6	NT	NT	5.6	
	Brevibacillus brevis	2	NT	ND-3.8[5]	ND-0.1	ND-11.2	16.3-43.1	NT	NT	6.8-8.8	
Baechu kimchi (Napa cabbage kimchi)	*Lactobacillus brevis*	6	NT	NT	NT	NT	NT	287-372	NT	NT	[53]
	Lactobacillus curvatus	4	NT	NT	NT	NT	NT	333-388	NT	NT	
	Leuconostoc mesenteroides	2	NT	NT	NT	NT	NT	282-322	NT	NT	
	Staphylococcus hominis	2	NT	NT	NT	NT	NT	287-296	NT	NT	
	Leuconostoc citreum	2	NT	NT	ND	18.1-18.2	ND	ND	NT	NT	[54]
	Leuconostoc lactis	4	NT	NT	15.6-16.2	17.6-19.1	ND	ND	NT	NT	
	Leuconostoc mesenteroides	3	NT	NT	ND	ND-18.8	ND	ND	NT	NT	
	Weissella cibaria	16	NT	NT	ND-17.7	ND-19.5	ND-72.9	ND-59.9	NT	NT	
	Weissella confusa	8	NT	NT	ND-17.1		ND-73.3	ND-56.6	NT	NT	
	Weissella paramesenteroides	1	NT	NT	ND		55.2	56.3	NT	NT	
Kkakdugi (diced radish kimchi)	Lactic acid bacteria	39	ND	ND	ND	ND	ND	287.23-386.17	ND	ND	[30]
Chonggak kimchi (ponytail radish kimchi)	Lactic acid bacteria	16	ND	ND	ND	ND	ND	260.93-339.56	ND	ND	
Pa kimchi (green onion kimchi)	*Lactobacillus brevis*	14	ND	ND-2.39	ND-362.44	ND-54.79	ND	ND-301.52	ND	ND	[31]
	Lactobacillus sakei	2	ND	1.00-3.96	ND	ND	ND	113.98-131.36	ND	ND	
Gat kimchi (mustard leaf kimchi)	*Enterococcus faecium*	2	ND	3.51-3.88	ND	ND	ND	259.10-269.57	ND	ND	
	Lactobacillus brevis	7	ND	ND-2.34	ND-320.42	ND-47.73	ND	ND-365.96	ND	ND	
	Leuconostoc mesenteroides	2	ND	1.47-1.91	ND	ND	ND	145.14-301.67	ND	ND	
Myeolchi-jeot (salted and fermented anchovy)	*Staphylococcus equorum*	39	NT	NT	ND-22.6	ND-29.6	ND-40.0	ND-29.7	NT	NT	[56]
Saeu-jeot (salted and fermented shrimp)	*Bacillus licheniformisr*	1	NT	NT	NT	NT	1699.3 ± 35.6[6]	NT	NT	NT	[57]
Myeolchi-jeot (salted and fermented anchovy)	*Serratia marcescens*	1	NT	NT	NT	NT	1987.2 ± 27.8	NT	NT	NT	
	Staphylococcus xylosus	1	NT	NT	NT	NT	2257.4 ± 30.7	NT	NT	NT	
	Aeromonas hydrophila	1	NT	NT	NT	NT	1655.5 ± 41.2	NT	NT	NT	
	Morganella morganii	1	NT	NT	NT	NT	2869.4 ± 49.0	NT	NT	NT	

[1] N: Number of samples examined; [2] TRP: tryptamine, PHE: β-phenylethylamine, PUT: putrescine, CAD: cadaverine, HIS: histamine, TYR: tyramine, SPD: spermidine, SPM: spermine; [3] NT: not tested; [4] ND: not detected; [5] Values are the minimum and maximum concentrations reported. The same number of digits is used after the decimal point in the values, as was presented in the corresponding references; [6] mean ± standard deviation. The same number of digits is used after the decimal point in the values, as was presented in the corresponding references.

The aforementioned studies reported BA production by isolated strains at widely varying concentrations, even among the same species. Lee et al. [31] suggested that the BA production by LAB isolated from kimchi may be strain-dependent. Differences in BA production are widely considered to be strain-dependent, and not species-dependent [59]. The claim is further substantiated by the evidence for horizontal gene transfer for decarboxylase genes [60–62]. For example, as tyrosine decarboxylation was observed only for some strains, even belonging to the same species of LAB, tyramine production is considered strain-specific rather than species-specific [63]. Nonetheless, BA production by isolated strains indicates a risk for BA accumulation during *Jeotgal* and kimchi fermentation. Consequently, the control of BA accumulation during the production of fermented foods necessitates the reduction of microbial BA production by control of fermentation conditions, utilization of starter cultures, and sanitary practices to prevent contamination by BA-producing microorganisms.

5. Strategies to Reduce Biogenic Amine Content in Kimchi Products

Despite the risks associated with BA accumulation, limited research has been conducted on reducing the BA content of kimchi products. Instead of directly reducing BA content in kimchi, several studies have reported various methods to reduce BA concentrations in the kimchi ingredients *Jeotgal* and *Aekjeot*. Kim et al. [64] reported that kimchi produced using fermented seafood products contained BA at significantly higher concentrations. Lee et al. [65] suggested that the BA concentration of kimchi products may be reduced by limiting the quantity of the fermented seafood products used during kimchi production. For example, Kang [66] reported the histamine content of kimchi without *Myeolchi-aekjeot* at safe levels, however, the addition of *Myeolchi-aekjeot* raised histamine content to unsafe concentrations above the recommended limit by a factor of approximately 6. The study also described the effect of heat treatment of *Myeolchi-aekjeot* on the histamine content of kimchi. Histamine concentrations in kimchi produced using heat-treated *Myeolchi-aekjeot* were reported at 546.14 ± 1.33 mg/kg, while non-treated kimchi contained 592.78 ± 3.43 mg/kg. The reported results indicate that microorganisms from *Myeolchi-aekjeot* contributed towards the production of histamine during kimchi fermentation. Also, as research shows that histamine is heat-stable [67], the lower BA content in kimchi produced using the heat-treated *Myeolchi-aekjeot* may be due to the sterilization of histamine-producing microorganisms [66]. In addition to the contribution of BA content in kimchi by *Myeolchi-aekjeot*, Lee et al. [31] suggested that microorganisms from *Myeolchi-aekjeot* may produce BA during kimchi fermentation. Utilizing substitute ingredients in lieu of *Myeolchi-aekjeot* and *Kkanari-aekjeot* may also be effective in reducing BA content in kimchi. As other *Jeotgal* products including *Ojingeo-jeot* (salted and fermented sliced squid), *Toha-jeot* (salted and fermented *toha* shrimp), *Jogae-jeot* (salted and fermented clam), *Baendaengi-jeot* (salted and fermented big-eyed herring), and *Eorigul-jeot* (salted and fermented oysters) have been found to contain individual BA content below 100 mg/kg [47], utilization of the fermented seafood products with low BA content for kimchi production is expected to reduce the overall BA content of kimchi products [29].

Research on using additives to reduce the BA content of fermented seafood products has also been reported. Mah et al. [68] conducted research to reduce BA production by microorganisms isolated from *Myeolchi-jeot*, introducing additives into assay media and *Myeolchi-jeot*. The results confirmed that compared to the control, garlic extract was the most effective inhibitor of bacterial growth and BA production by yielding lower in vitro production of putrescine, cadaverine, histamine, tyramine, and spermidine by 11.2%, 18.4%, 11.7%, 30.9%, and 17.4%, respectively. Further results revealed that compared to *Myeolchi-jeot* samples treated with ethanol (control), the addition of 5% garlic extract to *Myeolchi-jeot* (treatment) inhibited bacterial growth and consequently reduced overall BA production by up to 8.7%. In another study by Mah and Hwang [69], other additives were also used for the reduction of BA production by *Myeolchi-jeot* microorganisms in assay media and *Myeolchi-jeot*. Among the additives tested in assay media, glycine most effectively inhibited in vitro BA production by bacterial strains. In comparison to the control without additives, the addition of 10% glycine in assay media resulted in reductions in putrescine, cadaverine, histamine, tyramine, and spermidine production by

32.6%, 78.4%, 93.2%, 100.0%, and 100.0%, respectively. Compared to the *Myeolchi-jeot* samples salted at 20% NaCl, additional supplementation of 5% glycine reportedly reduced overall BA content by 73.4%. The results suggest that the addition of glycine as well as salt may improve the safety of fermented seafood products. It is noteworthy that despite the results showing effective BA reduction, the use of garlic extract or glycine may affect the flavor of the final product.

Aside from additives, other studies have utilized starter cultures to reduce BA content in *Jeotgal*. In a study by Mah and Hwang [70], some bacterial strains isolated from *Myeolchi-jeot* were found to reduce BA content in *Myeolchi-jeot*. The reported results showed that, of the 7 starter candidate strains, *S. xylosus* exhibited the highest histamine degradation capability as well as the ability to slightly degrade tyramine in assay media. In comparison to the uninoculated *Myeolchi-jeot* control, the addition of the starter culture reduced the production of putrescine, cadaverine, histamine, tyramine, and spermidine by 16.5%, 10.8%, 18.0%, 38.9%, and 45.6%, respectively. Jeong et al. [56] isolated strains from *Jeotgal* for use as potential starters and found that *S. equorum* strain KS1039 did not produce putrescine, cadaverine, histamine, and tyramine in vitro.

A limited number of studies have even attempted to directly reduce the BA content of kimchi through the inoculation of bacterial strains. Kim et al. [71] reported reductions in tryptamine, putrescine, cadaverine, histamine, and tyramine levels in *Baechu* kimchi fortified with *Leu. carnosum*, *Leu. mesenteroides*, *Lb. plantarum*, and *Lb. sakei* strains. Similarly, Jin et al. [30] reported that *Kkakdugi* and *Chonggak* kimchi inoculated with *Lb. plantarum* strains incapable of producing BA contained lower level of tyramine (but not the other BA) than the uninoculated control. Therefore, utilizing LAB strains unable to produce (and/or able to degrade) BA as kimchi starter cultures may likely reduce the total BA content during kimchi fermentation.

Although the aforementioned studies have shown both direct and indirect methods of reducing BA content in kimchi, current commercial kimchi production processes do not appear to utilize the BA reduction techniques. This might be due to the application of BA reduction methods such as the use of additives, starter cultures, and adjusting the quantity of fermented seafood products have been reported to affect the flavor of kimchi products [69,72,73]. Consequently, inconsistent product quality is reflected in the wide range of BA content of kimchi products, including concentrations that exceed recommended limits for safe consumption. The high BA content reported for various kimchi products indicates that modern production methods require further preventative measures to ensure the safety of the fermented vegetable products, including practical application of research-based BA reduction techniques described above. Commercial kimchi production may greatly benefit from utilizing the aforementioned and novel strategies including control of fermentation conditions, utilizing starter cultures, alternative ingredients, and/or ingredients with low BA content. Furthermore, the establishment and expansion of regulations limiting BA content in fermented foods remain necessary to safeguard consumers against the potential BA intoxication.

6. Conclusions

The current study evaluated the BA content of kimchi, a term used to describe a group of Korean fermented vegetable products. Some kimchi samples have been reported to contain high concentrations of BA which exceeded recommended limits. Consumption of the fermented foods with high BA content may have detrimental effects on the body. Several factors contribute to the high BA concentrations in kimchi, which include BA production by microorganisms during fermentation and BA content of ingredients such as *Jeotgal* and *Aekjeot*. As variables such as ingredients, microorganisms, and initial BA content of *Jeotgal* that influence kimchi fermentation differed extensively, the reported BA concentrations of kimchi products also varied widely, even among the same varieties. Due to the large variations among kimchi products, standardization of kimchi production appears to be necessary to limit BA content. Furthermore, though several studies have described methods to indirectly reduce BA concentrations in kimchi by reducing the BA content of ingredients *Jeotgal* and *Aekjeot*, limited research has been conducted on the direct reduction of BA content in kimchi products.

To ensure the safe consumption of kimchi products, further research on methods to reduce the BA concentrations below recommended limits appears to be necessary. In conjunction with BA reduction studies, implementation of regulations such as continuous monitoring during production remains necessary to control BA content in kimchi and *Jeotgal* products.

Supplementary Materials: The following are available online at http://www.mdpi.com/2304-8158/8/11/547/s1, Table S1: Biogenic amine content of fermented vegetable and seafood products from various countries.

Author Contributions: Conceptualization, Y.K.P. and J.-H.M.; Literature data collection, Y.K.P.; Writing—original draft, Y.K.P. and J.H.L.; Writing—review and editing, Y.K.P., J.H.L. and J.-H.M.; Supervision: J.-H.M.

Funding: This work was supported by the National Research Foundation of Korea (NRF) grant funded by the Korea government (MSIT) (no. 2019R1H1A2100972).

Acknowledgments: The authors thank Young Hun Jin, Junsu Lee, and Alixander Mattay Pawluk of Department of Food and Biotechnology at Korea University for technical assistance.

Conflicts of Interest: The authors declare no conflict of interest.

References

1. Food Information Statistics System. Available online: https://www.atfis.or.kr/article/M001050000/view.do?articleId=2821&boardId=3&page=&searchKey=&searchString=&searchCategory= (accessed on 3 October 2019).
2. Lee, C.-H.; Ahn, B.-S. Literature review on Kimchi, Korean fermented vegetable foods I. History of Kimchi making. *Korean J. Food Cult.* **1995**, *10*, 311–319.
3. Cheigh, H.-S. *Kimchi Culture and Dietary Life in Korea*, 1st ed.; Hyoil Publishing Co.: Seoul, Korea, 2002; pp. 304–312.
4. Choi, S.-K.; Hwang, S.-Y.; Jo, J.-S. Standardization of kimchi and related products (3). *Korean J. Food Cult.* **1997**, *12*, 531–548.
5. Sim, S.G.; Shon, H.S.; Sim, C.H.; Yoon, W.H. *Fermented Foods*, 1st ed.; Jin Ro Publishing Co.: Seoul, Korea, 2001; pp. 233–286.
6. Codex Alimentarius Commission. *Codex Standard for Kimchi, Codex Stan 223–2001*; Food and Agriculture Organization of the United Nations: Rome, Italy, 2001.
7. Park, K.-Y. The nutritional evaluation, and antimutagenic and anticancer effects of Kimchi. *Korean J. Food Nutr.* **1995**, *24*, 169–182.
8. Park, K.-Y. Increased health functionality of fermented foods. *Korean J. Food Nutr.* **2012**, *17*, 1–8.
9. Jung, E.H.; Ryu, J.P.; Lee, S.-I. A study on foreigner preferences and sensory characteristics of kimchi fermented for different periods. *Korean J. Food Cult.* **2012**, *27*, 346–353. [CrossRef]
10. Jung, J.Y.; Lee, S.H.; Jeon, C.O. Kimchi microflora: History, current status, and perspectives for industrial kimchi production. *Appl. Microbiol. Biotechnol.* **2014**, *98*, 2385–2393. [CrossRef]
11. Cho, E.-J.; Rhee, S.-H.; Lee, S.-M.; Park, K.-Y. In vitro antimutagenic and anticancer effects of kimchi fractions. *J. Cancer Prev.* **1997**, *2*, 113–121.
12. Kim, J.-H.; Ryu, J.-D.; Song, Y.-O. The effect of *kimchi* intake on free radical production and the inhibition of oxidation in young adults and the elderly people. *Korean J. Community Nutr.* **2002**, *7*, 257–265.
13. Askar, A.; Treptow, H. *Biogene Amine in Lebensmitteln: Vorkommen, Bedeutung und Bestimmung*, 1st ed.; Verlag Eugen Ulmer: Stuttgart, Germany, 1986; pp. 21–74.
14. Silla Santos, M.H. Biogenic amines: Their importance in foods. *Int. J. Food Microbiol.* **1996**, *29*, 213–231. [CrossRef]
15. Ten Brink, B.; Damink, C.; Joosten, H.M.L.J.; Huis in't Veld, J.H.J. Occurrence and formation of biologically active amines in foods. *Int. J. Food Microbiol.* **1990**, *11*, 73–84. [CrossRef]
16. Gilbert, R.J.; Hobbs, G.; Murray, C.K.; Cruickshank, J.G.; Young, S.E.J. Scombrotoxic fish poisoning: Features of the first 50 incidents to be reported in Britain (1976–9). *Br. Med. J.* **1980**, *281*, 71–72. [PubMed]
17. Del Rio, B.; Redruello, B.; Linares, D.M.; Ladero, V.; Fernandez, M.; Martin, M.C.; Ruas-Madiedo, P.; Alvarez, M.A. The dietary biogenic amines tyramine and histamine show synergistic toxicity towards intestinal cells in culture. *Food Chem.* **2017**, *218*, 249–255. [CrossRef] [PubMed]

18. Del Rio, B.; Redruello, B.; Linares, D.M.; Ladero, V.; Ruas-Madiedo, P.; Fernandez, M.; Martin, M.C.; Alvarez, M.A. Spermine and spermidine are cytotoxic towards intestinal cell cultures, but are they a health hazard at concentrations found in foods? *Food Chem.* **2018**, *269*, 321–326. [CrossRef] [PubMed]
19. Del Rio, B.; Redruello, B.; Linares, D.M.; Ladero, V.; Ruas-Madiedo, P.; Fernandez, M.; Martin, M.C.; Alvarez, M.A. The biogenic amines putrescine and cadaverine show in vitro cytotoxicity at concentrations that can be found in foods. *Sci. Rep.* **2019**, *9*, 120. [CrossRef] [PubMed]
20. Ender, F.; Čeh, L. Conditions and chemical reaction mechanisms by which nitrosamines may be formed in biological products with reference to their possible occurrence in food products. *Z. Lebensm. Unters. Forsch.* **1971**, *145*, 133–142. [CrossRef]
21. Mah, J.-H.; Yoon, M.-Y.; Cha, G.-S.; Byun, M.-W.; Hwang, H.-J. Influence of curing and heating on formation of N-nitrosamines from biogenic amines in food model system using Korean traditional fermented fish product. *Food Sci. Biotechnol.* **2005**, *14*, 168–170.
22. Taylor, S.L. Histamine food poisoning: Toxicology and clinical aspects. *Crit. Rev. Toxicol.* **1986**, *17*, 91–128. [CrossRef]
23. Smith, T.A. Amines in food. *Food Chem.* **1981**, *6*, 169–200. [CrossRef]
24. Mah, J.-H.; Park, Y.K.; Jin, Y.H.; Lee, J.-H.; Hwang, H.J. Bacterial production and control of biogenic amines in Asian fermented soybean foods. *Foods* **2019**, *8*, 85. [CrossRef]
25. Cho, T.-Y.; Han, G.-H.; Bahn, K.-N.; Son, Y.-W.; Jang, M.-R.; Lee, C.-H.; Kim, S.-H.; Kim, D.-B.; Kim, S.-B. Evaluation of biogenic amines in Korean commercial fermented foods. *Korean J. Food Sci. Technol.* **2006**, *38*, 730–737.
26. Kang, K.H.; Kim, S.H.; Kim, S.-H.; Kim, J.G.; Sung, N.-J.; Lim, H.; Chung, M.J. Analysis and risk assessment of N-nitrosodimethylamine and its precursor concentrations in Korean commercial kimchi. *J. Korean Soc. Food Sci. Nutr.* **2017**, *46*, 244–250. [CrossRef]
27. Tsai, Y.-H.; Kung, H.-F.; Lin, Q.-L.; Hwang, J.-H.; Cheng, S.-H.; Wei, C.-I.; Hwang, D.-F. Occurrence of histamine and histamine-forming bacteria in kimchi products in Taiwan. *Food Chem.* **2005**, *90*, 635–641. [CrossRef]
28. Shin, S.-W.; Kim, Y.-S.; Kim, Y.-H.; Kim, H.-T.; Eum, K.-S.; Hong, S.-R.; Kang, H.-J.; Park, K.-H.; Yoon, M.-H. Biogenic-amine contents of Korean commercial salted fishes and cabbage kimchi. *Korean J. Fish. Aquat. Sci.* **2019**, *52*, 13–18.
29. Mah, J.-H.; Kim, Y.J.; No, H.-K.; Hwang, H.-J. Determination of biogenic amines in *kimchi*, Korean traditional fermented vegetable products. *Food Sci. Biotechnol.* **2004**, *13*, 826–829.
30. Jin, Y.H.; Lee, J.H.; Park, Y.K.; Lee, J.-H.; Mah, J.-H. The occurrence of biogenic amines and determination of biogenic amine-producing lactic acid bacteria in *Kkakdugi* and *Chonggak* kimchi. *Foods* **2019**, *8*, 73. [CrossRef]
31. Lee, J.-H.; Jin, Y.H.; Park, Y.K.; Yun, S.J.; Mah, J.-H. Formation of biogenic amines in *Pa* (green onion) kimchi and *Gat* (mustard leaf) kimchi. *Foods* **2019**, *8*, 109. [CrossRef]
32. Halász, A.; Baráth, Á.; Holzapfel, W.H. The influence of starter culture selection on sauerkraut fermentation. *Z. Lebensm. Unters. Forsch.* **1999**, *208*, 434–438. [CrossRef]
33. Kalač, P.; Špička, J.; Křížek, M.; Steidlová, Š.; Pelikánová, T. Concentrations of seven biogenic amines in sauerkraut. *Food Chem.* **1999**, *67*, 275–280. [CrossRef]
34. Lee, K.J. Westerner's view of Korean food in modern period-centering on analyzing Westerners' books. *Korean J. Food Cult.* **2013**, *28*, 356–370. [CrossRef]
35. Taylor, S.L.; Leatherwood, M.; Lieber, E.R. Histamine in sauerkraut. *J. Food Sci.* **1978**, *43*, 1030–1032. [CrossRef]
36. Mouritsen, O.G. *Tsukemono*—Crunchy pickled foods from Japan: A case study of food design by gastrophysics and nature. *Int. J. Food Des.* **2018**, *3*, 103–124. [CrossRef]
37. Handa, A.; Kawanabe, H.; Ibe, A. Content and origin of nonvolatile amines in various commercial pickles. *J. Food Hyg. Soc. Jpn.* **2018**, *59*, 36–44. [CrossRef] [PubMed]
38. Kung, H.-F.; Lee, Y.-H.; Teng, D.-F.; Hsieh, P.-C.; Wei, C.-I.; Tsai, Y.-H. Histamine formation by histamine-forming bacteria and yeast in mustard pickle products in Taiwan. *Food Chem.* **2006**, *99*, 579–585. [CrossRef]
39. Oh, S.-C. Influences of squid ink added to low-salted squid *Jeot-gal* on its proteolytic characteristics. *J. Korean Oil Chem. Soc.* **2013**, *30*, 348–355. [CrossRef]

40. Park, D.-C.; Kim, E.-M.; Kim, E.-J.; Kim, Y.-M.; Kim, S.-B. The contents of organic acids, nucleotides and their related compounds in *kimchi* prepared with salted-fermented fish products and their alternatives. *Korean J. Food Sci. Technol.* **2003**, *35*, 769–776.
41. Park, C.L.; Kwon, Y.M. A study on the kimchi recipe in the early Joseon Dynasty through *[Juchochimjeobang]*. *J. Korean Soc. Food Cult.* **2017**, *32*, 333–360.
42. Cha, Y.-J.; Lee, Y.-M.; Jung, Y.-J.; Jeong, E.-J.; Kim, S.-J.; Park, S.-Y.; Yoon, S.-S.; Kim, E.-J. A nationwide survey on the preference characteristics of minor ingredients for winter *kimchi*. *Korean J. Food Nutr.* **2003**, *32*, 555–561.
43. Lee, C.-H.; Lee, E.-H.; Lim, M.-H.; Kim, S.-H.; Chae, S.-K.; Lee, K.-W.; Koh, K.-H. Characteristics of Korean fish fermentation technology. *Korean J. Food Cult.* **1986**, *1*, 267–278.
44. Ha, S.-D.; Kim, A.-J. Technological trends in safety of jeotgal. *Korean J. Food Nutr.* **2005**, *38*, 46–64.
45. Kim, S.-M.; Lee, K.-T. The shelf-life extension of low-salted Myungran-Jeot 1. The effects of pH control on the shelf-life of low-salted Myungran-Jeot. *Korean J. Fish. Aquat. Sci.* **1997**, *30*, 459–465.
46. Um, I.-S.; Seo, J.-K.; Kim, H.-D.; Park, K.-S. The quality of commercial salted and fermented anchovy *Engraulis japonicas* sauces produced in Korea. *Korean J. Fish. Aquat. Sci.* **2018**, *51*, 667–672.
47. Mah, J.-H.; Han, H.-K.; Oh, Y.-J.; Kim, M.-G.; Hwang, H.-J. Biogenic amines in Jeotkals, Korean salted and fermented fish products. *Food Chem.* **2002**, *79*, 239–243. [CrossRef]
48. Moon, J.S.; Kim, Y.; Jang, K.I.; Cho, K.-J.; Yang, S.-J.; Yoon, G.-M.; Kim, S.-Y.; Han, N.S. Analysis of biogenic amines in fermented fish products consumed in Korea. *Food Sci. Biotechnol.* **2010**, *19*, 1689–1692. [CrossRef]
49. Cho, Y.-J.; Lee, H.-H.; Kim, B.-K.; Gye, H.-J.; Jung, W.-Y.; Shim, K.-B. Quality evaluation to determine the grading of commercial salt-fermented fish sauce in Korea. *J. Fish. Mar. Sci. Educ.* **2014**, *26*, 823–830.
50. Joung, B.C.; Min, J.G. Changes in postfermentation quality during the distribution process of anchovy (*Engraulis japonicus*) fish sauce. *J. Food Prot.* **2018**, *81*, 969–976. [CrossRef]
51. Saaid, M.; Saad, B.; Hashim, N.H.; Ali, A.S.M.; Saleh, M.I. Determination of biogenic amines in selected Malaysian food. *Food Chem.* **2009**, *113*, 1356–1362. [CrossRef]
52. Rosma, A.; Afiza, T.S.; Wan Nadiah, W.A.; Liong, M.T.; Gulam, R.R.A. Microbiological, histamine and 3-MCPD contents of Malaysian unprocessed 'budu'. *Int. Food Res. J.* **2009**, *16*, 589–594.
53. Kim, M.-J.; Kim, K.-S. Tyramine production among lactic acid bacteria and other species isolated from kimchi. *LWT-Food Sci. Technol.* **2014**, *56*, 406–413. [CrossRef]
54. Jeong, D.-W.; Lee, J.-H. Antibiotic resistance, hemolysis and biogenic amine production assessments of *Leuconostoc* and *Weissella* isolates for kimchi starter development. *LWT-Food Sci. Technol.* **2015**, *64*, 1078–1084. [CrossRef]
55. Guan, L.; Cho, K.H.; Lee, J.H. Analysis of the cultivable bacterial community in *jeotgal*, a Korean salted and fermented seafood, and identification of its dominant bacteria. *Food Microbiol.* **2011**, *28*, 101–113. [CrossRef]
56. Jeong, D.-W.; Han, S.; Lee, J.-H. Safety and technological characterization of *Staphylococcus equorum* isolates from jeotgal, a Korean high-salt-fermented seafood, for starter development. *Int. J. Food Microbiol.* **2014**, *188*, 108–115. [CrossRef] [PubMed]
57. Lim, E.-S. Inhibitory effect of bacteriocin-producing lactic acid bacteria against histamine-forming bacteria isolated from *Myeolchi-jeot*. *Fish. Aquat. Sci.* **2016**, *19*, 42. [CrossRef]
58. Mah, J.-H.; Ahn, J.-B.; Park, J.-H.; Sung, H.-C.; Hwang, H.-J. Characterization of biogenic amine-producing microorganisms isolated from Myeolchi-jeot, Korean salted and fermented anchovy. *J. Microbiol. Biotechnol.* **2003**, *13*, 692–699.
59. Bover-Cid, S.; Hugas, M.; Izquierdo-Pulido, M.; Vidal-Carou, M.C. Amino acid-decarboxylase activity of bacteria isolated from fermented pork sausages. *Int. J. Food Microbiol.* **2001**, *66*, 185–189. [CrossRef]
60. Coton, E.; Coton, M. Evidence of horizontal transfer as origin of strain to strain variation of the tyramine production trait in *Lactobacillus brevis*. *Food Microbiol.* **2009**, *26*, 52–57. [CrossRef]
61. Lucas, P.M.; Wolken, W.A.M.; Claisse, O.; Lolkema, J.S.; Lonvaud-Funel, A. Histamine-producing pathway encoded on an unstable plasmid in *Lactobacillus hilgardii* 0006. *Appl. Environ. Microbiol.* **2005**, *71*, 1417–1424. [CrossRef]
62. Marcobal, A.; de las Rivas, B.; Moreno-Arribas, M.V.; Munoz, R. Evidence for horizontal gene transfer as origin of putrescine production in *Oenococcus oeni* RM83. *Appl. Environ. Microbiol.* **2006**, *72*, 7954–7958. [CrossRef]

63. Wolken, W.A.M.; Lucas, P.M.; Lonvaud-Funel, A.; Lolkema, J.S. The mechanism of the tyrosine transporter TyrP supports a proton motive tyrosine decarboxylation pathway in *Lactobacillus brevis*. *J. Bacteriol.* **2006**, *188*, 2198–2206. [CrossRef]
64. Kim, S.-H.; Kang, K.H.; Kim, S.H.; Lee, S.; Lee, S.-H.; Ha, E.-S.; Sung, N.-J.; Kim, J.G.; Chung, M.J. Lactic acid bacteria directly degrade N-nitrosodimethylamine and increase the nitrite-scavenging ability in kimchi. *Food Control* **2017**, *71*, 101–109. [CrossRef]
65. Lee, G.-I.; Lee, H.-M.; Lee, C.-H. Food safety issues in industrialization of traditional Korean foods. *Food Control* **2012**, *24*, 1–5. [CrossRef]
66. Kang, H.-W. Characteristics of *kimchi* added with anchovy sauce from heat and non-heat treatments. *Culin. Sci. Hosp. Res.* **2013**, *19*, 49–58.
67. Becker, K.; Southwick, K.; Reardon, J.; Berg, R.; MacCormack, J.N. Histamine poisoning associated with eating tuna burgers. *JAMA* **2001**, *285*, 1327–1330. [CrossRef] [PubMed]
68. Mah, J.-H.; Kim, Y.J.; Hwang, H.-J. Inhibitory effects of garlic and other spices on biogenic amine production in *Myeolchi-jeot*, Korean salted and fermented anchovy product. *Food Control* **2009**, *20*, 449–454. [CrossRef]
69. Mah, J.-H.; Hwang, H.-J. Effects of food additives on biogenic amine formation in *Myeolchi-jeot*, a salted and fermented anchovy (*Engraulis japonicus*). *Food Chem.* **2009**, *114*, 168–173. [CrossRef]
70. Mah, J.-H.; Hwang, H.-J. Inhibition of biogenic amine formation in a salted and fermented anchovy by *Staphylococcus xylosus* as a protective culture. *Food Control* **2009**, *20*, 796–801. [CrossRef]
71. Kim, S.-H.; Kim, S.H.; Kang, K.H.; Lee, S.; Kim, S.J.; Kim, J.G.; Chung, M.J. Kimchi probiotic bacteria contribute to reduced amounts of N-nitrosodimethylamine in lactic acid bacteria-fortified kimchi. *LWT-Food Sci. Technol.* **2017**, *84*, 196–203. [CrossRef]
72. Ku, K.H.; Sunwoo, J.Y.; Park, W.S. Effects of ingredients on the its quality characteristics during kimchi fermentation. *J. Korean Soc. Food Sci. Nutr.* **2005**, *34*, 267–276.
73. Jin, H.S.; Kim, J.B.; Yun, Y.J.; Lee, K.J. Selection of kimchi starters based on the microbial composition of kimchi and their effects. *J. Korean Soc. Food Sci. Nutr.* **2008**, *37*, 671–675. [CrossRef]

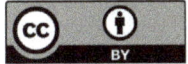

© 2019 by the authors. Licensee MDPI, Basel, Switzerland. This article is an open access article distributed under the terms and conditions of the Creative Commons Attribution (CC BY) license (http://creativecommons.org/licenses/by/4.0/).

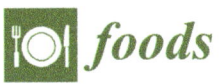

Article

Effect of Brine Concentrations on the Bacteriological and Chemical Quality and Histamine Content of Brined and Dried Milkfish

Chiu-Chu Hwang [1,*], Yi-Chen Lee [2], Chung-Yung Huang [2], Hsien-Feng Kung [3], Hung-Hui Cheng [4] and Yung-Hsiang Tsai [2,*]

1. Department of Hospitality Management, Yu Da University of Science and Technology, Miaoli 361027, Taiwan
2. Department of Seafood Science, National Kaohsiung University of Science and Technology, Kaohsiung 811213, Taiwan; lionlee@nkust.edu.tw (Y.-C.L.); cyhuang@nkust.edu.tw (C.-Y.H.)
3. Department of Pharmacy, Tajen University, Pingtung 907391, Taiwan; khfeng@mail.tajen.edu.tw
4. Mariculture Research Center, Fisheries Research Institute, Council of Agriculture, Tainan 724028, Taiwan; cheng.hunghui@msa.hinet.net
* Correspondence: omics1@ydu.edu.tw (C.-C.H.); yhtsai01@seed.net.tw (Y.-H.T.); Tel.: +886-37-651188-5600 (C.-C.H.); +886-7-3617141-23609 (Y.-H.T.); Fax: +886-7-3640634 (Y.-H.T.)

Received: 12 October 2020; Accepted: 31 October 2020; Published: 3 November 2020

Abstract: In this research, the occurrence of hygienic quality and histamine in commercial brined and dried milkfish products, and the effects of brine concentrations on the quality of brined and dried milkfish, were studied. Brined and dried milkfish products ($n = 20$) collected from four retail stores in Taiwan were tested to investigate their histamine-related quality. Among them, five tested samples (25%, 5/20) had histamine contents of more than 5 mg/100 g, the United States Food and Drug Administration guidelines for scombroid fish, while two (10%, 2/20) contained 69 and 301 mg/100 g of histamine, exceeding the 50 mg/100 g potential hazard level. In addition, the effects of brine concentrations (0%, 3%, 6%, 9%, and 15%) on the chemical and bacteriological quality of brined and dried milkfish during sun-drying were evaluated. The results showed that the aerobic plate count (APC), coliform, water activity, total volatile basic nitrogen (TVBN), and histamine content values of the brined and dried milkfish samples decreased with increased brine concentrations, whereas those of salt content and thiobarbituric acid (TBA) increased with increasing brine concentrations. The milkfish samples prepared with 6% NaCl brine had better quality with respect to lower APC, TVBN, TBA, and histamine levels.

Keywords: histamine; dried milkfish; hygienic quality; brine-salting

1. Introduction

Histamine is a biogenic amine in charge of histamine fish poisoning (HFP) or scombroid poisoning. Histamine fish poisoning is a food outbreak with allergy-like symptoms arising from ingesting mishandled scombroid fish that have high levels of histamine in their flesh [1]. Histamine is formed mainly through the decarboxylation of free histidine in fish muscles by histidine decarboxylases produced by a number of histamine-forming bacteria present in seafood [2]. HFP has occasionally been associated with the consumption of milkfish, marlin, mackerel, and tuna in Taiwan [2–6]. However, there is compelling evidence to implicate that other factors, such as other biogenic amines, can potentiate histamine toxicity, as spoiled fish containing histamine tends to be more toxic than the equivalent amount of pure histamine that is ingested orally [1,2]. Putrescine and cadaverine were shown to enhance histamine toxicity when present in spoiled fish by inhibiting the intestinal histamine metabolizing enzyme, including diamine oxidase [1,2].

Milkfish (*Chanos chanos*) is widely distributed throughout the Indo-Pacific region and is the second most important inland aquaculture fish in Taiwan [7,8]. This fish has been cultivated in Taiwan for more than 350 years. Taiwan's total milkfish production is approximately 50,000–60,000 tons each year [8]. Chiou et al. [9] demonstrated that histidine at 441 mg/100 g is the most prominent free amino acid (FAA) in the white muscles of milkfish and accounts for 80% of the total FAAs in the fish. Therefore, milkfish products have become most often associated with HFP in Taiwan, including dried milkfish [6], milkfish sticks [10], and milkfish surimi [11]. In addition, our research team determined that 78% of commercial dry-salting and dried milkfish products have histamine contents greater than the 5 mg/100 g recommended value of the United States Food and Drug Administration's (USFDA) guidelines, while 43.7% of the fish samples were found to exceed 50 mg/100 g of histamine [12].

In general, there are two major salting methods for milkfish preservation, namely, dry-salting and brine-salting. In Taiwan, the traditional processes of dry-salting and dried milkfish include scaling, back-cutting, degutting, and dry-salting with 3–12% NaCl (w/w) followed by sun-drying for 5–7 days [12]. However, the consumption of high salt levels from seafood can result in several chronic diseases, such as hypertension and cardiovascular diseases [13]. Brine-salting for fish processing may be a better method to reduce salt uptake and water loss and, thus, to reach a higher weight yield and better quality in salted fish compared to dry-salting [14]. Therefore, in recent years, brine- and light-salting milkfish has gained popularity with Taiwanese people. However, the quality of brined and dried fish is influenced by the brine concentrations and dry methods used for drying the fish [15].

There is no information of the occurrence of hygienic quality and histamine in brined and dried milkfish products, and the formation of histamine and the quality of brined and dried milkfish produced with different brine concentrations. Therefore, the main aim of this study was to monitor the bacteriological and chemical quality, including histamine content, in 20 brined and dried milkfish samples sold in retail stores in southern Taiwan. This work also aimed to examine the effects of different brine concentrations (0%, 3%, 6%, 9%, and 15%) on the bacteriological and chemical quality and histamine contents in brined and dried milkfish products during sun-drying for five days.

2. Materials and Methods

2.1. Materials

Twenty brined and dried milkfish products were collected from four retail stores in southern Taiwan, including store A (six samples), store B (five samples), store C (five samples), and store D (four samples). All brined and dried milkfish products were home-made by the farmer or manufacturer and delivered to the store for sale. Trackback information indicated that the samples collected from store A and D were processed using higher brine concentration (>10%) and longer sun-drying days (5–7 days); on the other hand, the samples of store B and C were processed using lower brine concentration (<6%) and shorter sun-drying days (3–5 days). In general, the processing of brined and dried milkfish include scaling, back-cutting, degutting, and brine-salting with 3–15% NaCl concentrations at room temperature for 1-2 h, followed by sun-drying for 3–7 days. After the samples were purchased, they were wrapped in aseptic bags, placed in an ice box, and instantly delivered to the laboratory for analysis within 6 h. The dorsal part of the commercial dried milkfish samples were cut and taken for microbiological and chemical determinations.

Sixty fresh milkfish (weights of 546 ± 11.6 g, lengths of 31.9 ± 1.2 cm) were purchased from the fish market of the city of Kaohsiung in Taiwan and transported to our laboratory within half an hour in an ice box. Once the fish samples arrived at the laboratory, they were manually scaled, back-cut, gutted, washed with clean water, and then drained.

2.2. Reagents

Histamine dihydrochloride, trichloroacetic acid, 2-thiobarbituric acid, and butylated hydroxytoluene were purchased from Sigma-Aldrich (St. Louis, MO, USA). Acetonitrile (LC grade) and dansyl chloride (GR grade) were purchased from E. Merck (Darmstadt, Germany).

2.3. Brine-Salting and Drying of Milkfish

The back-cut milkfish were brine-salted with concentrations of 3%, 6%, 9%, or 15% NaCl with a fish-to-brine ratio of 1:2 for 60 min at 20 °C, and unsalted milkfish were used as controls. After brine-salting, all milkfish samples were placed under sun light at 30–33 °C for seven hours each day for five days. Sampling analyses were conducted at days 1, 3, and 5 for sun-drying. The experiments were conducted in triplicate for each brine concentration and sampling time. The dorsal part of the fish samples was used for analysis.

2.4. Determination of pH Value, Moisture Content, Water Activity, and Salt Content

Ten grams of the samples was weighted and homogenized with a mixer (FastPrep-24, MP Biomedicals, Solon, OH, USA) for 2 min with 20 mL of deionized water to make a thick slurry. The pH of this slurry was determined using a digital pH meter (Mettler Toledo FE20/EL20, Schwerzenbach, Switzerland). The moisture of each sample (1–3 g) was measured using the oven-dry method at 105.0 ± 1.0 °C for drying, followed by the determination of the sample weight until a constant weight was achieved. Water activity was determined by an Aqualab 4TE (Decagon Devices, Pullman, WA, USA) at 25 °C. The salt (NaCl) content was determined using Mohr's titration method [16].

2.5. Determination of Total Volatile Basic Nitrogen (TVBN) and Thiobarbituric Acid (TBA)

The TVBN values were measured using Conway's dish method as described by Cobb et al. [17]. Five grams of the minced samples was homogenized with 45 mL of 6% trichloroacetic acid (TCA; Sigma-Aldrich, St. Louis, MO, USA). After the extract was filtered, saturated K_2CO_3 was added to the filters. The released TVBN was absorbed by boric acid and then titrated with 0.02 N HCl, while the TVBN value was expressed in milligrams per 100 g fish sample. The TBA values were determined by the modified method of Faustman et al. [18]. Briefly, 20 g of dried milkfish sample was added into a tube containing 180 mL of deionized water and then homogenized with a mixer for 3 min. Twelve milliliters of 0.1 M TBA reagent in 0.2% HCl and 0.15 mL of 0.2% butylated hydroxytoluene (BHT) in 95% ethanol were added into 2 mL of the homogenate and then mixed well. The mixtures were heated in a water bath at 90 °C for 20 min and then filtered, and the absorbance of the filtrates was detected using a spectrophotometer (UV-1201, Shimazu, Tokyo, Japan) at 532 nm. The TBA values in the fish samples are expressed in milligrams of malondialdehyde (MDA) per kilogram.

2.6. Microbiological Analysis

Twenty-five grams of the minced samples was homogenized with 225 mL of sterile 0.85% (w/v) physiological saline in a sterile blender at a 1200 rpm speed for 2 min. The homogenate was serially diluted with a sterile physiological saline for 1:10 (v/v) dilutions. With regard to spread plate counting, 0.1 mL of the dilutes was spread on aerobic plate count (APC) agar (Difco, BD, Sparks, MD, USA) with 0.5% NaCl and then incubated at 30 °C for 24–48 h. After the bacterial colonies grown on the plate were counted, the data were expressed as $\log_{10}$ colony forming units (CFUs) per gram. The levels of coliform and *Escherichia coli* in the milkfish samples were performed according to the three-tube most probable number (MPN) method as described by the FDA [19].

2.7. Histamine Analysis

Histamine dihydrochloride (82.8 mg) was dissolved in 50 mL of 0.1 M HCl and used as the working solution, and the final concentration of histamine (free base) was 1.0 mg/mL. Five grams of the ground milkfish samples were homogenized with 20 mL of 6% cold trichloroacetic acid (TCA) using a Polytron PT-MR 3100 homogenizer for 3 min. The homogenates were collected via centrifugation at 4500× g for 8 min at 7 °C and filtered through Advantec Toyo No. 2 filter paper. The filtrates were diluted up to 50 mL with a 6% TCA solution. For the derivatization reaction of histamine, 1 mL aliquots of the TCA extract of each sample and histamine standard solution were derivatized with dansyl chloride using the method of Chen et al. [3] with some modifications. Briefly, 0.2 mL of 2 M sodium hydroxide and 0.3 mL of saturated sodium bicarbonate were added to 1 mL aliquots of the TCA extract of each sample and the histamine standard solution. The solution was added to 2 mL of 1% dansyl chloride solution dissolved in acetone, mixed by a vortex mixer, and left to stand at 40 °C for 45 min. After the reaction, 100 µL of ammonia was added to terminate the derivatization reaction. Acetonitrile was added to a final volume of 5 mL and the solution was centrifuged (10,000× g, 5 min, 4 °C). After the supernatants were filtered through 0.22 µm membrane filters, 20 µL of the filtrates were injected into high-performance liquid chromatography (HPLC). The histamine levels in each milkfish sample were analyzed by HPLC (Hitachi, Tokyo, Japan) equipped with a LiChrospher 100 RP-18 reversed-phase column (5 µm, 125 × 4.6 mm, E. Merck, Damstadt, Germany) and a UV-Vis detector (Model L-4000, Hitachi, wavelength at 254 nm). The mobile phase consisted of eluent A (acetonitrile) and eluent B (water). At the beginning, eluents A and B at a ratio of 50:50 (v/v) were applied for 19 min, followed by a linear gradient with an increase of eluent A up to 90% during the next minute. In the final 10 min, the eluent A and B mix was set to a linear decrease to 50:50 (v/v). The flow rate was 1.0 mL/min. Validation of the histamine analysis method including inter- and intra-day repeatability (expressed as % and relative standard deviation, RSD) was determined by fortifying homogenized dried milkfish meats with 1.0, 5.0, and 10 mg/100 g of standard histamine. Each spiked amount was extracted and derivatized with dansyl chloride using the above procedure in triplicate, including a blank test to evaluate the average recovery.

2.8. Statistical Analysis

One-way analysis of variance (ANOVA) and Tukey's pairwise comparison tests were performed within the 95% confidence interval. Pearson correlation was carried out to determine relationships between pH, moisture, water activity, salt content, TVBN, APC, coliform, and histamine contents in the brined and dried milkfish samples. All statistical analyses were carried out using the Statistical Package for Social Sciences (SPSS) Version 16.0 for Windows (SPSS Inc., Chicago, Il, USA), and $p < 0.05$ was used to consider significant deviation.

3. Results and Discussion

3.1. Chemical and Bacteriological Quality of the Brined and Dried Milkfish Samples

For all 20 brined and dried milkfish samples collected from the four retail stores, the pH, moisture, water activity, salt content, TVBN, APC, coliform, and histamine ranged from 5.67 to 6.05, 38.27% to 69.78%, 0.89 to 0.98, 0.16% to 4.37%, 8.86 to 19.88 mg/100 g, 3.51 to 8.25 log CFU/g, <3 to >2400 MPN/g, and 0.16 to 301 mg/100 g, respectively (Table 1). *E. coli* was not detected in any milkfish samples. Store A samples had significantly lower ($p < 0.05$) mean water activity (0.94) than did samples collected from the other three stores, while the mean salt content (3.23%) in store A samples was higher ($p < 0.05$) than the others (Table 1). Moreover, the mean TVBN and APC values in store B samples (16.06 mg/100 g and 6.62 log CFU/g, respectively) and store D samples (16.82 mg/100 g and 6.33 log CFU/g, respectively) were markedly higher ($p < 0.05$) than those samples obtained from the other two stores, while the mean coliform level (356 MPN/g) in store D samples were higher than that of the other stores (Table 1). The highest mean histamine content of 79 mg/100 g was obtained from five samples from store B, followed by store D with a mean of 4.9 mg/100 g of histamine.

Table 1. pH, moisture, water activity, salt content, total volatile basic nitrogen (TVBN), aerobic plate count (APC), coliform, *Escherichia coli*, and histamine values in brined and dried milkfish products.

Sample Sources	Number of Samples	pH	Moisture (%)	Water Activity	Salt Content (%)	TVBN (mg/100 g)	APC (log CFU/g)	Coliform (MPN/g)	E. coli (MPN/g)	Histamine (mg/100 g)
A	6	5.74–5.83 (5.78 ± 0.04) A	38.27–65.37 (51.78 ± 9.28) B	0.89–0.97 (0.94 ± 0.03) B	2.47–4.37 (3.23 ± 0.78) A	8.86–17.36 (12.79 ± 3.25) B	3.51–7.65 (5.50 ± 1.05) B	<3–70 (42 ± 25) B	<3	0.34–4.9 (1.3 ± 1.8) C
B	5	5.67–6.05 (5.76 ± 0.17) A	52.31–60.18 (55.41 ± 3.23) AB	0.97–0.98 (0.98 ± 0.01) A	0.16–1.88 (0.80 ± 0.77) C	13.86–19.32 (16.06 ± 2.08) A	5.87–8.03 (6.62 ± 0.83) A	<3–40 (25 ± 13) B	<3	0.62–301 (79 ± 57) A
C	5	5.80–5.95 (5.87 ± 0.07) A	54.68–69.78 (64.17 ± 5.95) A	0.97–0.98 (0.98 ± 0.01) A	0.61–1.02 (0.86 ± 0.18) C	10.85–13.93 (12.35 ± 1.39) B	4.18–5.92 (5.32 ± 0.66) B	<3–240 (90 ± 130) B	<3	0.16–0.31 (0.20 ± 0.11) C
D	4	5.75–5.82 (5.78 ± 0.03) A	51.07–54.12 (52.46 ± 1.26) B	0.95–0.96 (0.96 ± 0.01) AB	1.47–1.80 (1.68 ± 0.15) B	15.40–19.88 (16.82 ± 2.66) A	5.80–8.25 (6.33 ± 0.60) A	20–>2400 (356 ± 47) A	<3	0.24–19 (4.9 ± 4.8) B

The values in parentheses represent the mean ± standard deviation (SD). Values in the same column with different letters are statistically different ($p < 0.05$). CFU, colony forming unit; MPN, most probable number.

In this study, the proportion of the 20 brined and dried milkfish samples that did not meet the 6.47 log CFU/g Taiwanese regulatory standard for APC was 35% (7/20). Therefore, brined and dried milkfish manufacturers may need to be more careful with hygienic handling or processing in their preparation of brined and dried milkfish products. The distribution of histamine contents in the brined and dried samples is shown in Table 2. Five samples (25%, 5/20) failed to meet the 5 mg/100 g level of histamine, the allowable limit by the USFDA for scombroid fish and/or products, while two (10%) had 69 and 301 mg/100 g of histamine, greater than the potential toxicity level (50 mg/100 g). According to information by Bartholomev et al. [20], which showed that fish with histamine levels >100 mg/100 g could result in illness and health hazards if ingested by humans, one sample with 301 mg/100 g of histamine could have caused disease symptoms if consumed (Table 2). In contrast, our previous research showed that 78.1% (25 samples) and 43.7% (14 samples) of 32 dry-salted and dried milkfish products contained more than 5 mg/100 g and 50 mg/100 g of histamine, respectively [21].

Table 2. Distribution of the histamine content in the 20 brined and dried milkfish products.

Content of Histamine (mg/100 g)	Brined and Dried Milkfish Products	
	Number of Samples	% of Samples
<4.9	15	75
5.0–49.9	3	15
50.0–99.9	1	5
>100	1	5
Total	20	100

High levels of histamine have been found in various types of milkfish implicated in HFP. Our research group detected 61.6 mg/100 g of histamine in dried milkfish products that were implicated in an incident of HFP [6]. Two fried milkfish sticks implicated in a poisoning incident contained 86.6 mg/100 g and 235.0 mg/100 g of histamine [10]. The high content of histamine (i.e., 91.0 mg/100 g) in a suspected milkfish surimi product could be the etiological factor for this fish-borne poisoning in Taiwan [11]. Therefore, it is also very important for people, especially those from the Indo-Pacific region, such as the Philippines, Indonesia, and Taiwan, to be aware that milkfish products could become a hazardous food item, causing histamine poisoning.

Pearson correlation was conducted to determine if there existed any relationship among the pH, moisture, water activity (a_w), salt content, TVBN, APC, coliform, and histamine contents of the tested 20 samples. In general, positive correlations existed between moisture and a_w (r, correlation coefficient = 0.81, $p < 0.05$), TVBN and APC ($r = 0.76$, $p < 0.05$), APC and histamine ($r = 0.71$, $p < 0.05$), and histamine and TVBN ($r = 0.76$, $p < 0.05$). However, negative correlations were noted between moisture and salt content ($r = -0.73$, $p < 0.05$), and a_w and salt content ($r = -0.76$, $p < 0.05$).

3.2. Effect of Brine Concentrations on the Quality of Brined and Dried Milkfish

Changes in the moisture and water activity (a_w) of the milkfish samples pre-immersed in different brine concentrations (i.e., 0%, 3%, 6%, 9%, and 15%) during a sun-drying period of five days are shown in Figure 1. The initial moisture of the fish samples was 70.3%, while the moisture of all fish samples rapidly decreased with increasing drying time. At the end of the drying period, the moisture content in all of the samples ranged from 44.2% to 46.9%, and no significant differences ($p > 0.05$) were observed among the samples of the various brine concentrations and control samples (Figure 1A). For all fish samples with an initial a_w value of 0.985, the a_w values gradually decreased with an increase in the drying time and reduced to 0.967 in the control sample, 0.959 in the 3% NaCl sample, 0.950 in the 6% NaCl sample, 0.945 in the 9% NaCl sample, and 0.942 in the 15% NaCl sample at the end of the sun-drying period (Figure 1B). It was found that the milkfish samples with higher brine concentrations had lower a_w values ($p < 0.05$).

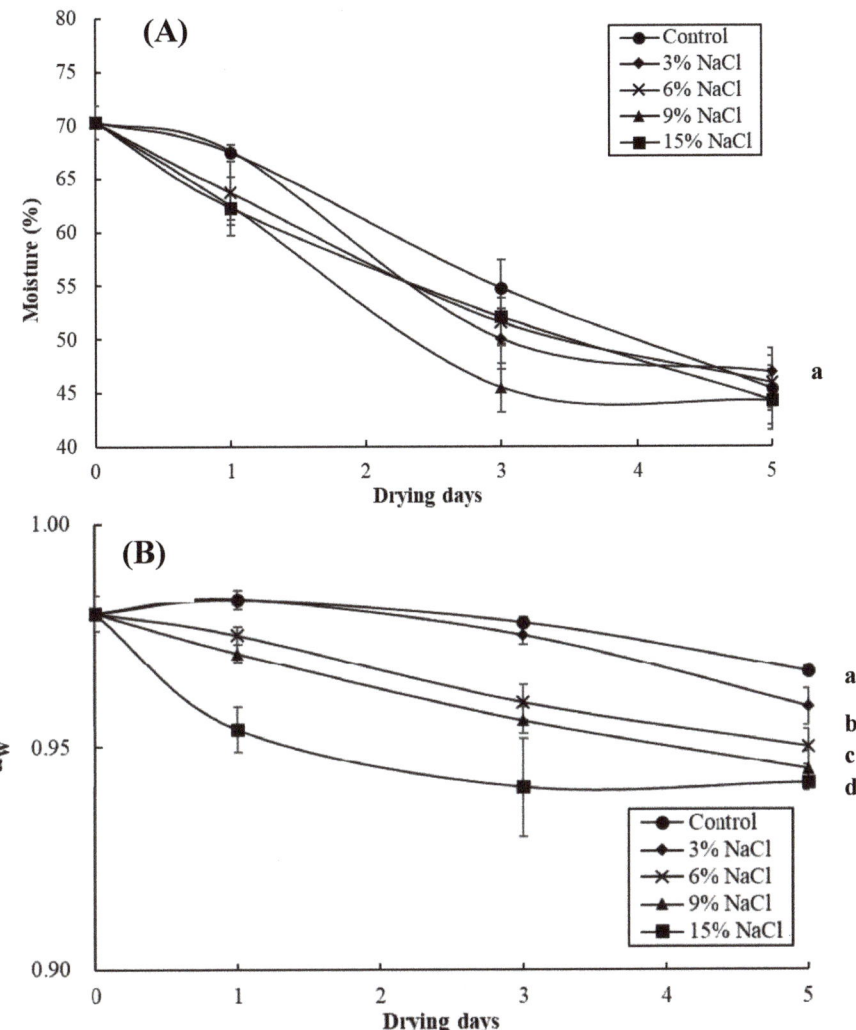

Figure 1. Changes in the moisture (**A**) and water activity (a_w) (**B**) in the milkfish samples as a result of brine-salting with 0% (control), 3%, 6%, 9%, and 15% NaCl during sun-drying. Each value represents the mean ± SD of three replications. Different lower letters indicate significant differences ($p < 0.05$) within the data at the end of the sun-drying period.

Changes in the pH and salt content of the milkfish samples pre-immersed in different brine concentrations (i.e., 0%, 3%, 6%, 9%, and 15%) over a sun-drying period of five days are presented in Figure 2. The pH values of the milkfish samples slightly increased from the initial reading of 5.41 to 5.69 for the control sample, 5.70 for the 3% and 6% NaCl samples, 5.87 for the 9% NaCl sample, and 5.89 for the 15% NaCl sample at the end of the sun-drying period. The increase in the pH for all of the group samples may be due to the formation of basic components, including ammonia, trimethylamine, and other amines by bacterial spoilage [22]. Moreover, the final pH values of the 9% and 15% NaCl samples were higher ($p < 0.05$) than those of the control and the 3% and 6% NaCl samples (Figure 2A). As shown in Figure 2B, the salt content in the fish sample slightly increased from 0.05% to 0.13% in the control sample, 0.20% to 0.70% in the 3% NaCl sample, 0.51% to 1.17% in the

6% NaCl sample, 0.85% to 2.24% in the 9% NaCl sample, and 1.62% to 2.87% in the 15% NaCl sample after give days of sun-drying. The results also show that the milkfish samples pre-immersed in a higher brine concentration had a higher salt content ($p < 0.05$).

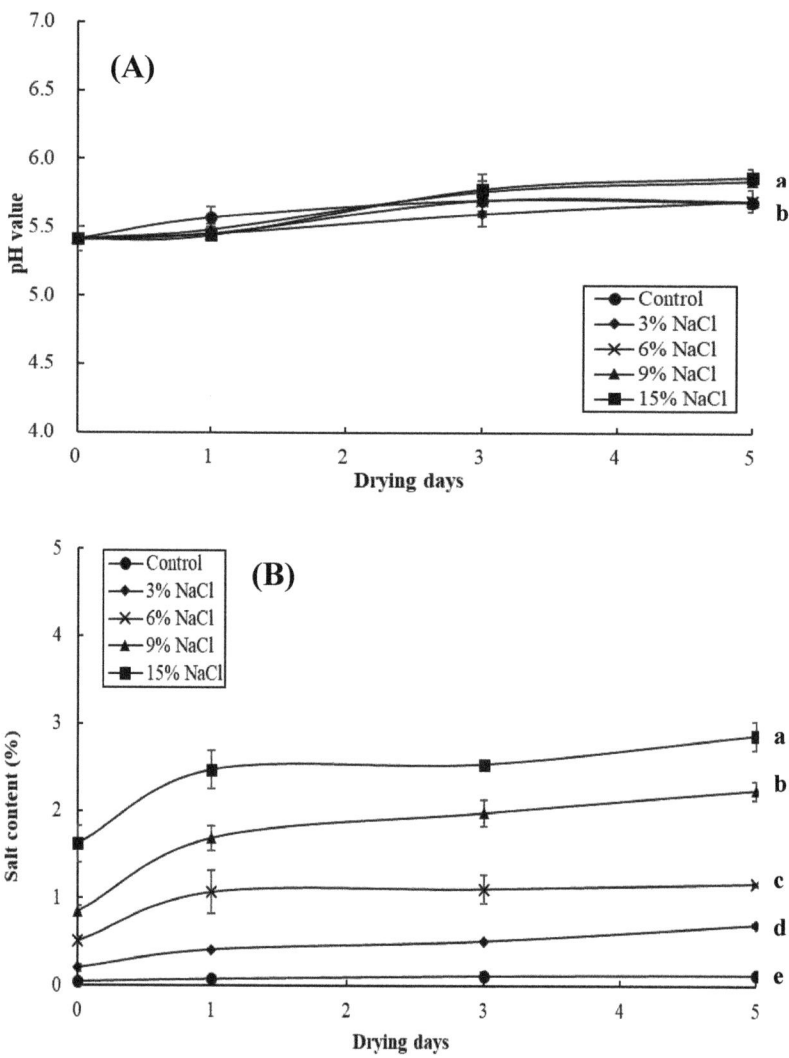

Figure 2. Changes in the pH (**A**) and salt content (**B**) of the milkfish samples as a result of brine-salting with 0% (control), 3%, 6%, 9%, and 15% NaCl during sun-drying. Each value represents the mean ± SD of three replications. Different lower letters indicate significant differences ($p < 0.05$) within the data at the end of the sun-drying period.

Figure 3 shows the changes in the TVBN and TBA values in the milkfish samples pre-immersed in different brine concentrations (i.e., 0%, 3%, 6%, 9%, and 15%) during a sun-drying period of five days. Initially, the milkfish samples had 13.7 mg/100 g of TVBN, and subsequently, the TVBN content in all fish samples increased gradually while drying, reaching 34.0 mg/100 g for the control sample, 30.5 mg/100 g for the 3% NaCl sample, 29.76 mg/100 g for the 6% NaCl sample, 27.0 mg/100 g for the 9% NaCl sample, and 26.9 mg/100 g for the 15% NaCl sample at the end of the sun-drying period. Thus, the highest TVBN level was detected in the control sample, followed by the 3% and 6% NaCl samples, and the lowest levels were observed for the 9% and 15% NaCl samples ($p < 0.05$) (Figure 3A). Connell [23] revealed that the increase in TVBN is due to the production of volatile basic compounds, including ammonia, trimethylamine and dimethylamine, via decomposition by autolytic enzymes and spoilage bacteria. Moreover, Nooralabettu [15] demonstrated that the addition of NaCl addition in Bombay duck can decrease autolytic enzyme activity in fish meat. An increase in salt content above 1% in fish can have an inhibitory effect on the bacteria associated with fish spoilage [24]. Consequently, the high content of TVBN in the unsalted samples (i.e., the control sample) obtained in this study was probably due to the increasing decomposition by enzymes and spoilage bacteria with the lack of salt's inhibitory effect.

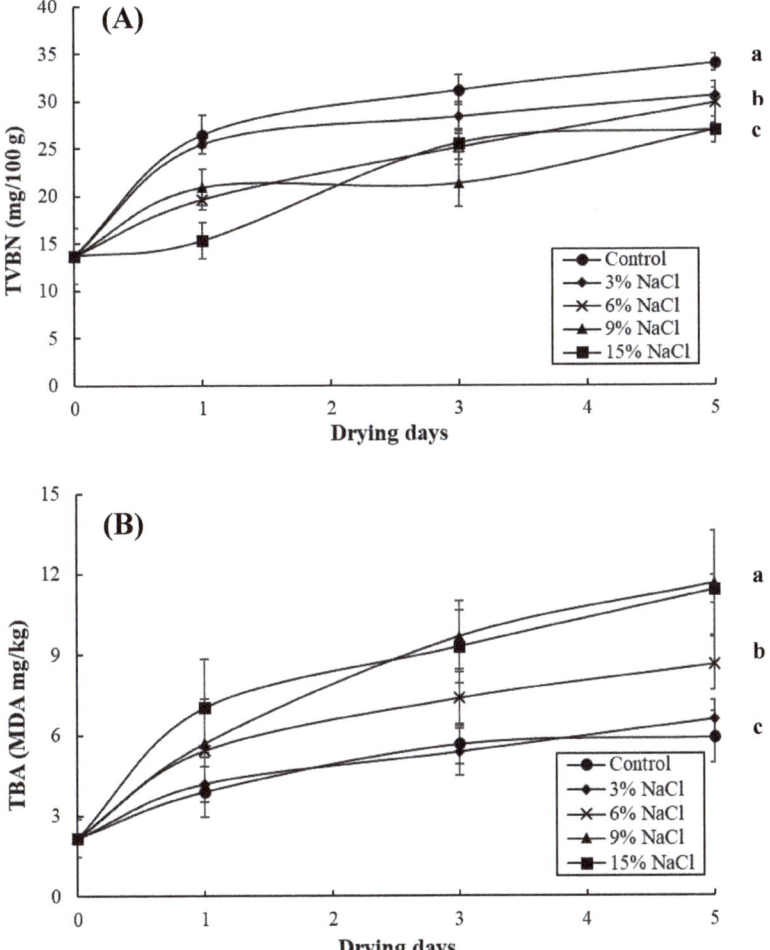

Figure 3. Changes in total volatile basic nitrogen (TVBN) (**A**) and thiobarbituric acid (TBA) (**B**) in the milkfish samples as a result of brine-salting with 0% (control), 3%, 6%, 9%, and 15% NaCl during sun-drying. Each value represents the mean ± SD of three replications. Different lower letters indicate significant differences ($p < 0.05$) within the data at the end of the sun-drying period.

Thiobarbituric acid (TBA), a measure of MDA as a secondary lipid oxidation product, is one of the most widely used indicators for the assessment of food lipid oxidation [25]. Initially, the TBA values for the control and brined samples were 2.18 MDA mg/kg. The value of TBA in all of the samples increased during the sun-drying period, reaching 5.9 MDA mg/kg for the control sample, 6.5 MDA mg/kg for the 3% NaCl sample, 8.6 MDA mg/kg for the 6% NaCl sample, 11.5 MDA mg/kg for the 9% NaCl sample, and 11.4 MDA mg/kg for the 15% NaCl sample at the end of the sun-drying period. In contrast to TVBN, the highest levels of TBA were observed in the 9% and 15% NaCl samples, followed by the 6% NaCl sample, and the lowest TBA level was detected in the control and 3% NaCl samples ($p < 0.05$) (Figure 3B). Yanar et al. [26] also reported that hot-smoked tilapia samples treated with a 15% brine concentration contained very high levels of TBA. Sodium chloride can promote lipid oxidation, while sodium ions may replace iron from myoglobin, thereby resulting in free iron ions for the catalysis of lipid oxidation [26,27]. Therefore, the results in this study reveal that the high TBA values in the samples prepared with 9% and 15% brine concentrations may be attributed to the addition of NaCl by accelerating the rate of lipid oxidation. In addition, when seafood is dried by exposure to sunlight, lipids can be oxidized and low molecular weight carbonyl components can be produced [28]. The results of this study are in agreement with a previous study reporting that the TBA values of dried yellow corvina increased rapidly during sun-drying [28].

Figure 4 shows the changes in APC and coliform bacteria in the milkfish samples pre-immersed in different brine concentrations (i.e., 0%, 3%, 6%, 9%, and 15%) over a sun-drying period of five days. The APC numbers of the milkfish sample gradually increased from the initial population of 3.21 to 6.88 log CFU/g for the control sample, 6.81 log CFU/g for the 3% NaCl sample, 6.15 log CFU/g for the 6% NaCl sample, 6.0 log CFU/g for the 9% NaCl sample, and 5.86 log CFU/g for the 15% NaCl sample at the end of the sun-drying period. Thus, the APC bacteria detected in the control and 3% NaCl samples were markedly higher ($p < 0.05$) than those of other brine concentration samples (Figure 4A) and exceeded the 6.47 log CFU/g Taiwanese regulatory standard. Similar to the APC population, the growth of coliform in this fish samples was considerably faster in the unsalted (control) sample than in the other brined samples ($p < 0.05$). The coliform counts in the control, 3%, 6%, 9%, and 15% NaCl samples increased to 3.51, 2.87, 2.75, 2.70, and 2.41 log MPN/g, respectively, at the end of the sun-drying period (Figure 4B). These results are in agreement with our previous report, in which the APC and coliform levels of dry-salted and sun-dried milkfish samples decreased with increasing salt concentrations [21]. A similar finding was also reported by Yang et al. [14], who found that higher brine-salting could inhibit the growth of bacteria in grass carp. Moreover, higher brine concentrations (>6%) in the milkfish samples obviously had a repressive action on microbiological growth in this study, indicating that salt content is able to inactivate or inhibit bacteria.

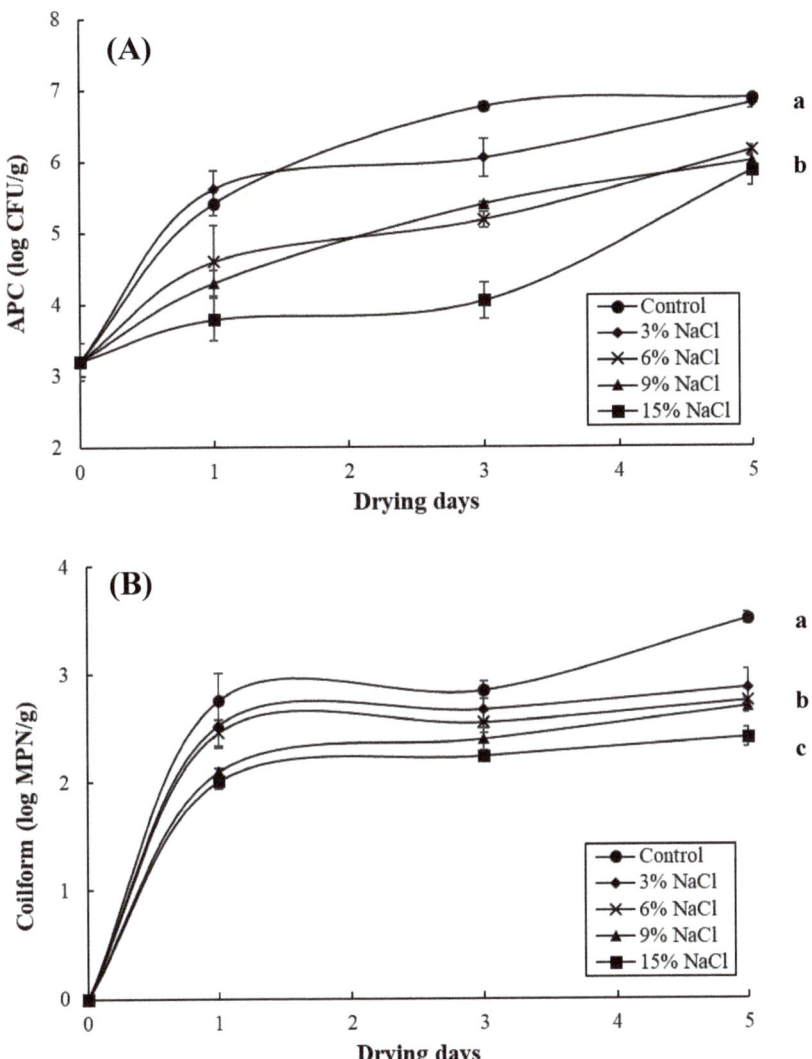

Figure 4. Changes in aerobic plate count (APC) (**A**) and coliform (**B**) in the milkfish samples as a result of brine-salting with 0% (control), 3%, 6%, 9%, and 15% NaCl during sun-drying. Each value represents the mean ± SD of three replications. Different lower letters indicate significant differences ($p < 0.05$) within the data at the end of the sun-drying period.

Figure 5 shows that the histamine content in the control sample increased gradually during the sun-drying period, reaching 4.8 mg/100 g by the end. On the other hand, the histamine contents in the 3%, 6%, 9%, and 15% NaCl samples only slightly increased during the sun-drying period, reaching 2.8, 2.0, 0.79, and 0.27 mg/100 g, respectively, by the end. In conclusion, the histamine content observed in the control sample was markedly higher ($p < 0.05$) than that of the other brine concentrations samples (Figure 5). These results agree with the previous research of Hwang et al. [21], where high contents of histamine at 67 mg/100 g were found in unsalted dried milkfish samples via sun-drying. The low levels of histamine (<2.8 mg/100 g) detected in the salted samples (>3% NaCl) in this study may be due to the growth reduction of histamine-forming bacteria by the preservative effect of salt, indicating that the addition of salt could be effective in reducing or inhibiting histamine accumulation. In our previous study, high levels of a$_w$, moisture, TVBN, APC, and histamine were detected in unsalted dried milkfish samples produced by sun-drying; therefore, dried milkfish producers should be aware that dried milkfish with low salt and sun-drying periods could become a vehicle for histamine poisoning [21]. Similarly, since high levels of TVBN (>30 mg/100g), APC (>6.81 log CFU/g), and histamine (>2.8 mg/100 g) were observed in the unsalted and 3% NaCl samples during the sun-drying period, brined and dried milkfish manufacturers should pay attention to the fact that dried milkfish brined with a low amount of salt (<3% NaCl) and a sun-drying period could lead to worse hygienic quality and potential hazards, such as food poisoning. However, the samples with higher brine concentrations (>9% NaCl) had higher TBA values (>11.4 MDA mg/kg) (Figure 3B). With regard to an assessment of APC, TBA, TVBN, and histamine, this study suggests that dried milkfish brined with a 6% NaCl addition has better chemical and bacteriological quality.

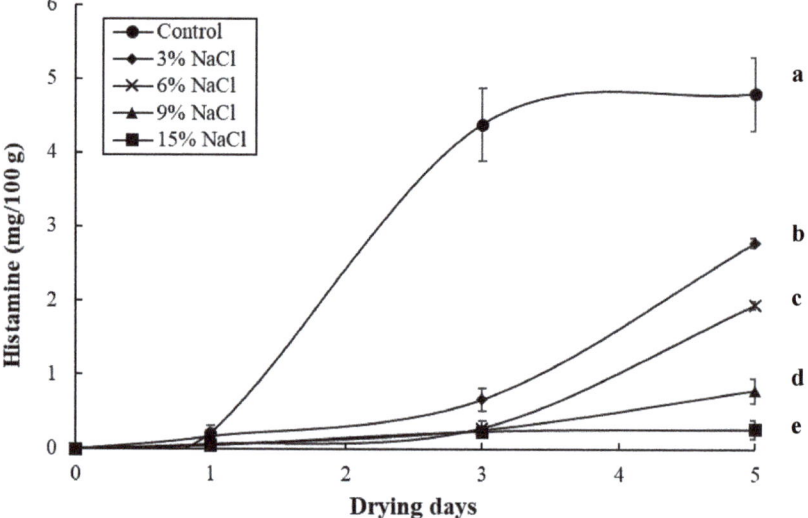

Figure 5. Changes in the histamine of milkfish samples as a result of brine-salting with 0% (control), 3%, 6%, 9%, and 15% NaCl during sun-drying. Each value represents the mean ± SD of three replications. Different lower letters indicate significant differences ($p < 0.05$) within the data at the end of the sun-drying period.

Pearson correlation was conducted to determine if there existed any relationship among the moisture, a$_w$, pH, salt content, TVBN, TBA, APC, coliform, and histamine contents of the samples at the end of the sun-drying period. In general, positive correlations existed between APC and a$_w$ ($r = 0.95$, $p < 0.05$), APC and histamine ($r = 0.88$, $p < 0.05$), coliform and a$_w$ ($r = 0.93$, $p < 0.05$), coliform and histamine ($r = 0.90$, $p < 0.05$), a$_w$ and TVBN ($r = 0.88$, $p < 0.05$), salt content and TBA ($r = 0.85$, $p < 0.05$), a$_w$ and histamine ($r = 0.89$, $p < 0.05$), and histamine and TVBN ($r=0.86$, $p < 0.05$). However, negative correlations were noted between salt content and APC ($r = -0.89$, $p < 0.05$), salt content and coliform ($r = -0.90$, $p < 0.05$), salt content and a$_w$ ($r = -0.92$, $p < 0.05$), a$_w$ and TBA ($r = -0.90$, $p < 0.05$), and salt content and histamine ($r = -0.95$, $p < 0.05$).

4. Conclusions

This study, aimed at investigating the hygienic quality of 20 brined and dried milkfish products, revealed that the APC numbers in seven samples (35%) exceeded the 6.47 log CFU/g Taiwanese regulatory standard. Moreover, 25% of the tested samples had histamine contents greater than the

5 mg/100 g recommended by the USFDA in their guideline levels, and 10% (2/20) of the fish samples had >50 mg/100 g of histamine. After the consumption of these samples, histamine fish poisoning could occur. In addition, the chemical and bacteriological quality of the brined and dried milkfish pre-immersed in various brine concentrations during a sun-drying period were observed in this study. Although the samples prepared with higher brine concentrations presented a retarded APC growth rate and a reduced formation of TVBN and histamine, as compared with the control sample, they produced higher TBA values. It is suggested that 6% NaCl for brined milkfish is the optimal condition for maintaining the quality of brined and dried milkfish. Our results could suggest that application of brine concentration information is effective in controlling quality and enhancing the safety of brined and dried milkfish products.

Author Contributions: Conceptualization, C.-C.H., Y.-C.L., and Y.-H.T.; methodology, C.-C.H., Y.-H.T., and H.-H.C.; analysis, C.-C.H., Y.-C.L., and H.-F.K.; data curation, Y.-C.L., H.-F.K., and C.-C.H.; writing—original draft preparation, C.-C.H. and Y.-H.T.; writing—review and editing, C.-C.H., Y.-H.T., and C.-Y.H.; supervision, Y.-C.L. and H.-F.K.; project administration, C.-C.H.; funding acquisition, C.-C.H. and Y.-H.T. All authors read and agreed to the published version of the manuscript.

Funding: This work was supported by the Ministry of Science and Technology, R.O.C. (Contract No. MOST 107-2635-E-412-001).

Acknowledgments: The authors gratefully acknowledge Shinn-Lih Yeh, a director of Mariculture Research Center, Fisheries Research Institute with providing equipment, Su-Sing Liu with the operation and maintenance of the equipment, and partly financial support from higher education sprout project of National Kaohsiung University of Science and Technology.

Conflicts of Interest: The authors declare no conflict of interest.

References

1. Hugerford, J.M. Scombroid poisoning: A review. *Toxicon* **2010**, *56*, 231–243. [CrossRef] [PubMed]
2. Chen, H.C.; Kung, H.F.; Chen, W.C.; Lin, W.F.; Hwang, D.F.; Lee, Y.C.; Tsai, Y.H. Determination of histamine and histamine-forming bacteria in tuna dumpling implicated in a food-borne poisoning. *Food Chem.* **2008**, *106*, 612–618. [CrossRef]
3. Chen, H.C.; Huang, Y.R.; Hsu, H.H.; Lin, C.S.; Chen, W.C.; Lin, C.M.; Tsai, Y.H. Determination of histamine and biogenic amines in fish cubes (*Tetrapturus angustirostris*) implicated in a food-borne poisoning. *Food Control* **2010**, *21*, 13–18. [CrossRef]
4. Chang, S.C.; Kung, H.F.; Chen, H.C.; Lin, C.S.; Tsai, Y.H. Determination of histamine and bacterial isolation in swordfish fillets (*Xiphias gladius*) implicated in a food borne poisoning. *Food Control* **2008**, *19*, 16–21. [CrossRef]
5. Tsai, Y.H.; Kung, H.F.; Lee, T.M.; Chen, H.C.; Chou, S.S.; Wei, C.I.; Hwang, D.F. Determination of histamine in canned mackerel implicated in a food borne poisoning. *Food Control* **2005**, *16*, 579–585. [CrossRef]
6. Tsai, Y.H.; Kung, H.F.; Chen, H.C.; Chang, S.C.; Hsu, H.H.; Wei, C.I. Determination of histamine and histamine-forming bacteria in dried milkfish (*Chanos chanos*) implicated in a food-borne poisoning. *Food Chem.* **2007**, *105*, 1289–1296. [CrossRef]
7. Hsieh, S.L.; Chen, Y.N.; Kuo, C.M. Physiological responses, desaturase activity, and fatty acid composition in milkfish (*Chanos chanos*) under cold acclimation. *Aquaculture* **2003**, *220*, 903–918. [CrossRef]
8. Chiang, F.S.; Sun, C.H.; Yu, J.M. Technical efficiency analysis of milkfish (*Chanos chanos*) production in Taiwan-an application of the stochastic frontier production function. *Aquaculture* **2004**, *230*, 99–116. [CrossRef]
9. Chiou, T.K.; Shiau, C.Y.; Chai, T.J. Extractive nitrogenous components of cultured milkfish and tilapia. *Nippon Suisan Gakk.* **1990**, *56*, 1313–1317. [CrossRef]
10. Lee, Y.C.; Kung, H.F.; Wu, C.H.; Hsu, H.M.; Chen, H.C.; Huang, T.C.; Tsai, Y.H. Determination of histamine in milkfish stick implicated in a foodborne poisoning. *J. Food Drug Anal.* **2016**, *24*, 63–71. [CrossRef]
11. Hwang, C.C.; Kung, H.F.; Lee, Y.C.; Wen, S.Y.; Chen, P.Y.; Tsen, D.I.; Tsai, Y.H. Histamine fish poisoning and histamine production by *Raoultella ornithinolytica* in milkfish surimi. *J. Food Prot.* **2020**, *83*, 874–880. [CrossRef]
12. Hsu, H.H.; Chuang, T.C.; Lin, H.C.; Huang, Y.R.; Lin, C.M.; Kung, H.F.; Tsai, Y.H. Histamine content and histamine-forming bacteria in dried milkfish (*Chanos chanos*) products. *Food Chem.* **2009**, *114*, 933–938. [CrossRef]

13. Gallart-Jornet, L.; Rustad, T.; Barat, J.M.; Fito, P.; Escriche, I. Effect of superchilled storage on the freshness and salting behaviour of Atlantic salmon (*Salmo salar*) fillets. *Food Chem.* **2007**, *103*, 1268–1281. [CrossRef]
14. Yang, W.; Shi, W.; Qu, Y.; Wang, Z.; Shen, S.; Tu, L.; Huang, H.; Wu, H. Research on the quality changes of grass carp during brine salting. *Food Sci. Nutri.* **2020**, *8*, 2968–2983. [CrossRef]
15. Nooralabettu, K.P. Effect of sun drying and artificial drying of fresh, salted Bombay duck (*Harpodon neherius*) on the physical characteristics of the product. *J. Aquat. Food Prod. Technol.* **2008**, *17*, 99–116. [CrossRef]
16. AOAC. *Official Methods of Analysis of AOAC International*, 21st ed.; AOAC International: Arlington, VA, USA, 2019.
17. Cobb, B.F.; Alaniz, I.; Thompson, C.A. Biochemical and microbial studies on shrimp: Volatile nitrogen and amino nitrogen analysis. *J. Food Sci.* **1973**, *38*, 431–435. [CrossRef]
18. Faustman, C.; Spechtm, S.M.; Malkus, L.A.; Kinsman, D.M. Pigment oxidation in ground veal: Influence of lipid oxidation, iron and zinc. *Meat Sci.* **1992**, *31*, 351–362. [CrossRef]
19. FDA. *Bacteriological Analytical Manual*; AOAC International: Arlington, VA, USA, 1998.
20. Bartholomev, B.A.; Berry, P.R.; Rodhouse, J.C.; Gilhouse, R.J. Scombrotoxic fish poisoning in Britain: Features of over 250 suspected incidents from 1976 to 1986. *Epidemiol. Infect.* **1987**, *99*, 775–782. [CrossRef]
21. Hwang, C.C.; Lin, C.M.; Kung, H.F.; Huang, Y.L.; Hwang, D.F.; Su, Y.C.; Tsai, Y.H. Effect of salt concentrations and drying methods on the quality and formation of histamine in dried milkfish (*Chanos chanos*). *Food Chem.* **2012**, *135*, 839–844. [CrossRef]
22. Arulkumar, A.; Paramasiam, S.; Rameshthangam, P.; Rabie, M.A. Changes on biogenic, volatile amines and microbial quality of the blue swimmer crab (*Portunus pelagicus*) muscle during storage. *J. Food Sci. Technol.* **2017**, *54*, 2503–2511. [CrossRef]
23. Connell, J.J. Methods of assessing and selecting for quality. In *Control of Fish Quality*, 3rd ed.; Fishing News Books: Oxford, UK, 1990; pp. 122–150.
24. Mohamed, S.B.; Mendes, R.; Slama, R.B.; Oliveira, P.; Silva, H.A.; Bakhrouf, A. Changes in bacterial counts and biogenic amines during the ripening of salted anchovy (*Engraulis encrasicholus*). *J. Food Nutr. Res.* **2016**, *5*, 318–325.
25. Fernandez, J.; Perez-Alvarez, J.A.; Fernandez-Lopez, J.A. Thiobarbituric acid test for monitoring lipid oxidation in meat. *Food Chem.* **1997**, *59*, 343–353. [CrossRef]
26. Yanar, Y.; Celik, M.; Akamca, E. Effects of brine concentration on shelf-life of hot-smoked tilapia (*Oreochromis niloticus*) stored at 4 °C. *Food Chem.* **2006**, *97*, 244–247. [CrossRef]
27. Kanner, J.; Harel, S.; Jaffe, R. Lipid peroxidation in muscle food as affected by NaCl. *J. Agri. Food Chem.* **1991**, *39*, 1017–1021. [CrossRef]
28. Gwak, H.; Eun, J.B. Changes in the chemical characteristics of *Gulbi*, salted and dried yellow Corvenia, during drying at different temperatures. *J. Aquat. Food Prod. Technol.* **2010**, *19*, 274–283. [CrossRef]

Publisher's Note: MDPI stays neutral with regard to jurisdictional claims in published maps and institutional affiliations.

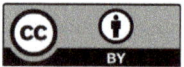

© 2020 by the authors. Licensee MDPI, Basel, Switzerland. This article is an open access article distributed under the terms and conditions of the Creative Commons Attribution (CC BY) license (http://creativecommons.org/licenses/by/4.0/).

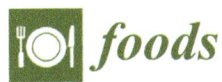

Article

Biogenic Amine Contents and Microbial Characteristics of Cambodian Fermented Foods

Dalin Ly [1,2,*], Sigrid Mayrhofer [1], Julia-Maria Schmidt [1], Ulrike Zitz [1] and Konrad J. Domig [1]

1. Institute of Food Science, Department of Food Science and Technology, BOKU - University of Natural Resources and Life Sciences Vienna, Muthgasse 18, A-1190 Vienna, Austria; sigrid.mayrhofer@boku.ac.at (S.M.); jm_schmidt@gmx.net (J.-M.S.); ulrike.zitz@boku.ac.at (U.Z.); konrad.domig@boku.ac.at (K.J.D.)
2. Faculty of Agro-Industry, Department of Food Biotechnology, RUA - Royal University of Agriculture, Dangkor District, P.O. BOX 2696 Phnom Penh, Cambodia
* Correspondence: dalin.ly@boku.ac.at or dalinely@rua.edu.kh; Tel.: +43-1-47654-75455; Fax: +43-1-47654-75459

Received: 30 January 2020; Accepted: 11 February 2020; Published: 15 February 2020

Abstract: Naturally fermented foods are an important part of the typical diet in Cambodia. However, the food safety status of these products has not been widely studied. The aim of this study was, therefore, to provide an overview of the quality of these foods in relation to microbiology and biogenic amines. Additionally, the obtained results were compared to the habits and practices of Cambodians in handling this type of food. A total of 57 fermented foods (42 fishery and 15 vegetable products) were collected from different retail markets in the capital of Cambodia. Pathogenic *Salmonella* spp., *Listeria* spp., and *Listeria monocytogenes* were not detected in 25 g samples. Generally, less than 10^2 cfu/g of *Staphylococcus aureus*, *Escherichia coli*, *Pseudomonas* spp., Enterobacteriaceae, and molds were present in the fermented foods. *Bacillus cereus* group members (<10^2 to 2.3×10^4 cfu/g), lactic acid bacteria (<10^2 to 1.1×10^7 cfu/g), halophilic and halotolerant bacteria (<10^2 to 8.9×10^6 cfu/g), sulfite-reducing *Clostridium* spp. (<10^2 to 3.5×10^6 cfu/g), and yeasts (<10^2 to 1.1×10^6 cfu/g) were detected in this study. Still, the presence of pathogenic and spoilage microorganisms in these fermented foods was within the acceptable ranges. Putrescine, cadaverine, tyramine, and histamine were detected in 100%, 89%, 81%, and 75% of the tested products, respectively. The concentrations of histamine (>500 ppm) and tyramine (>600 ppm) were higher than the recommended maximum levels in respectively four and one of 57 fermented foods, which represents a potential health risk. The results suggest that the production process, distribution, and domestic handling of fermented foods should be re-evaluated. Further research is needed for the establishment of applicable preservation techniques in Cambodia.

Keywords: Cambodian fermented foods; microbial characteristics; biogenic amines; food quality; food safety

1. Introduction

Cambodia is an agricultural country that has a tropical climate with two distinct monsoon seasons (dry and rainy seasons). Thus, the availability of certain products is not stable through the year, and food preservation and storage are required to maintain the food supply [1]. Since food spoilage is mainly caused by microorganisms, preventing their access to susceptible foods is one method of food preservation. Another one is the inhibition of microbial growth through fermentation, salting, drying, or smoking, as it is common in Cambodia [2,3]. The storage time of food depends on factors that affect the growth of spoilage microorganisms like intrinsic food characteristics (e.g., pH, a_w, composition) and extrinsic parameters (e.g., temperature, relative humidity, atmospheric gases). Due to higher ambient temperatures and moisture, food spoils faster in the tropics. As a result, it is not surprising that food security issues are reported in densely populated tropical cities [2]. However, the majority of the Cambodian population lives in rural areas where poverty is high and access to drinking water, electricity, and sanitation is limited [4].

Fermented foods are an important part of the typical diet in Cambodia [1]. Since Cambodia has an extensive network of waterways, freshwater fish, along with marine, fermented and preserved fish, is a major component of the diet of most Cambodians [5]. Fermented fishery products are consumed daily as main dishes, side dishes, or condiments/seasonings [5]. Additionally, they are applied as flavor enhancers due to their delicacy and high nutritional properties [6,7]. Vegetables also play an essential role in daily dishes for their nutrient content. The availability of certain fresh vegetables, however, does not last throughout the year. Depending on the varieties of domestic raw vegetables, many types of fermented vegetables have emerged in Cambodia with the popularity of traditional fermentation [8]. In the meantime, these foods have become a common part of the Cambodian diet [1,8].

Cambodian fermented foods are produced through knowledge that is passed on from generation to generation and from person to person [1]. The great majority of fermented products are locally produced by smallholders, many of them women, and sold in traditional wet markets where women also predominate as retailers [9]. Most of them are illiterate and have a poor knowledge about hygiene practices. Additionally, the awareness of food safety is limited in Cambodia. The quality of these foods is influenced by raw materials, processing methods, and climate, but there is no quality control of these determinants as well as of the finished products in Cambodia [1]. Fermented foods are generally not labelled with an appropriate shelf-life and usually stored at room temperature until they are completely consumed [1]. Fermented fishery products are usually cooked before consumption. However, fish paste and sauce can also be eaten raw and are often mixed with chili or lemon juice [1]. In contrast, fermented vegetables are normally considered as ready-to-eat (RTE) foods. As a result, it is not surprising that foodborne outbreaks are common in Cambodia [8]. But there is no coordinated food surveillance program and little analytical data regarding microbiological or chemical contamination of food are present [10]. Nevertheless, food safety is a key priority of the Cambodian government [11], and efforts to improve foodborne disease surveillance and food safety are being undertaken [10].

Escherichia coli, *Cronobacter sakazakii*, *Enterobacter* spp., opportunistic non-Enterobacteriaceae, *Staphylococcus* spp., and *Listeria* spp. have already been detected in fermented vegetables in Cambodia [8,12]. Furthermore, potentially pathogenic bacteria such as *Bacillus*, *Clostridium*, and *Staphylococcus* were found in traditional Cambodian fermented fish products [5]. Next to microbiological contamination, chemical substances can lead to acute poisoning or even long-term diseases such as cancer [13]. The most prevalent ones are biogenic amines (BAs) and biotoxins [14]. BAs are low molecular weight organic molecules, formed by microbial decarboxylation of their precursor amino acids or by transamination of aldehydes and ketones by amino acid transaminases [15]. Beside spoilage, preservative technological processes such as fermentation, salting, and ripening may increase BA formation in food. As BAs are thermostable, they cannot be inactivated by thermal treatment [13]. The most common BAs found in foods and beverages are histamine (HIS), tyramine (TYR), putrescine (PUT), and cadaverine (CAD) [16,17]. Low levels of BAs in food are not considered as a serious risk. However, when high amounts of BAs are consumed, various physiological effects may occur, namely, hypotension (in the case of HIS, PUT, and CAD) or hypertension (in the case of TYR), nausea, headache, rash, dizziness, cardiac palpitation, and even intracerebral hemorrhage and death in very severe cases [18]. BAs with more severe acute effects for human health are HIS and TYR [19]. PUT and CAD have low toxicological properties on their own, but they can act as precursor of carcinogenic N-nitrosamines when nitrite is present. These two BAs also potentiate the effects of HIS and TYR by inhibiting their metabolizing enzymes [19]. HIS is the only BA with regulatory limits [20]. In addition to their potential toxicity, BAs are also used to evaluate the hygienic quality of foods, as their levels in food can be an indirect indicator of excessive microbial proliferation [19].

Baseline surveillance data are essential to monitor the disease burden of fermented foods in Cambodia. To obtain such data, the physicochemical properties (pH, a_w, and salt content) as well as the presence of certain microorganisms (spoilage and pathogenic bacteria) and the concentrations of the BAs HIS, TYR, PUT, and CAD were determined in 57 Cambodian fermented food samples within this study. The main purpose of this manuscript is to give an overview of the quality of Cambodian fermented foods, to correlate physicochemical parameters with BA contents, and to describe the prevailing habits and practices of Cambodians in dealing with this type of food.

2. Materials and Methods

2.1. Sample Collection

Fifty-seven samples of naturally fermented foods (42 raw fermented fish and 15 RTE fermented vegetable products) were randomly purchased from wet markets in Phnom Penh, the capital city of Cambodia. These products originated from various provinces of the country. Fermented fishery samples included fish sauce (teuktrey; $n = 7$), fish paste (prahok; $n = 12$), shrimp paste (kapi; $n = 6$), fermented fish (paork chav; $n = 7$; mam trey; $n = 3$), sour fermented fish (paork chou; $n = 3$), and salted fish (trey proheum; $n = 4$). Fermented vegetables such as salty fermented radish (chaipov brey; $n = 3$), sweet fermented radish (chaipov paem; $n = 3$), fermented melon (trasork chav; $n = 3$), fermented mustard (spey chrourk; $n = 3$), and fermented papaya (mam lahong; $n = 3$) were bought on the next day. Detailed information about each fermented product is provided in Table 1. After purchasing, the samples were immediately packed into plastic boxes and stored at their storage temperature. One day later, the samples were transported to Vienna by airplane. At the Department of Food Science and Technology, Vienna, the samples were checked shortly after arrival and kept in their original containers at 4 °C until analysis. All samples were analyzed within the usual shelf-life of the products [21].

2.2. Physicochemical Properties Analysis

2.2.1. Determination of pH and Water Activity (a_w)

The pH value was determined by penetrating the spear tip of the Blueline 21 pH electrode (Schott AG, Mainz, Germany) into the samples. The pH values were then measured using a digital pH meter (Schott Lab 870, Mainz, Germany).

The a_w value was measured using the digital water activity meter Rotronic Hygropalm HP23-AW-A (Rotronic, Zurich, Switzerland) after equilibration at room temperature (~25 °C).

2.2.2. Determination of Salt Content (NaCl)

The salt content was analyzed by potentiometric precipitation titration of chloride-ions with the 877 Titrino plus-Titrator equipped with a calomel electrode (Metrohm AG, Herisau, Switzerland). The protocol was performed according to the producer with minor modifications. Depending on the expected salt content, 1 to 10 g ± 0.01 g (a) of the samples was weighed into a glass beaker and filled with distilled water to 200 g ± 0.01 g (b). Subsequently, the samples were homogenized for 2 min at 9500 rpm using an Ultra Turrax T25 (IKA, Germany). Fifty grams ± 0.01 g (c) of the homogenized samples was weighed into a new glass beaker, and 50 mL of distilled water was added. Afterwards, 2 mL (2 M) HNO_3 was added. The samples were then titrated with 0.1 M $AgNO_3$. With the obtained results, the salt content of the original samples was calculated as % (w/w) NaCl = $V \times M \times 0.0584 \times 100/m$; where V and M are the volume and molarity of the $AgNO_3$ standard solution used. The initial sample weight is m, which was calculated considering the sample preparation: $m = a \times c/b$. The test was conducted in duplicate.

Table 1. Detailed information of fermented food products.

Product Type	English Name	Local Name of Fish/Vegetable Species [a]	Scientific Family Name of Fish/Vegetable Species	Major Ingredients	Usage	Market Origin
Fermented Fishery Products						
Teuktrey (n = 7)	Fish sauce	Trey Kakeum Trey Kamong Trey Riel Trey Kanchanhchras Trey Linh Trey Kralong	Engraulidae Scombridae Cyprinidae Ambassis Cyprinidae Cyprinidae	Freshwater/sea fish, salt	Side dish, Condiment, Seasoning	Chamkadaung, Oreusey
Prahok (n = 12)	Fish paste	Trey Achkok Trey Riel Trey Chhkork Trey Phourk Trey Kampleanh	Cyprinidae Cyprinidae Cyprinidae Channidae Osphronemidae	Freshwater fish, salt	Main dish, Side dish, Condiment, Seasoning	Deumkor, Oreusey, Chamkadaung
Kapi (n = 6)	Shrimp paste	-	-	Tiny marine shrimp, salt	Side dish, Condiment, Seasoning	Kandal, Chas, Oreusey
Paork chav (n = 7)	Fermented fish	Trey Por Trey Pra Trey Chhkork	Pangasiidae Pangasiidae Cyprinidae	Freshwater fish, brown glutinous rice, salt	Main dish, Side dish	Thmey, Oreusey
Paork chou (n = 3)	Sour fermented fish	Trey Sleuk Reusey	Engraulidae	Freshwater fish, rice, salt	Main dish, Side dish	Chamkadaung, Oreusey
Mam trey (n = 3)	Fermented fish	Trey Bondol Ampow	Clupeidae	Freshwater fish, palm sugar, salt	Main dish, Side dish	Thmey
Trey proheum (n = 4)	Salted fish	Trey Pra, Trey Proma	Pangasiidae, Sciaenidae,	Freshwater fish, salt	Main dish, Seasoning	Thmey
Fermented Vegetables						
Chaipov brey (n = 3)	Salty fermented radish	Chaitav	Brassicaceae	Chinese white radish, salt	Side dish, Seasoning, Appetizer	Kandal Chas Oreusey
Chaipov paem (n = 3)	Sweet fermented radish	Chaitav	Brassicaceae	Chinese white radish, sugar	Main dish, Side dish, Appetizer	Kandal Chas Oreusey
Trasork chav (n = 3)	Fermented melon	Trasork	Cucurbitaceae	Baby melon, salt, purple sticky rice	Side dish	Thmey
Spey chnourk (n = 3)	Fermented mustard	Speythom	Brassicaceae	Chinese mustard, salt	Side dish	Phumreusey Limcheanghak
Mam lahong (n = 3)	Fermented papaya	Lahong	Caricaceae	Green papaya, tiny fermented fish, salt, herb	Side dish	Phumreusey Limcheanghak

[a] Name in Cambodian.

2.3. Microbiological Analysis

From each fermented product, a 10 g sample was aseptically collected, transferred to a stomacher bag, and homogenized (Stomacher 400 Circulator, Seward, UK) with 90 mL of buffered peptone water for 45 s at 230 rpm. Appropriate dilutions of the samples were prepared using the same diluent, and 0.1 or 1 mL aliquots of each dilution were applied on various selective media using the spread plate method or pour plate method. Lactic acid bacteria (LAB) were anaerobically grown on DeMan Rogosa Sharpe agar (MRS, Merck, Darmstadt, Germany) at 30 °C for 72 h according to ISO 15214 [22]. Enterobacteriaceae were enumerated using the pour plate method with an additional overlay on Violet Red Bile Dextrose agar (VRBD, Merck, Darmstadt, Germany) and an incubation at 37 °C for 24 h according to ISO 21528-2 [23]. *Pseudomonas* spp. were detected by plating appropriate dilutions on Cephalothin-Sodium Fusidate-Cetrimide agar (CFC, Oxoid, Hampshire, UK) and incubation at 25 °C for 44 h based on ISO 13720 [24]. Yeasts and molds were determined according to ISO 21527-2 [25] using the spread plate method on Dichloran Glycerol agar (DG18, Merck, Darmstadt, Germany). The plates were incubated at 25 °C for 5–7 d and counted on the 5th and 7th day of incubation. Selected yeast colonies were confirmed by methylene blue staining and microscopy [26]. Halophilic and halotolerant bacteria were counted after an incubation at 30 °C for 2–4 d on Tryptone Soya agar (TS, Oxoid, Hampshire, UK) supplemented with 10% NaCl (Roth, Karlsruhe, Germany) [27]. *Staphylococcus aureus* was enumerated on Baird Parker agar (BP, Merck, Darmstadt, Germany), which was incubated at 37 °C for 24 h based on ISO 6888-1/AMD 1 [28]. The plates were evaluated again after an additional 24 h incubation. The confirmation of colonies was performed using Gram-stain and DNase agar (Oxoid, Hampshire, UK) according to Kateete et al. [29]. The number of presumptive *Bacillus cereus* group members was investigated by spreading dilutions on Mannitol Yolk Polymyxin agar (MYP, Merck, Darmstadt, Germany) and incubating plates at 30 °C for 18–48 h. The evaluation was also performed after 18 h and 48 h of incubation. Colonies were confirmed by endospore staining [30]. *E. coli* was enumerated by pour plating on Tryptone Bile Glucuronic medium (TBX, Oxoid, Hampshire, UK) with an incubation at 44 °C for 18–24 h based on ISO 16649-2 [31]. The presence of sulfite-reducing *Clostridium* spp. (SRC) was analyzed by pour plating with an additional overlay on Sulfite-Cycloserin agar (SC, Oxoid, Hampshire, UK). Plates were anaerobically incubated at 37 °C for 20 h. Confirmation tests were performed using Lactose-Gelatine medium (Conda, Madrid, Spain) and Motility-Nitrate medium (Conda, Madrid, Spain) according to ISO 7937 [32]. The presence of *Salmonella* spp. was investigated using the VIDAS UP (BioMerieux, Crappone, France) *Salmonella* (SPT) system, whereas that of *Listeria* spp. and *L. monocytogenes* was tested by the VIDAS LDUO (BioMerieux, Crappone, France) system. VIDAS SPT and VIDAS LDUO are based on an enzyme-linked fluorescent immunoassay. The preparation of the samples was similar to the previous method, but 25 g of the sample was weighted in instead of 10 g. After pre-enrichment (*Listeria* spp.) and enrichment (*L. monocytogenes*, *Salmonella* spp.) steps, which were carried out according to the manufacturer's manual, the assay steps were performed automatically by the instrument.

2.4. Determination of Biogenic Amines (BAs)

The concentrations of BAs in the supernatant were analyzed by reverse-phase HPLC (Waters 2695 Separations Module, Waters, MA, USA) according to the method of Šimat et al. and Saarinen et al. [33,34]. Briefly, 1 g of the homogenized sample was extracted overnight with 5 mL of 0.4 M perchloric acid (Merk, Darmstadt, Germany). Then, the sample was centrifuged at 5000 rpm for 10 min and the supernatant was kept for further analysis. For derivatization, 80 µL of 2 M NaOH (Roth, Karlsruhe, Germany), 120 µL of saturated sodium bicarbonate solution (Merck, Darmstadt, Germany), and 400 µL of derivatization reagent (1% dansyl chloride in acetone; prepared daily; Fluka, Seelze, Germany) were added to 400 µL of sample solution. The sample was mixed and incubated for 45 min at 40 °C. Afterwards, 60 µL of 1 M ammonia solution (Roth, Karlsruhe, Germany) was added, mixed, and incubated in the dark for 60 min at room temperature. Finally, 940 µL acetonitrile (Roth, Karlsruhe, Germany) was added. The sample was mixed and centrifuged for 10 min at 13,400 rpm. A RP-18 column (Li Chro CART 250-4, 5 µm,

Merck, Darmstadt, Germany) with a LiChroCART 4-4 Guard Column (RP-18, 5 µm) (Merk, Darmstadt, Germany) and a manu-CART NT cartridge holder (Merck, Darmstadt, Germany) was used for separation. The flow rate was 1 mL/min, the column temperature was 40 °C, and the injection volume was 20 µL. The mobile phase A consisted of 0.1 M ammonium acetate (Roth, Karlsruhe, Germany) and the mobile phase B was 100% acetonitrile. The following gradient was used for the separation: time = 0 min, 50% A and 50% B; time = 19 min, 10% A and 90% B; time = 20 min, 50% A and 50% B; time = 28 min, 50% A and 50% B. The detection was performed by UV–vis (Waters 2489 UV-visible detector, Waters, MA, USA) at a wavelength of 254 nm. Heptylamine (Fluka, Seelze, Germany) was used as an internal standard that was well separated from other compounds. The specificity of the method was checked using standard mixtures of 12 BA chemicals, which included spermine tetrahydrochloride, spermidine trihydrochloride, ethanolamine, isopropylamine, histamine dihydrochloride, putrescine (1,4-diaminobutan dihydrochloride), methylamine hydrochloride, agmatine sulfate, cadaverine (1,5-diaminopentan dihydrochloride), tyramine hydrochloride, dimethylamine hydrochloride, and pyrrolidine. Except for the last four chemicals, which were from Sigma-Aldrich (St. Louis, MO, USA), all chemicals were from Fluka. Standard stock solutions of BAs were prepared at 500 mg/L in 0.01 M perchloric acid. The stock solutions were diluted with 0.4 M perchloric acid to obtain series of working standard solutions (0.25, 1, 5, 10, and 15 mg/L). The derivatization procedure was the same as for the samples. All compounds were separated and could be identified by their retention times. The linearity of the method was tested by analyzing the series of working standard solutions. The correlation coefficients for the linear regression lines were better than 0.99 for all compounds. The limit of detection (LOD = 3x standard deviation of y-residuals of low concentrations/slope of calibration curve) of all BAs ranged between 0.5 and 1.5 ppm, and the limit of quantification (LOQ = 10x standard deviation of y-residuals of low concentrations/slope of calibration curve) ranged between 1.5 and 4.8 ppm. PUT, CAD, HIS, and TYR were analyzed in duplicate.

2.5. Statistical Analysis

Result units of quantitative microbiological analyses were cfu/g. The physicochemical parameters and BA concentrations results were analyzed with statistical analyses using the Statistical Package for the Social Sciences (SPSS, Version 20.0.0 for Windows, 2011; IBM Co., Somers, NY, USA). Data were analyzed for the degree of variation by calculating the mean and standard deviations (SDs) of the results. The significance of differences was evaluated using analysis of variance (ANOVA). A *p* value of less than 0.05 was considered statistically significant. The least-squares difference (LSD) test was used to determine the significance of differences in the physicochemical parameters and BA contents among the samples. The relationship value was determined using the Pearson correlation coefficient.

3. Results

3.1. Physicochemical Characteristics in Fermented Foods

Physicochemical parameters such as pH, a_w, and salt content were measured and compared to discuss possible causes for the different BA levels. Table 2 shows the physicochemical parameters of the tested fermented products. The pH values in fermented fishery samples were in the range of 4.4 to 7.6. Lower pH values were found in paork chav (fermented fish), while higher values were detected in kapi (shrimp paste) and trey proheum (salted fish). The a_w values of the fermented fishery products ranged from 0.69 to 0.84. The lowest a_w value (0.69) was detected in kapi (shrimp paste) and the highest (0.84) in paork chav (fermented fish). The salt contents were in the range of 6% to 34%, with the lowest value (6%) found in trey proheum (salted fish) and the highest (34%) in prahok (fish paste). In the fermented vegetables, the pH values were between 3.6 and 5.5. Lower pH values were found in spey chrourk (fermented mustard, 3.6–3.9) and mam lahong (fermented papaya, 3.7–3.8), while the highest value was detected in chaipov brey (salty fermented radish) (4.6). The a_w values in these fermented products were between 0.75 and 0.97. The highest salt concentration (25%) was found in chaipov brey (salty fermented radish), while the lowest (2%) was detected in spey chrourk (fermented mustard) (Table 2).

Table 2. Physicochemical characteristics (pH, a_w, % NaCl) of fermented food products.

Product Types	English Name	Physicochemical Characteristics (Mean ± SD)		
		pH	a_w	Salt Content (%)
Fermented Fishery Products				
Teuktrey ($n = 7$)	Fish sauce	4.8–6.3 [#] (5.5 ± 0.6 [¥]) [a]	0.72–0.82 (0.76 ± 0.04) [a]	19–25 (22 ± 2) [a]
Prahok ($n = 12$)	Fish paste	5.3–5.7 (5.5 ± 0.1) [a]	0.71–0.80 (0.73 ± 0.02) [ab]	15–34 (21 ± 5) [a]
Kapi ($n = 6$)	Shrimp paste	6.6–7.3 (7.0 ± 0.2) [b]	0.69–0.72 (0.71 ± 0.01) [b]	13–28 (19 ± 7) [a]
Paork chav ($n = 7$)	Fermented fish	4.4–5.1 (4.8 ± 0.3) [c]	0.74–0.84 (0.80 ± 0.03) [c]	9–14 (11 ± 2) [b]
Paork chou ($n = 3$)	Sour fermented fish	4.9–5.1 (5.0 ± 0.1) [c]	0.74–0.76 (0.75 ± 0.01) [a]	13–15 (14 ± 1) [b]
Mam trey ($n = 3$)	Fermented fish	4.9–5.6 (5.3 ± 0.4) [ac]	0.76–0.78 (0.77 ± 0.01) [ac]	8–14 (10 ± 3) [b]
Trey proheum ($n = 4$)	Salted fish	6.3–7.6 (6.8 ± 0.6) [b]	0.78–0.83 (0.80 ± 0.02) [c]	6–17 (12 ± 5) [b]
Fermented Vegetables				
Chaipov brey ($n = 3$)	Salty fermented radish	4.4–4.8 (4.6 ± 0.2) [g]	0.75–0.76 (0.75 ± 0.01) [g]	24–25 (24 ± 0.4) [g]
Chaipov paem ($n = 3$)	Sweet fermented radish	3.9–5.5 (4.5 ± 0.9) [gh]	0.78–0.87 (0.82 ± 0.04) [h]	10–18 (13 ± 4) [h]
Trasork chav ($n = 3$)	Fermented melon	4.1–4.4 (4.3 ± 0.2) [gh]	0.76–0.83 (0.80 ± 0.03) [h]	9–13 (10 ± 2) [h]
Spey chrourk ($n = 3$)	Fermented mustard	3.6–3.9 (3.7 ± 0.2) [h]	0.96–0.97 (0.97 ± 0.01) [i]	2–5 (4 ± 1) [i]
Mam lahong ($n = 3$)	Fermented papaya	3.7–3.8 (3.7 ± 0.1) [h]	0.91–0.94 (0.92 ± 0.01) [i]	3–4 (3 ± 1) [i]

[#] Ranged values (minimum to maximum). [¥] Mean ± SD (standard deviation). Values with different superscript letters in the same column indicate significant differences at $p < 0.05$ by LSD test. Statistical analysis of fermented fish and vegetable samples was conducted separately.

Based on the statistical analysis (ANOVA) of fermented fishery products, there were significant differences ($p < 0.05$) between the physicochemical parameters of teuktrey (fish sauce) and those of paork chav (fermented fish) and trey proheum (salted fish). There was no statistically significant difference ($p > 0.05$) among the samples of teuktrey (fish sauce) and prahok (fish paste), and of paork chav (fermented fish), paork chou (sour fermented fish), and mam trey (fermented fish). Statistical analysis of fermented fish and vegetables samples was conducted separately. Regarding the fermented vegetable products, the physicochemical values of chaipov brey (salty fermented radish) were significantly different from that of spey chrourk (fermented mustard) and mam lahong (fermented papaya) ($p < 0.05$), while no significant difference was found among chaipov paem (sweet fermented radish) and trasork chav (fermented melon) ($p > 0.05$) (Table 2).

3.2. Presence of Microorganisms

Counts of LAB ($<10^2$ to 1.1×10^6 cfu/g), halophilic and halotolerant bacteria ($<10^2$ to 8.9×10^6 cfu/g), Enterobacteriaceae ($<10^2$ cfu/g), *Pseudomonas* spp. ($<10^2$ cfu/g), yeasts ($<10^2$ to 1.1×10^6 cfu/g), and molds ($< 10^2$ to 2.3×10^2 cfu/g) from the different types of fermented fish tested are indicated in Table 3. Table 3 also presents the results regarding the *B. cereus* group members ($<10^2$ to 2.3×10^4 cfu/g), SRC ($<10^2$ to 3.5×10^6 cfu/g), *S. aureus*, and *E. coli* ($<10^2$ cfu/g, respectively).

The microbial profiles found in fermented vegetables are displayed in Table 3 as well. The LAB counts were in the range of $<10^2$ to 1.1×10^7 cfu/g. The highest LAB counts were detected in spey chrourk (fermented mustard) and mam lahong (fermented papaya). Halophilic and halotolerant bacteria were found in numbers ranging from 2×10^2 to 5.5×10^4 cfu/g. The counts of *B. cereus* group members ranged from $<10^2$ to 1.2×10^4 cfu/g. SRC and yeasts were detected in the range of $< 10^2$ to 1.5×10^3 cfu/g and $<10^2$ to 2.6×10^5 cfu/g in the tested vegetable samples, respectively (Table 3). The counts of all other microorganisms were $<10^2$ cfu/g.

Table 3. Microbial profiles found in fermented food products.

Product Type	English Name	LAB [a]	Halophilic & Halotolerant Bacteria	Microorganisms (cfu/g)						
				Entero-Bacteriaceae	Pseudomonas spp.	Yeasts	Molds	B. cereus Group Members	SRC [b]	S. aureus	E. coli

Product Type	English Name	LAB [a]	Halophilic & Halotolerant Bacteria	Entero-Bacteriaceae	Pseudomonas spp.	Yeasts	Molds	B. cereus Group Members	SRC [b]	S. aureus	E. coli
Fermented Fishery Products											
Teuktrey ($n = 7$)	Fish sauce	$<10^2$	$<10^2$	$<10^2$	$<10^2$	$<10^2$	$<10^2$	$<10^2$	$<10^2$	$<10^2$	$<10^2$
Prahok ($n = 12$)	Fish paste	$<10^2$–1.5×10^2	10^2–9.5×10^3	$<10^2$	$<10^2$	$<10^2$	$<10^2$	$<10^2$–1.6×10^3	2.4×10^2–2.8×10^6	$<10^2$	$<10^2$
Kapi ($n = 6$)	Shrimp paste	$<10^2$–2.8×10^3	5.2×10^3–5×10^5	$<10^2$	$<10^2$	$<10^2$	$<10^2$	$<10^2$–6.8×10^3	2×10^2–1.3×10^5	$<10^2$	$<10^2$
Paork chav ($n = 7$)	Fermented fish	$<10^2$–1.6×10^3	1.2×10^3–2.6×10^5	$<10^2$	$<10^2$	$<10^2$–1.1×10^6	$<10^2$	10^2–2.3×10^4	$<10^2$–9×10^4	$<10^2$	$<10^2$
Paork chou ($n = 3$)	Sour fermented fish	$<10^2$	2×10^2–9×10^3	$<10^2$	$<10^2$	$<10^2$–2.7×10^4	$<10^2$	$<10^2$–3.5×10^3	4×10^2–1.2×10^4	$<10^2$	$<10^2$
Mam trey ($n = 3$)	Fermented fish	$<10^2$–1.2×10^3	10^3–5.1×10^4	$<10^2$	$<10^2$	$<10^2$	$<10^2$	1.1×10^2–1.2×10^4	1.9×10^3–3.5×10^6	$<10^2$	$<10^2$
Trey proheum ($n = 4$)	Salted fish	$<10^2$–1.1×10^6	2.3×10^4–8.9×10^6	$<10^2$	$<10^2$	$<10^2$	$<10^2$	$<10^2$–2.6×10^2	$<10^2$–1.6×10^5	$<10^2$	$<10^2$
Fermented Vegetables											
Chaipov brey ($n = 3$)	Salty fermented radish	$<10^2$	3×10^3–1.6×10^4	$<10^2$	$<10^2$	$<10^2$	$<10^2$	$<10^2$	$<10^2$	$<10^2$	$<10^2$
Chaipov paem ($n = 3$)	Sweet fermented radish	$<10^2$	1.7×10^4–5.5×10^4	$<10^2$	$<10^2$	$<10^2$	$<10^2$	$<10^2$–2.2×10^2	$<10^2$–3×10^2	$<10^2$	$<10^2$
Trasork chav ($n = 3$)	Fermented melon	$<10^2$	2×10^2–8×10^3	$<10^2$	$<10^2$	$<10^2$	$<10^2$	$<10^2$	$<10^2$	$<10^2$	$<10^2$
Spey chrourk ($n = 3$)	Fermented mustard	$<10^2$–1.1×10^7	7.3×10^2–2×10^4	$<10^2$	$<10^2$	$<10^2$–2.6×10^3	$<10^2$	2×10^2–1.2×10^4	$<10^2$	$<10^2$	$<10^2$
Mam lahung ($n = 3$)	Fermented papaya	$<10^2$–5.8×10^6	2×10^2–1.1×10^3	$<10^2$	$<10^2$	1.7×10^2–2.6×10^5	$<10^2$	$<10^2$–1.6×10^2	3.2×10^2–1.5×10^3	$<10^2$	$<10^2$

[a] Lactic acid bacteria; [b] sulfite-reducing clostridia.

3.3. Quantification of Biogenic Amines (BAs) in Fermented Foods

Table 4 shows the BA contents of 57 fermented product samples. The detection limits in this study were <0.5 ppm (PUT, CAD, and TYR) and <2 ppm for HIS. The results indicate that PUT was detected in quantifiable amounts in all tested fishery samples (100%), while CAD, TYR, and HIS concentrations were quantified in approximately 95%, 88%, and 86% of these products, respectively. PUT and CAD were the most frequently detected BAs in the tested samples. The highest concentrations of PUT (830 ppm), CAD (2035 ppm), HIS (840 ppm), and TYR (691 ppm) were detected in paork chav (fermented fish). PUT concentrations in 42 fishery samples were in the range between 23 to 830 ppm, with the lowest (23 ppm) presented in paork chou (sour fermented fish) and the highest (830 ppm) found in paork chav (fermented fish). The concentrations of HIS in the quantifiable fishery products (86%) ranged from 32 to 840 ppm (Table 4). The current results show that, overall, less than 50 ppm HIS was determined in all kapi (shrimp paste) samples. The concentrations of TYR in the quantifiable fishery samples (88%) ranged from 10 to 691 ppm (Table 4). In general, lower levels of TYR were detected in kapi (shrimp paste) and paork chou (sour fermented fish) than in other fermented fishery products in this study.

Table 4. Contents of biogenic amines in fermented food products.

Product Type	English Name	Biogenic Amines (ppm)			
		PUT *	CAD	HIS	TYR
Fermented Fishery Products					
Teuktrey ($n = 7$)	Fish sauce	75–404 [#] (233 ± 126 [¥]) [ab]	99–766 (368 ± 231) [abc]	40–253 (155 ± 74) [ab]	39–342 (144 ± 110) [ab]
Prahok ($n = 12$)	Fish paste	191–649 (360 ± 150) [b]	119–899 (522 ± 231) [abc]	35–408 (179 ± 115) [abc]	76–594 (218 ± 159) [ab]
Kapi ($n = 6$)	Shrimp paste	29–294 (112 ± 99) [ac]	ND [#]–270	ND–46	ND–57
Paork chav ($n = 7$)	Fermented fish	33–830 (386 ± 337) [b]	38–2035 (672 ± 782) [bc]	32–840 (422 ± 264) [c]	10–691 (299 ± 294) [b]
Paork chou ($n = 3$)	Sour fermented fish	23–92 (49 ± 37) [a]	26–69 (43 ± 24) [a]	46–559 (260 ± 267) [bc]	ND–82
Mam trey ($n = 3$)	Fermented fish	37–569 (378 ± 296) [bc]	23–1470 (930 ± 788) [c]	33–732 (320 ± 366) [bc]	ND–196
Trey proheum ($n = 4$)	Salted fish	72–278 (153 ± 99) [ab]	187–485 (297 ± 130) [ab]	ND–183	53–118 (79 ± 30) [a]
Fermented Vegetables					
Chaipov brey ($n = 3$)	Salty fermented radish	12–18 (15 ± 3) [g]	ND–12	ND	ND
Chaipov paem ($n = 3$)	Sweet fermented radish	11–16 (14 ± 3) [g]	ND–10	ND	ND
Trasork chav ($n = 3$)	Fermented melon	28–107 (70 ± 40) [g]	ND–23	ND–18	7–30 (15 ± 13) [g]
Spey chrouk ($n = 3$)	Fermented mustard	33–197 (95 ± 89) [g]	16–51 (29 ± 19) [g]	34–103 (66 ± 35) [g]	22–86 (44 ± 36) [gh]
Mam lahong ($n = 3$)	Fermented papaya	72–184 (119 ± 58) [g]	22–118 (68 ± 48) [g]	33–72 (49 ± 20) [g]	38–63 (53 ± 13) [h]

* PUT, putrescine; CAD, cadaverine; HIS, histamine; TYR, tyramine; [#] Ranged values (minimum to maximum) [¥] Mean ± SD; [#] ND, not detected (Limit of detection < 0.5 ppm for PUT, CAD, and TYR; <2 ppm for HIS). Values with different superscript letters in the same column indicate significant differences at $p < 0.05$ by LSD test. Statistical analysis of fermented fish and vegetable samples was conducted separately.

The four types of BAs were also analyzed for the safety evaluation of fermented vegetables from Cambodia. The BA levels varied among the collected RTE fermented vegetables (Table 4). PUT, CAD, TYR, and HIS were detected in 100%, 73%, 60%, and 47% of the fermented vegetables, respectively. The ranges of the quantifiable BAs were from 11 to 197 ppm for PUT, 10 to 118 ppm for CAD, 18 to 103 ppm for HIS, and 7 to 86 ppm for TYR (Table 4). The results clearly show that most BA concentrations in the five types of fermented vegetables were less than 100 ppm. Even no HIS and TYR could be detected in chaipov brey (salty fermented radish) and chaipov paem (sweet fermented radish) samples (Table 4).

According to one-way ANOVA and LSD tests of 42 fermented fisheries samples, statistically significant differences ($p < 0.05$) were found among the detected concentrations of PUT, CAD, HIS, and TYR in each product type. The statistical analysis of 15 fermented vegetable samples showed no statistical difference ($p > 0.05$) among concentrations of PUT, CAD, and HIS, while TYR concentrations were statistically different ($p < 0.05$) (Table 4).

Analyzing the correlation between total BA contents and the physicochemical parameters pH, a_w, and salt content (%) in 42 fermented fishery products, a weak positive relationship between total BAs and a_w values ($r = 0.22$, $p > 0.05$; $n = 42$), and a weak negative with pH values ($r = -0.22$, $p > 0.05$; $n = 42$) were found. There was no correlation among total BAs and salt content ($r = 0.00$, $p > 0.05$; $n = 42$) (Figure S1A–C). Furthermore, the linear functions between total BA contents and parameters of pH ($r = -0.57$, $p < 0.05$; $n = 15$) and salt content ($r = -0.81$, $p < 0.05$; $n = 15$) were characterized by a moderate and strong negative correlation coefficient, respectively, while a strong positive correlation between total BAs and a_w value ($r = 0.79$, $p < 0.05$; $n = 15$) were determined in fermented vegetable products (Figure S2A–C).

4. Discussion

4.1. Physicochemical Characteristics in Fermented Foods

Based on the physicochemical results, types of fermented fishery products were more different than those of fermented vegetables. Nevertheless, the pH values of this study are in good agreement with those of fermented fish products in Thailand, Vietnam, Laos, Myanmar, China, Korea, Japan, Malaysia, and Taiwan [5,35–38]. The results of the salt concentration analysis are also consistent with previous data for fermented fish products [5,38], shrimp paste [6], and fish sauce [37]. The a_w values of fermented fish products were comparable to fermented fish products from other countries, for example, Thai shrimp paste (0.65–0.72) and Indonesian fermented fish (0.75–0.93) [39,40].

The pH values found in the fermented vegetables were between 3.6 and 5.5 (Table 2). This is in agreement with a previous study, which reported that the pH of Cambodian fermented vegetables ranged from 3.6 to 6.5, depending on the raw materials and processing techniques [8]. Chaipov brey (salty fermented radish) was found to have the highest salt value (25%) of the fermented vegetables. Salty fermented radish with high salt concentrations (20–25%) has also been reported elsewhere [8]. As salt reduces a_w, the lowest a_w values were also determined in these samples (0.75–0.76) (Table 2).

Growth of microorganisms in foods are mainly influenced by the a_w and pH [41]. The addition of salt, in turn, has an inhibitory effect on the growth of microorganisms due to its impacts on the a_w value [42].

4.2. Microbiological Parameters in Fermented Foods

Microorganisms associated with fermented foods are commonly present on the external surface and in the pre- and post-harvest environment of raw materials. Additionally, they exist in the gill and gut of seafood [14].

Regarding *Bacillus* spp. and *Clostridium* spp., our results are comparable to those of Chuon et al., who also analyzed Cambodian traditional fermented fish sauce, fish paste, and shrimp paste [5]. Such traditionally home-prepared salted or fermented products are often associated with foodborne botulism [43]. However, routine testing for *C. botulinum* to ensure food safety is not recommended [43]. Instead, SRC have been proposed to identify risks from *C. botulinum* [43]. In addition to *C. botulinum*, *C. perfringens*—the most important of the SRC—poses a frequent problem and challenge in fish industry [44]. It is estimated that 10^5 to 10^8 cfu/g *C. perfringens* are capable of generating toxinfection [44]. Foodborne diseases that have *C. perfringens* as causative agent are related to inadequate storage, processing, and food service operations [44]. Nevertheless, no *C. perfringens* could be confirmed within this study. It is known that $>10^5$ cfu/g *B. cereus* group members are potentially harmful for human consumption [45]. None of the fermented products exceeded this limit (Table 3). The survival of *B. cereus* in low numbers in several fermented products, including those based on fish and vegetables, has already been described [46]. The inactivation of this pathogen could be attributed to the presence of organic acids or higher salt concentrations [46]. Moreover, no *S. aureus* could be quantified ($<10^2$ cfu/g) in the tested samples, which is in contradiction to a previous study [5]. In addition, it is reported that *S. aureus* is uniquely resistant to adverse conditions such as low a_w values (0.83), high salt contents, and pH stress. Thus, most strains can grow over an a_w and pH range of 0.83 to >0.99 and 4.5–9.3, respectively [47]. Although 11 of all 57 food products tested (19.3%) had an a_w value in the range specified above, 10 of them (e.g., all trasork chav (fermented melon), spey chrourk (fermented mustard), and mam lahong (fermented papaya), and one chaipov paem (sweet fermented radish) product had a pH < 4.5 (Table 2). Overall, *S. aureus* could only have grown in one sample. Although *L. monocytogenes* appears to be relatively tolerant to acidic conditions, no representatives of this species as well as of other *Listeria* species were verified, which may be due to the low a_w (<0.9) of most food samples tested (90%). Also, less than 10^2 cfu/g of *Pseudomonas* spp., Enterobacteriaceae, and *E. coli* were detected in all products examined (Table 3). Furthermore, no *Salmonella* spp. could be determined using the VIDAS system. These Gram-negative bacteria are often inhibited by a salt concentration >10%, an a_w value <0.95, a pH value <3.8 or >9.0 (depending on the acidulant), and the fermentation process itself [48]. LAB are not only responsible for the fermentation, they also significantly contribute to the flavor, texture, and nutritional value of fermented products [48], produce effective antimicrobial agents, and are the primary preservation factor in fermented fish products [49]. However, LAB are generally only tolerant to moderate salt concentrations (10%–18%). Consequently, their counts decrease as the salt concentration increases [50]. Forty-three samples (~75%) of all fermented products tested in this study contained more than 10% salt (Table 3). LAB were only present in high numbers in samples with less than 10% salt (Table 2 and 3).

Since typical spoilage bacteria are generally non- or only slightly halotolerant (e.g., pseudomonads, enterobacteria), the extensive use of salt is another technological process for food preservation besides fermentation [51]. Up to 25% and 34% salinity was respectively determined for fermented vegetable and fishery products in this study. Classifying the various products according to their salt content (e.g., 0–10%, 11–20%, >20%, data not shown), the numbers of halophilic and halotolerant bacteria generally decreased with increasing salinity.

The unfavorable conditions for bacterial growth (high salt content, a low pH or a_w) may result in higher yeasts and mold numbers. These microorganisms are quite salt-tolerant [51]. As recommended by the European Food Safety Authority (EFSA), the accepted limit for molds in foods is $<10^3$ cfu/g [52]. As shown in Table 3, all 57 fermented food products were acceptable regarding molds. It has been reported that $<10^6$ cfu/g of yeasts are acceptable in RTE foods placed on the market [53]. An unsatisfactorily higher yeasts count ($>10^6$ cfu/g) was only found in one paork chav (fermented fish) sample, which could lead to spoilage by acid and gas production [45,53]. However, the limit was just exceeded marginally (Table 3).

According to different organizations and previous studies [45,52–56], the detected counts of the investigated microorganisms in this study are satisfactory. Thus, the fermented foods tested are suitable for human consumption regarding the microbiological quality.

4.3. Formation of BAs in Fermented Foods

A deviation in BA concentrations within a specific food category is probably due to intrinsic food characteristics such as pH and a_w values, nutrients, and microbiota, as well as extrinsic factors including storage time, temperature, and manufacturing processes [57–59]. This may explain the wide variation of BA concentrations between the fermented fishery products and even within the same tested product type. Shalaby (1996) stated that BA levels differ not only between different food varieties but also within the same variety [57]. However, no significant difference was observed in fermented vegetables within this study.

Fish species associated with a high amount of histidine belong to the families *Scombridae, Clupeidae, Engraulidae, Coryphenidae, Pomatomidae*, and *Scombreresosidae* [60]. As seen in Table 1, the fish species of some fermented fish products belong to the families *Engraulidae* and *Scombridae* for teuktrey (fish sauce), *Engraulidae* for paork chou (fermented fish) and *Clupeidae* for mam trey (fermented fish). Hence, these products contained higher HIS amounts (Table 4). In contrast, low HIS and TYR contents are reported in crustaceans such as shrimp [61]. Corresponding values were determined for six kapi (shrimp paste) samples within this study. Fresh fruits and vegetables such as melon, cabbage, radishes, and cucumber contain lower HIS levels; however, papaya is considered as a HIS liberator [62]. Mustard is generally an allergen, and sometimes listed as moderately high in HIS [63]. Accordingly, HIS has been found in all fermented spey chrouk (fermented mustard) and mam lahong (fermented papaya) samples, but only in one trasork chav (fermented melon) and in no chaipov (fermented radish) sample within this study. TYR has been detected in more fermented vegetable samples than HIS, although in lower concentrations. TYR and CAD have been described in few vegetables in relatively low concentrations [64]. In contrast, it has been reported that PUT is the most common BA found in food of plant origin. It is particularly abundant in vegetables [64,65] and fermented products [60]. As seen in Table 4, this BA was the only one that was verified in all fermented vegetable samples with relatively high values.

The possible involvement of molds and yeasts in BA (especially CAD and PUT) accumulation is still discussed [19]. However, it is known that different genera, species, and strains of Gram-positive and Gram-negative bacteria are able to produce BAs by the action of microbial decarboxylases [66]. In particular, Enterobacteriaceae were identified as HIS-producing bacteria, but also halophilic and halotolerant bacteria (among other representatives of the families Enterobacteriaceae, Pseudomonadaceae, and the genera *Photobacterium*, *Vibrio*, and *Staphylococcus*), LAB, *Bacillus* spp., and *Clostridium* spp. were said to be capable of HIS formation [14,57,67]. According to Rodriguez-Jerez et al., microbial species with the capacity to form HIS and those with the capacity to form other BAs are similar [68]. Thus, Enterobacteriaceae were also reported to produce PUT, CAD, and to a lesser extent TYR. These BAs have also been detected when testing various *Bacillus* strains [67]. However, TYR should be mainly formed by LAB (*Lactobacillus*, *Enterococcus*) during fermentation [16]. Next to strains of the genera *Clostridium*, *Pseudomonas*, and *Staphylococcus*, LAB (*Enterococcus*, *Lactococcus*) are also involved in the production of PUT. It should be kept in mind that decarboxylase activities are often related to strains rather than to species or genera [69]. The capabilities of such strains, in turn, vary depending on the type and even batch of food product from which the strains are isolated [67].

The main factors affecting microbial activities in food are temperature, salt concentration, and pH [19]. Most fermented foods in this study had a pH value within the range of 3.0 to 6.0 (79%, Table 2), providing an acidic environment. The transcription of many decarboxylase genes is induced by a low pH value, which improves the fitness of the microbial cells subjected to acidic stress [19]. As the decarboxylation of amino acids is a mechanism of BA-forming bacteria to counteract acidic stress and to adapt to environmental conditions, their decarboxylase activity increases, resulting in higher BA concentrations [7,58]. Hence, it contributed to higher BA contents (Table 4). This effect could be confirmed within this study, as weak and moderate negative correlations ($r = -0.22$ and -0.57) were respectively found between the total BA contents and pH values for fermented fishery and fermented vegetable products. A strong negative linear fit ($r = -0.81$) could be detected between total BAs and salt content in fermented vegetables, whereas there was no correlation between these parameters in fermented fishery products (Figures S1 and S2). In general, increasing salt concentrations contribute to the reduction of BA accumulation in foods, mainly reducing the metabolic activities of decarboxylase-positive microorganisms [19] as it may have been the case for the fermented vegetables. However, a possible enhancing effect of NaCl on the BA production has also been described [19]. Thus, stressed cells seem to activate the decarboxylating pathways in the framework of more complex response systems [19] being probably more present in fermented fishery than vegetable products. In contrast, the rate of BA accumulation decreases with the decrease of a_w values due to the water loss [19]. Correspondingly, a positive correlation should be observed between total BA contents and a_w values. In fact, weak and strong positive relationships were determined for fermented fishery ($r = 0.22$) and vegetable ($r = 0.79$) products, respectively.

The ability of microorganisms to produce BAs is limited by low temperature [19]. Within this study, samples were stored at 4°C until investigation. However, fermented fishery and vegetable products are usually stored at room temperature in Cambodia due to the given conditions. Thus, even higher BA amounts could be expected for these products in this country. Paork chav (fermented fish) and other fermented fish products are stored at room temperature up to a year [21]. In the case of fermented vegetables, the salt content seems to be particularly relevant for the storage time. Thus, vegetables with 5–6% salt should be sold as soon as possible, while chaipov brey (salty fermented radish) samples with high salt concentrations (20–25%) have a longer storage time [8]. In this regard, higher BA values were detected in fermented vegetables with lower salt contents (2–5%).

4.4. BAs and Food Safety

Table 5 shows the distribution of the tested fermented food products according to the different allowable limits. Several organizations have set legal maximum limits on HIS concentrations in fermented foods that should ensure safe human consumption if the limits are not exceeded. Such organizations are the US Food and Drug Administration (FDA) with 50 ppm, FAO/WHO with 200 ppm for fish and fishery products, respectively, and EFSA with 400 ppm for fishery products that have undergone enzyme maturation treatment in brine [60,70,71]. The HIS level in fish sauce has been regulated in particular by the Codex Alimentarius Commission (CAC) and EFSA, with a maximum allowable limit of 400 ppm [55,72]. Correspondingly, the contents of HIS in all teuktrey (fish sauce) products did not exceed 400 ppm (Table 5). Thus, the levels of HIS in teuktrey (fish sauce) products in the current study can be regarded as safe for human consumption according to EFSA and CAC. Due to numerous outbreaks with toxic HIS concentrations ≥500 ppm [60], one paork chou (sour fermented fish), one mam trey (fermented fish), and two paork chav (fermented fish) products, representing about 7% (4/57) of the fermented products (Table 5), could pose a health risk. Although a food safety criterion is only set for HIS, HIS is not the only BA responsible for health hazards. Healthy individuals should also not be exposed to TYR values of 600 ppm or more by meal as recommended by EFSA [60]. The concentrations of TYR in all tested products were less than 600 ppm (Table 4), except for one paork chav (fermented fish) sample, which may constitute a health hazard [60]. Nevertheless, this sample is still fine according to Prester et al., who suggested a dietary value of up to 800 ppm of TYR as acceptable. More than 1080 ppm are toxic for adults [61].

Table 5. Distribution of fermented foods with quantifiable histamine contents.

Product Type	English Name	Histamine Contents (ppm)					
		≤50	>50 to 200	>200 to 400	>400 to <500	≥500	Total
Fermented Fishery Products—Number of Quantifiable Samples							
Teuktrey (n = 7)	Fish sauce	1 (14%)	3 (43%)	3 (43%)			7
Prahok (n = 12)	Fish paste	1 (9%)	7 (58%)	3 (25%)	1 (8%)		12
Kapi (n = 6)	Shrimp paste	6 (100%)					6
Paork chav (n = 7)	Fermented fish	1 (14%)		2 (29%)	2 (29%)	2 (29%)	7
Paork chou (n = 3)	Sour fermented fish	1 (33%)	1 (33%)			1 (33%)	3
Mam trey (n = 3)	Fermented fish	1 (33%)	1 (33%)			1 (33%)	3
Trey proheum (n = 4)	Salted fish	2 (50%)	2 (50%)				4
Total		13 (31%)	14 (33%)	8 (19%)	3 (7%)	4 (10%)	42 (100%)
Fermented Vegetables—Number of Quantifiable Samples							
Chaipov brey (n = 3)	Salty fermented radish	3 (100%)					3
Chaipov paem (n = 3)	Sweet fermented radish	3 (100%)					3
Trasork chav (n = 3)	Fermented melon	3 (100%)					3
Spey chrourk (n = 3)	Fermented mustard	1 (33%)	2 (67%)				3
Mam lahong (n = 3)	Fermented papaya	2 (67%)	1 (33%)				3
Total		12 (80%)	3 (20%)				15 (100%)

TYR concentrations from <0.4 to 270.6 ppm in commercially Chinese fish sauces [73], from 77.5 to 381.1 ppm in Korean anchovy sauces [74], and from 0 to 1178 ppm in commercial fish sauces the Far East sold at German markets [75] were reported. Hence, the concentrations of TYR in teuktrey (fish sauce) from retail markets in Cambodia were generally within or even below these concentrations (Table 4).

It has also been reported that the acute toxicity levels of TYR and CAD are respectively greater than 2000 ppm and the oral toxicity level of PUT is 2000 ppm [15]. It is known that TYR has a stronger and more rapid cytotoxic effect than HIS [76]. Unlike HIS and TYR, the pharmacological activities of PUT and CAD seem to be less potent. Nonetheless, both amines show in vitro cytotoxicity at concentrations easily reached in inherently BA-rich foods [77] and enhance the toxicity of HIS and TYR [19]. In the tested teuktrey (fish sauce) products, the highest levels of PUT (404 ppm) and CAD (766 ppm) were higher than those in fish sauce sold at Malaysian markets (242.8 ppm PUT and 704.7 ppm CAD) [78] and Chinese markets (276.6 ppm PUT and 606.3 ppm CAD) [73] but much lower than the levels in imported fish sauce products sold at German markets (1257 ppm PUT and 1429 ppm CAD) [75], Austrian markets (510 ppm PUT and 1540 ppm CAD) [65], and other European markets (1220 ppm PUT and 1150 ppm CAD) [60]. Extremely high PUT and CAD contents characterize inferior fish sauces, which may be due to the minor production hygiene, less salt content (<20%), the type of fish species, and storage condition [19,61]. Nevertheless, a health risk from consuming such a fish sauce is likely to be excluded due to the relatively small average intake [75]. Interestingly, the PUT concentrations of fish sauce samples were generally lower than the associated CAD concentrations (Table 4). The complexity of fish protein, which releases more lysine (precursor of CAD) during the fermentation of fish sauce, resulting in increased CAD concentrations could be the reason [78]. The current results also show that the highest PUT and CAD values in fish and shrimp pastes were higher than those in paste products in Taiwan [35] and in the Maldives [79]. Generally, BAs were detected in low levels in the tested fermented vegetables, which should not cause any risk when consumed. These results were consistent with previous studies [60,80], which reported that fermented vegetables should be considered as low-risk products in terms of BAs.

4.5. BAs and Food Quality

The HIS content alone may be a reliable indicator of food safety, but not of food quality. TYR and CAD are used as spoilage index [81]. Other authors have considered PUT and CAD as spoilage indicators [82]. Furthermore, PUT and CAD increase with longer storage times [19] and give strong unpleasant decaying odors at very low concentrations [75]. Therefore, the PUT and CAD concentration could be used as quality indicator [19], and their accumulation should be avoided [15,77]. These BAs are also included in the biogenic amine index (BAI) [83]. The BAI, the sum of HIS, TYR, PUT, and CAD, is more indicative of food quality, as these BAs are mostly produced at the end of shelf-life, indicating spoilage [83,84]. This index was also established to facilitate the evaluation and comparison of the BA concentrations in food. However, the usefulness of the BAI as quality index depends on many factors, mainly concerning the nature of the product (e.g., fresh or fermented food). Owing to the number of different factors (e.g., fermentation, maturation, starters), BA amounts vary much more in fermented products [13]. Thus, the BAI has proven to be more satisfactory for fresh products, and there is a BAI for freshwater fish of 50 ppm [85], while it is missing for fermented fishery products. The only BAI for a fermented food product was given by Wortberg and Woller [84] for Bologna sausages at 500 ppm. The higher BAI mainly results from the fermentation process and/or ripening. Using this limit, about one-third (31%) of the fermented fishery products in this study had a BAI of less than 500 ppm, while two-thirds (69%) had a higher BAI (>500 ppm), indicating a poor hygienic quality (Figure S3). Of the fermented vegetables, about 13% (2/15) had a BAI higher than 300 ppm (Figure S4). This value corresponds to the sum of HIS, TYR, PUT, and CAD, which should not be exceeded by acceptable sauerkraut [57].

In view of these results, the production process, distribution, and domestic handling of fermented products should be re-evaluated under strict hygienic practices together with the hazard analysis critical control point (HACCP) approach in order to minimize the content of BAs and microbiological contamination. The storage of food by cooling or freezing requires electricity that is not available to all Cambodians. Therefore, preservation techniques, such as the use of antimicrobial substances and/or autochthonous starter cultures, which are characterized by the absence of any BA formation ability or the presence of a BA detoxification activity, should be tested for their possible application on an industrial and small scale.

5. Conclusions

The presence of microorganisms in the examined fermented samples presented no health risk since pathogenic and spoilage microorganisms were in acceptable ranges. Nevertheless, one paork chou (sour fermented fish), one mam trey (fermented fish), and two paork chav (fermented fish) products represent a health risk because of the high level of HIS (>500 ppm). One of the paork chav (fermented fish) samples additionally exceeded the recommended TYR maximum (>600 ppm) per meal. The totals of all BAs tested were higher than the recommended corresponding BAI values in about 69% of the tested fermented fishery and 13% of the vegetable products. This may indicate a poor hygienic quality for these products. Hence, the production process, distribution, and domestic handling of fermented products in Cambodia should be re-evaluated in order to minimize the content of BAs and microbiological contamination. Further research is required to establish preservation techniques that could be applied on an industrial and small-scale in Cambodia.

Supplementary Materials: The following are available online at http://www.mdpi.com/2304-8158/9/2/198/s1, Figure S1: Linear fitting between total biogenic amines and physicochemical parameters, including pH (A), water activity (B), and salt content (C), in fermented fishery products (n = 42). Each dot indicates a data set obtained from a single sample, Figure S2. Linear fitting between total biogenic amines and physicochemical parameters, including pH (A), water activity (B), and salt content (C), in fermented vegetable products (n = 15). Each dot indicates a data set obtained from a single sample, Figure S3. Biogenic amine index (BAI) evaluated for 42 samples of fermented fishery products. The bold horizontal line describes the limit value of 500 ppm, which is used to distinguish between fermented fishery products of good and poor hygienic quality, Figure S4. Biogenic amine index (BAI) evaluated for 15 samples of fermented vegetable products. The bold horizontal line describes the limit value of 300 ppm, which is used to distinguish between fermented vegetable products of good and poor hygienic quality.

Author Contributions: Conceptualization, D.L., K.J.D., and S.M.; Analysis, D.L.; Investigation, J.-M.S.; Resources, U.Z. and K.J.D.; Writing—original draft, D.L.; Writing—Review and Editing, D.L., S.M., and K.J.D.; Supervision, K.J.D. and S.M. All authors have read and agreed to the published version of the manuscript.

Funding: This study was financed by the European Commission for the Erasmus Mundus Action 2 under the ALFABET project (the reference number: 552071) and partially funded by the Schlumberger Foundation Faculty for the Future Program for supporting the first author to pursue a Ph.D.

Acknowledgments: Special thanks is given to Vibol San for his valuable contribution. This work was supported by the European Commission for the Erasmus Mundus scholarship under the ALFABET project Reference number: 552071 and partially funded by the Schlumberger Foundation, Faculty for the Future Program for supporting the first author to pursue a Ph.D.

Conflicts of Interest: The authors confirm that they have no conflict of interest with respect to the work described in this manuscript.

References

1. Ly, D.; Mayrhofer, S.; Domig, K.J. Significance of traditional fermented foods in the lower Mekong subregion: A focus on lactic acid bacteria. *Food Biosci.* **2018**, *26*, 113–125. [CrossRef]
2. Hammond, S.T.; Brown, J.H.; Burger, J.R.; Flanagan, T.P.; Fristoe, T.S.; Mercado-Silva, N.; Nekola, J.C.; Okie, J.G. Food Spoilage, Storage, and Transport: Implications for a Sustainable Future. *BioScience* **2015**, *65*, 758–768. [CrossRef]
3. Hubackova, A.; Kucerova, I.; Chrun, R.; Chaloupkova, P.; Banout, J. Development of solar drying model for selected Cambodian fish species. *Sci World J.* **2014**, *2014*, 439431. [CrossRef]
4. Collignon, B.; Gallegos, M.; Kith, R. *Global Evaluation of UNICEF's Drinking Water Supply Programming in Rural Areas and Small Towns 2006–2016: Country Case Study Report—Cambodia*; Unicef: Cambodia, 2017; p. 71.
5. Chuon, M.R.; Shiomoto, M.; Koyanagi, T.; Sasaki, T.; Michihata, T.; Chan, S.; Mao, S.; Enomoto, T. Microbial and chemical properties of Cambodian traditional fermented fish products. *J. Sci. Food Agric.* **2014**, *94*, 1124–1131. [CrossRef] [PubMed]

6. Faithong, N.; Benjakul, S.; Phatcharat, S.; Binsan, W. Chemical composition and antioxidative activity of Thai traditional fermented shrimp and krill products. *Food Chem.* **2010**, *119*, 133–140. [CrossRef]
7. Waché, Y.; Do, T.-L.; Do, T.-B.-H.; Do, T.-Y.; Haure, M.; Ho, P.-H.; Kumar Anal, A.; Le, V.-V.-M.; Li, W.-J.; Licandro, H.; et al. Prospects for food fermentation in South-East Asia, topics from the tropical fermentation and biotechnology network at the end of the AsiFood Erasmus+project. *Front. Microbiol.* **2018**, *9*. [CrossRef]
8. Chrun, R.; Hosotani, Y.; Kawasaki, S.; Inatsu, Y. Microbioligical hazard contamination in fermented vegetables sold in local markets in Cambodia. *Biocontrol Sci.* **2017**, *22*, 181–185. [CrossRef]
9. Grace, D. Food Safety in Low and Middle Income Countries. *Int. J. Environ. Res. Public Health* **2015**, *12*, 10490–10507. [CrossRef]
10. FAO/WHO. Cambodia Country Report on Food Safety. In Proceedings of the FAO/WHO Regional Conference on Food Safety for Asia and the Pacific, Seremban, Malaysia, 24–27 May 2004.
11. Cheng, M.; Spengler, M. *How (Un)Healthy and (Un)Safe is Food in Cambodia?* Konrad-Adenauer-Foundation Cambodia: Phnom Penh, Cambodia, 2016; p. 11.
12. Soeung, R.; Phen, V.; Buntong, B.; Chrun, R.; LeGrand, K.; Young, G.; Acedo, A.L. Detection of coliforms, *Enterococcus* spp. and *Staphylococcus* spp. in fermented vegetables in major markets in Cambodia. *Acta Hortic.* **2017**, 139–142. [CrossRef]
13. Ruiz-Capillas, C.; Herrero, A.M. Impact of Biogenic Amines on Food Quality and Safety. *Foods* **2019**, *8*, 62. [CrossRef]
14. Visciano, P.; Schirone, M.; Tofalo, R.; Suzzi, G. Biogenic amines in raw and processed seafood. *Front. Microbiol.* **2012**, *3*, 188. [CrossRef] [PubMed]
15. Biji, K.B.; Ravishankar, C.N.; Venkateswarlu, R.; Mohan, C.O.; Gopal, T.K. Biogenic amines in seafood: A review. *J. Food Sci. Technol.* **2016**, *53*, 2210–2218. [CrossRef]
16. Spano, G.; Russo, P.; Lonvaud-Funel, A.; Lucas, P.; Alexandre, H.; Grandvalet, C.; Coton, E.; Coton, M.; Barnavon, L.; Bach, B.; et al. Biogenic amines in fermented foods. *Eur. J. Clin. Nutr.* **2010**, *64*, S95–S100. [CrossRef] [PubMed]
17. Prester, L.; Orct, T.; Macan, J.; Vukusic, J.; Kipcic, D. Determination of biogenic amines and endotoxin in squid, musky octopus, Norway lobster, and mussel stored at room temperature. *Arh. Hig. Rada Toksikol.* **2010**, *61*, 389–397. [CrossRef]
18. Rawles, D.D.; Flick, G.J.; Martin, R.E. Biogenic amines in fish and shellfish. *Adv. Food Nutr. Res.* **1996**, *39*, 329–365. [CrossRef]
19. Gardini, F.; Özogul, Y.; Suzzi, G.; Tabanelli, G.; Özogul, F. Technological factors affecting biogenic amine content in foods: A review. *Front. Microbiol.* **2016**, *7*, 1–18. [CrossRef]
20. Suzzi, G.; Torriani, S. Biogenic amines in fermented foods. *Front. Microbiol.* **2015**, *6*, 472. [CrossRef]
21. Ly, D.; Mayrhofer, S.; Agung Yogeswara, I.B.; Nguyen, T.-H.; Domig, K.J. Identification, Classification and Screening for γ-Amino-butyric Acid Production in Lactic Acid Bacteria from Cambodian Fermented Foods. *Biomolecules* **2019**, *9*, 768. [CrossRef]
22. ISO 15214. *Microbiology of Food and Animal Feeding Stuffs—Horizontal Method for the Enumeration of Mesophilic Lactic Acid Bacteria—Colony-Count Technique at 30 °C*; International Organization for Standardization: Geneva, Switzerland, 1998; p. 7.
23. ISO 21528–2. *Microbiology of Food and Animal Feeding Stuffs—Horizontal Methods for the Detection and Enumeration of Enterobacteriaceas—Part. 2: Colony-Count Method*; International Organization for Standardization: Geneva, Switzerland, 2004; p. 15.
24. ISO 13720. *Meat and Meat Products—Enumeration of Presumptive Pseudomonas spp.*; International Organization for Standardization: Geneva, Switzerland, 2010; p. 7.
25. ISO 21527–2. *Microbiology of Food and Animal Feeding Stuffs—Horizontal Method for the Enumeration of Yeasts and Moulds—Part. 2: Colony Count Technique in Products with Water Activity Less Than or Equal to 0,95*; International Organization for Standardization: Geneva, Switzerland, 2008; p. 9.
26. Kwolek-Mirek, M.; Zadrag-Tecza, R. Comparison of methods used for assessing the viability and vitality of yeast cells. *Fems Yeast Res.* **2014**, *14*, 1068–1079. [CrossRef]
27. Essghaier, B.; Fardeau, M.L.; Cayol, J.L.; Hajlaoui, M.R.; Boudabous, A.; Jijakli, H.; Sadfi-Zouaoui, N. Biological control of grey mould in strawberry fruits by halophilic bacteria. *J. Appl. Microbiol.* **2009**, *106*, 833–846. [CrossRef]

28. ISO 6888–1/AMD 1. *Microbiology of Food and Animal Feeding Stuffs—Horizontal Method for the Enumeration of Coagulase-Positive Staphylococci (Staphylococcus Aureus and Other Species)—Part. 1: Technique Using Baird-Parker Agar Medium—Amendment 1: Inclusion of Precision Data*; International Organization for Standardization: Geneva, Switzerland, 2003; p. 9.
29. Kateete, D.P.; Kimani, C.N.; Katabazi, F.A.; Okeng, A.; Okee, M.S.; Nanteza, A.; Joloba, M.L.; Najjuka, F.C. Identification of *Staphylococcus aureus*: DNase and Mannitol salt agar improve the efficiency of the tube coagulase test. *Ann. Clin. Microbiol. Antimicrob.* **2010**, *9*, 23. [CrossRef] [PubMed]
30. Robinow, C.F. Observations on the structure of *Bacillus* spores. *J. Gen. Microbiol.* **1951**, *5*, 439–457. [CrossRef] [PubMed]
31. ISO 16649-2. *Microbiology of Food and Animal Feeding Stuffs—Horizontal Method for the Enumeration of Beta-Glucuronidase-Positive Escherichia Coli—Part. 2: Colony-Count Technique at 44 Degrees C Using 5-Bromo-4-Chloro-3-Indolyl Beta-D-Glucuronide*; International Organization for Standardization: Geneva, Switzerland, 2001; p. 8.
32. ISO 7937. *Microbiology of Food and Animal Feeding Stuffs—Horizontal Method for the Enumeration of Clostridium Perfringens—Colony-Count Technique*; International Organization for Standardization: Geneva, Switzerland, 2004; p. 16.
33. Šimat, V.; Dalgaard, P. Use of small diameter column particles to enhance HPLC determination of histamine and other biogenic amines in seafood. *LWT Food Sci. Technol.* **2011**, *44*, 399–406. [CrossRef]
34. Saarinen, M.T. Determination of biogenic amines as dansyl derivatives in intestinal digesta and feces by reversed phase HPLC. *Chromatographia* **2002**, *55*, 297–300. [CrossRef]
35. Tsai, Y.-H.; Lin, C.-Y.; Chien, L.-T.; Lee, T.-M.; Wei, C.-I.; Hwang, D.-F. Histamine contents of fermented fish products in Taiwan and isolation of histamine-forming bacteria. *Food Chem.* **2006**, *98*, 64–70. [CrossRef]
36. Lopetcharat, K.; Park, J.W. Characteristics of fish sauce made from pacific whiting and surimi by-products during fermentation storage. *J. Food Sci.* **2002**, *67*, 511–516. [CrossRef]
37. Park, J.-N.; Fukumoto, Y.; Fujita, E.; Tanaka, T.; Washio, T.; Otsuka, S.; Shimizu, T.; Watanabe, K.; Abe, H. Chemical composition of fish sauces produced in southeast and east Asian countries. *J. Food Compos. Anal.* **2001**, *14*, 113–125. [CrossRef]
38. Kobayashi, T.; Taguchi, C.; Kida, K.; Matsuda, H.; Terahara, T.; Imada, C.; Moe, N.K.; Thwe, S.M. Diversity of the bacterial community in Myanmar traditional salted fish *yegyo ngapi*. *World J. Microbiol. Biotechnol.* **2016**, *32*, 166. [CrossRef]
39. Daroonpunt, R.; Uchino, M.; Tsujii, Y.; Kazami, M.; Oka, D.; Tanasupawat, S. Chemical and physical properties of Thai traditional shrimp paste (Ka-pi). *J. Appl. Pharm. Sci.* **2016**, 58–62. [CrossRef]
40. Purnomo, H.; Suprayitno, E. Physicochemical characteristics, sensory acceptability and microbial quality of *Wadi Betok* a traditional fermented fish from South Kalimantan, Indonesia. *Int. Food Res. J.* **2013**, *20*, 933–939.
41. Lee, D.S. Packaging and the microbial shelf life of food. In *Food Packaging and Shelf Life: A Practical Guide*; Robertson, G.L., Ed.; CRC Press-Taylor and Francis Group: Boca Raton, FL, USA, 2010; pp. 55–79.
42. Doyle, M.E.; Glass, K.A. Sodium Reduction and Its Effect on Food Safety, Food Quality, and Human Health. *Compr. Rev. Food Sci. Food Saf.* **2010**, *9*, 44–56. [CrossRef]
43. ICMSF. Fish and Seafood Products. In *Microorganisms in Foods 8: Use of Data for Assessing Process Control and Product Acceptance*, 2nd ed.; Swanson, K.M., Ed.; Springer: New York, NY, USA, 2011; pp. 107–133. [CrossRef]
44. Cortés-Sánchez, A.D.J. *Clostridium perfringens* in foods and fish. *Regul. Mech. Biosyst.* **2018**, *9*, 112–117. [CrossRef]
45. Health Protection Agency. *Guidelines for Assessing the Microbiological Safety of Ready-To-Eat Foods*; Health Protection Agency: London, UK, 2009; pp. 1–33.
46. Panagou, E.Z.; Tassou, C.C.; Vamvakoula, P.; Saravanos, E.K.; Nychas, G.J. Survival of Bacillus cereus vegetative cells during Spanish-style fermentation of conservolea green olives. *J. Food Prot.* **2008**, *71*, 1393–1400. [CrossRef] [PubMed]
47. Bennett, R.W. Staphylococcal enterotoxin and its rapid identification in foods by enzyme-linked immunosorbent assay-based methodology. *J. Food Prot.* **2005**, *68*, 1264–1270. [CrossRef]
48. Ijong, G.G.; Ohta, Y. Physicochemical and microbiological changes associated with Bakasang processing—A traditional Indonesian fermented fish sauce. *J. Sci. Food Agric.* **1996**, *71*, 69–74. [CrossRef]

49. Aarti, C.; Khusro, A.; Arasu, M.V.; Agastian, P.; Al-Dhabi, N.A. Biological potency and characterization of antibacterial substances produced by *Lactobacillus pentosus* isolated from Hentak, a fermented fish product of North-East India. *Springerplus* **2016**, *5*, 1743. [CrossRef]
50. Besas, J.R.; Dizon, E.I. Influence of salt concentration on histamine formation in fermented Tuna Viscera (*Dayok*). *Food Nutr. Sci.* **2012**, *3*, 201–206. [CrossRef]
51. Larsen, H. Halophilic and halotolerant microorganisms-an overview and historical perspective. *Fems Microbiol. Lett.* **1986**, *39*, 3–7. [CrossRef]
52. EFSA. *Working Document on Microbial Contaminant Limits for Microbial PEST control Products*; OECD Environment, Health and Safety Publications: Paris, France, 2012; pp. 1–53.
53. Food Safety Authority of Ireland. *Guidance Note No. 3: Guidelines for the Interpretation of Results of Microbiological Testing of Ready-To-Eat Foods Placed on the Market (Revision 2)*; FSAI: Dublin, Ireland, 2016; pp. 1–41.
54. Centre for Food Safety. *Microbiological Guidelines for Food for Ready-To-Eat Food in General and Specific Food Items*; Centre for Food Safety, Food and Environmental Hygiene Department: Hong Kong, China, 2014; pp. 1–38.
55. EFSA. Commission regulation (EC) No 2073/2005 of 15 November 2005 on microbiological criteria for foodstuffs. *Off. J. Eur. Union* **2005**, *338*, 1–26.
56. Gilbert, R.; Louvois, J.D.; Donovan, T.; Little, C.; Nye, K.; Ribeiro, C.; Richards, J.; Roberts, D.; Bolton, F. Guidelines for the microbiological quality of some ready-to-eat foods sampled at the point of sale. *Commun. Dis. Public Health* **2000**, *3*, 163–167.
57. Shalaby, A.R. Significance of biogenic amines to food safety and human health. *Food Res. Int.* **1996**, *29*, 675–690. [CrossRef]
58. Silla Santos, M.H. Biogenic amines: Their importance in foods. *Int. J. Food Microbiol.* **1996**, *29*, 213–231. [CrossRef]
59. Fardiaz, D.; Markakis, P. Amines in fermented fish paste. *J. Food Sci.* **1979**, *44*, 1562–1563. [CrossRef]
60. EFSA. Scientific opinion on risk based control of biogenic amine formation in fermented foods. *EFSA J.* **2011**, *9*, 2393. [CrossRef]
61. Prester, L. Biogenic amines in fish, fish products and shellfish: A review. *Food Addit. Contam. Part A Chem. Anal. Control Expo. Risk Assess.* **2011**, *28*, 1547–1560. [CrossRef]
62. Food Intolerance Network. Histamine Levels in Foods. Available online: https://www.food-intolerance-network.com/food-intolerances/histamine-intolerance/histamine-levels-in-food.html (accessed on 25 November 2019).
63. Healing Histamine. High Histamine Foods I Still Eat. Available online: https://healinghistamine.com/supposedly-high-histamine-foods-i-still-eat/ (accessed on 25 November 2019).
64. Sanchez-Perez, S.; Comas-Baste, O.; Rabell-Gonzalez, J.; Veciana-Nogues, M.T.; Latorre-Moratalla, M.L.; Vidal-Carou, M.C. Biogenic Amines in Plant-Origin Foods: Are They Frequently Underestimated in Low-Histamine Diets? *Foods* **2018**, *7*, 205. [CrossRef]
65. Rauscher-Gabernig, E.; Gabernig, R.; Brueller, W.; Grossgut, R.; Bauer, F.; Paulsen, P. Dietary exposure assessment of putrescine and cadaverine and derivation of tolerable levels in selected foods consumed in Austria. *Eur. Food Res. Technol.* **2012**, *235*, 209–220. [CrossRef]
66. Ladero, V.; Calles-Enríquez, M.; Fernández, M.; Alvarez, A.M. Toxicological effects of dietary biogenic amines. *Curr. Nutr. Food Sci.* **2010**, *6*, 145–156. [CrossRef]
67. Mah, J.H.; Park, Y.K.; Jin, Y.H.; Lee, J.H.; Hwang, H.J. Bacterial Production and Control of Biogenic Amines in Asian Fermented Soybean Foods. *Foods* **2019**, *8*, 85. [CrossRef]
68. Rodriguez-Jerez, J.J.; Lopez-Sabater, E.I.; Roig-Sagues, A.X.; Mora-Ventura, M.T. Histamine, Cadaverine and Putrescine Forming Bacteria from Ripened Spanish Semipreserved Anchovies. *J. Food Sci.* **1994**, *59*, 998–1001. [CrossRef]
69. Bover-Cid, S.; Hugas, M.; Izquierdo-Pulido, M.; Vidal-Carou, M.C. Amino acid-decarboxylase activity of bacteria isolated from fermented pork sausages. *Int. J. Food Microbiol.* **2001**, *66*, 185–189. [CrossRef]
70. FDA. *Fish and Fishery Products Hazards and Controls Guidance*, 4th ed.; Health and Human Services, Public Health Service, Food and Drug Administration, Center for Food Safety and Applied Nutrition, Office of Food Safety: College Park, MD, USA, 2011; pp. 113–152.

71. Food and Agriculture Organization of the United Nations/World Health Organization (FAO/WHO). *Joint FAO/WHO Expert Meeting on the Public health Risks of Histamine and other Biogenic Amines from Fish and Fishery Products*; Joint FAO/WHO Expert Meeting Report; FAO/WHO: Rome, Italy, 2012; pp. 1–111.
72. Codex Alimentarius Commission (CAC). *Standard for Fish Sauce, CXS 302-2011 (Amended in 2012, 2013, 2018)*; FAO/WHO: Rome, Italy, 2011.
73. Jiang, W.; Xu, Y.; Li, C.; Dong, X.; Wang, D. Biogenic amines in commercially produced Yulu, a Chinese fermented fish sauce. *Food Addit. Contam. Part B Surveill.* **2014**, *7*, 25–29. [CrossRef] [PubMed]
74. Moon, J.S.; Kim, Y.; Jang, K.I.; Cho, K.-J.; Yang, S.-J.; Yoon, G.-M.; Kim, S.-Y.; Han, N.S. Analysis of biogenic amines in fermented fish products consumed in Korea. *Food Sci. Biotechnol.* **2010**, *19*, 1689–1692. [CrossRef]
75. Stute, R.; Petridis, K.; Steinhart, H.; Biernoth, G. Biogenic amines in fish and soy sauces. *Eur. Food Res. Technol.* **2002**, *215*, 101–107. [CrossRef]
76. Linares, D.M.; del Rio, B.; Redruello, B.; Ladero, V.; Martin, M.C.; Fernandez, M.; Ruas-Madiedo, P.; Alvarez, M.A. Comparative analysis of the *in vitro* cytotoxicity of the dietary biogenic amines tyramine and histamine. *Food Chem.* **2016**, *197*, 658–663. [CrossRef]
77. Del Rio, B.; Redruello, B.; Linares, D.M.; Ladero, V.; Ruas-Madiedo, P.; Fernandez, M.; Martin, M.C.; Alvarez, M.A. The biogenic amines putrescine and cadaverine show in vitro cytotoxicity at concentrations that can be found in foods. *Sci. Rep.* **2019**, *9*, 120. [CrossRef]
78. Zaman, M.Z.; Bakar, F.A.; Selamat, J.; Bakar, J. Occurrence of biogenic amines and amines degrading bacteria in fish sauce. *Czech J. Food Sci.* **2010**, *28*, 440–449. [CrossRef]
79. Naila, A.; Flint, S.; Fletcher, G.C.; Bremer, P.J.; Meerdink, G. Biogenic amines and potential histamine—Forming bacteria in Rihaakuru (a cooked fish paste). *Food Chem.* **2011**, *128*, 479–484. [CrossRef]
80. Andersson, R.E. Biogenic amines in lactic acid-fermented vegetables. *Lebensm. Wiss. Technol.* **1988**, *21*, 68–69.
81. Galgano, F.; Favati, F.; Bonadio, M.; Lorusso, V.; Romano, P. Role of biogenic amines as index of freshness in beef meat packed with different biopolymeric materials. *Food Res. Int.* **2009**, *42*, 1147–1152. [CrossRef]
82. Li, M.; Tian, L.; Zhao, G.; Zhang, Q.; Gao, X.; Huang, X.; Sun, L. Formation of biogenic amines and growth of spoilage-related microorganisms in pork stored under different packaging conditions applying PCA. *Meat Sci.* **2014**, *96*, 843–848. [CrossRef] [PubMed]
83. Jairath, G.; Singh, P.K.; Dabur, R.S.; Rani, M.; Chaudhari, M. Biogenic amines in meat and meat products and its public health significance: A review. *J. Food Sci. Technol.* **2015**, *52*, 6835–6846. [CrossRef]
84. Wortberg, W.; Woller, R. Quality and freshness of meat and meat products as related to their content of biogenic amines. *Fleischwirtschaft* **1982**, *62*, 1457–1463.
85. Venugopal, V. Postharvest quality changes and safety hazards. In *Seafood Processing: Adding Value Through Quick Freezing, Retortable Packaging and Cook-Chilling*; Venugopal, V., Ed.; CRC Press, Taylor and Francis Group: Boca Raton, FL, USA, 2006; pp. 23–60.

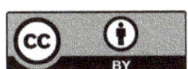

© 2020 by the authors. Licensee MDPI, Basel, Switzerland. This article is an open access article distributed under the terms and conditions of the Creative Commons Attribution (CC BY) license (http://creativecommons.org/licenses/by/4.0/).

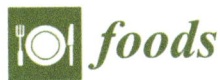

Article

Identification of a Lactic Acid Bacteria to Degrade Biogenic Amines in Chinese Rice Wine and Its Enzymatic Mechanism

Tianjiao Niu [1,2], Xing Li [1], Yongjie Guo [2] and Ying Ma [1,*]

[1] School of Chemistry and Chemical Engineering, Harbin Institute of Technology, Harbin 150090, China
[2] Mengniu Hi-tech Dairy (Beijing) Co., Ltd., Beijing 101107, China
* Correspondence: maying@hit.edu.cn

Received: 28 June 2019; Accepted: 31 July 2019; Published: 2 August 2019

Abstract: A *L. plantarum*, CAU 3823, which can degrade 40% of biogenic amines (BAs) content in Chinese rice wine (CRW) at the end of post-fermentation, was selected and characterized in this work. It would be an optimal choice to add 10^6 cfu/mL of selected strain into the fermentation broth to decrease the BAs while keeping the character and quality of CRW. Nine amine oxidases were identified from the strain and separated using Sephadex column followed by LC-MS/MS analysis. The purified amine oxidase mixture showed a high monoamine oxidase activity of 19.8 U/mg, and more than 40% of BAs could be degraded. The biochemical characters of the amine oxidases were also studied. This work seeks to provide a better solution to degrade BAs in CRW prior to keeping the character and quality of CRW and a better understanding of the degradability of the strain to the BAs.

Keywords: biogenic amines; *L. plantarum*; amines oxidase; Chinese rice wine; industrial fermentation

1. Introduction

Biogenic amines (BAs) are low molecular weight organic compounds that have been identified as toxicological agents in various foods, such as fishery products, dairy, meat, wine, and so on [1,2]. The ingestion of foods containing relatively high concentrations of BAs could lead to several health hazards, such as headaches, hypotension, respiratory distress, heart palpitations and digestive problems, particularly when alcohol is present [3,4]. Histamine, which is well-known because of its implication in many food poisoning cases, has a potent vasodilatory action that could cause important drops in blood pressure [5]. Tyramine, as one of the vasoconstrictor amines, can provoke a release of noradrenaline resulting in an increase of arterial pressure [5]. Even though there are no accurate regulations for BAs, several countries including France, Germany and Australia have set regulations and limits for histamine and many wine importers in the EU require a BA analysis [4,6]. The presence of BAs is considered a marker of poor wine quality and bad winemaking practices [4,7].

BAs are synthesized in fermented food by decarboxylation of corresponding amino acids by microorganisms [1]. According to the previous studies, BAs could be formed by lactic acid bacteria in wine [8,9], Chinese rice wine [10] and Korean rice wine [1]. As a traditional alcoholic beverage, Chinese rice wine (CRW), which has been popular in China for thousands of years [11], has high nutritional values, and thus, it has been used as an ingredient in traditional Chinese medicine [12]. Since the brewing process of CRW is the typical open semisolid-state fermentation, lots of microorganisms (molds, yeast, bacteria) are brought in the glutinous rice with the addition of Chinese koji [3,13], and the system is favorable to BAs generation combining with the high amount of free amino acids [2]. The abundant bacteria in CRW, mainly originating from Chinese koji, the surroundings and the surfaces of the equipment, could be one of the main reasons for the formation of BAs [10].

Histamine, tyramine, putrescine, cadaverine and phenylethylamine are the most representative BAs detected in the wine [6]. Histamine and tyramine have been considered as the most toxic products in wine, and putrescine and cadaverine could potentiate these effects [4]. The formation of BAs was traditionally controlled by avoiding the growth of spoilage bacteria, decreasing the amino acid precursors and inoculating starter cultures with negative decarboxylase activity [6,7]. Driven by greater awareness of the importance of food quality and safety by consumers, the methods for degradation of BAs in fermented foods have been explored. Biological enzymatic degradation of BAs would be a safe and economic way while avoiding the production difficulties. Two *Lactobacillus plantarum* strains (named NDT 09 and NDT 16) isolated from red wine were able to degrade 22% of tyramine and 31% of putrescine, respectively [14]. Three different strains of *Brevibacterium linens* were utilized to eliminate tyramine and histamine in cheese [6], and the strain *K. varians* LTH 1540, it was also found, could degrade tyramine during sausage ripening [15]. Two lactic acid bacteria were used to degrade 50%–54% of histamine in fish silage [16]. However, the relationship between BAs degradation and microbiological enzymes of the strains has not been explored yet.

In this work, a *Lactobacillus plantarum* was obtained from CRW which could degrade BAs. The optimal industrial conditions of the selected strain were analyzed, and the microbiological amine oxidase enzymes were identified and biochemically characterized. Our results could receive considerable interest by providing a green industrial strategy to control the BAs contents in the rice wine and improve the safety consumption of the fermented foodstuffs.

2. Materials and Methods

2.1. Materials

Man Rogosa Sharpe agar (MRS) medium was obtained from Oxoid. Ltd. (Basingstoke, Hants, UK). The BA standards were purchased from Sigma-Aldrich (St. Louis, MO, USA). Bacterial genomic DNA extraction kit was obtained from Tiangen (Beijing, China). Ultra-pure water was obtained from a Millipore purification system (>18.3 MΩ·cm). Formic acid, methanol and acetonitrile used in the preparation of the mobile phase were of LC-MS grade. All other chemicals used were of analytical grade.

2.2. Strains Screening and Identification

Fermentation broths were collected at the later stage from a typical rice wine production process in Shaoxing (Zhejiang, China). The suspension was filtered through four layers of sterile gauze to remove the unliquefied rice and sealed in a sterile plastic bottle. One gram of fermentation broths was diluted 10-fold by a 0.85% NaCl solution and routinely subcultured 5 to 10 times on MRS medium to obtain purified clones. The screening medium designed was based on the method of Landete [17] to obtain the bacteria that could decrease biogenic amine content. These strains isolated were kept frozen at −20 °C in a sterilized mixture of culture medium and glycerol (50:50, v/v) according to the methods described by García-Ruiz [18], and further identified by 16S rRNA gene sequencing.

2.3. HPLC Determination of Biogenic Amines

Eight biogenic amines of Histamine (HIS), tyramine (TYR), putrescine (PUT), cadaverine (CAD), phenylethylamine (PHE), tryptamine (TRY), spermine (SPM) and spermidine (SPD) were analyzed according to the method of Callejon, Sendra [13] with slight modifications. The individual strains were cultured on MRS, and 10^7 cfu/mL were inoculated with the MRS liquid medium contaminated with 50 mg/L of each amine at pH 5.5. After 48 h incubation at 30 °C, the reaction was stopped by adding HCl. Samples were centrifuged at 8000 rpm for 15 min and the supernatant was pipetted into a screw-capped vial. The pre-column derivatization procedure using dansyl chloride as derivatization reagent was performed according to the report of Yongmei, Xin [12]. The samples were filtered through 0.22 μm millipore syringe filters and analyzed by RP-HPLC using on LC-20A HPLC system (Shimadzu,

Kyoto, Japan) with an Agilent C18 column (250 mm × 4.6 mm, 300 A pores, 5 μm particles, Agilent Technologies, Inc., Santa Clara, CA, USA). The column temperature was kept at 30 °C and the detection wavelength was 254 nm with a flow rate of 1.0 mL/min by using water (A) and methanol (B) as eluents. The gradient elution program consisting of a linear gradient from 65% to 70% B in 7 min followed by from 70% to 80% B in 13 min and 3 min isocratic elution.

The percentage of BAs degradation was calculated based on the HPLC data as following,

$$\text{BAs degradation (\%)} = (C_{control} - C_{strain})/C_{control}$$

where $C_{control}$ was the concentration of the BAs in the control medium and C_{strain} was the concentration of the BAs in the medium incubated with the strain.

2.4. Bacterial Growth Analysis

The bacterial growth was measured according to the methods described by Cui [19]. Briefly, the isolated lactic acid bacteria (LAB) strains were diluted to 10^5 cfu/mL in MRS liquid medium, and the pH and optical density ($OD_{600\ nm}$) of medium was checked at 28 °C, 33 °C and 37 °C for 36 h, respectively.

2.5. The Bacterial Starter Application in Pilot Scale Fermentation

A pilot fermentation was performed according to the methods described by Zhang, Xue [10] with modifications (Figure 1). Glutinous rice (12 kg) was soaked at 18 °C for 20 h and steamed for 30 min. After naturally cooling to room temperature (about 25 °C), the steamed rice was transferred into a 33 L wide-mouth bottle to which 14.5 kg water, 1.5 kg Chinese koji (unique saccharifying agent including molds, yeasts and bacteria, obtained from COFCO Shaoxin wine Co., Ltd., Shaoxin, China) were added. The main fermentation was carried out at 33 °C for 4 days with intermittent oxygen filling, and post-fermentation was then carried out at 28 °C for 20 days. The isolated strain with 10^5 (low level), 10^6 (middle level) and 10^7 (high level) cfu/mL was added into the CRW at the main fermentation and post-fermentation stage, respectively. After filter pressing, clarification, wine frying and sterilization (90 °C for 3 min), finished Chinese rice wines were obtained. Ten milliliters of fermentation broths were taken from different fermentation stages, including addition of starter (AS); main fermentation (MF); post-fermentation 5d (PF5d); post-fermentation 10d (PF10d); and post-fermentation 20d (PF20d)), to analysis the changes in the BAs contents by using the HPLC method. According to the previous studies [20,21], pH, alcohol content, total sugar, total acid, non-sugar solid and amino acid nitrogen of CRW were analyzed by using official methods (Chinese National Standard GB/T 13662-2008). Sensory evaluation of CRW was conducted by 30 panelists (15 males and 15 females) who have professional training certificates. The procedure was conducted in a sensory laboratory following GB/T 13662-2008 and ISO 4121. A total of 11 sensory attributes of appearance (color and turbidity), aroma (alcohol, fruit and cereal), taste (sweet, sour and bitter), mouthfeel (astringency, continuation and full body) and harmony were chosen to characterize the sensory properties using quantitative descriptive analysis involving a 0–9 ten-point linear scale (0: none; 1–2: very weak; 3–4: ordinary; 5–6: moderate; 7–8: strong; 9: very strong).

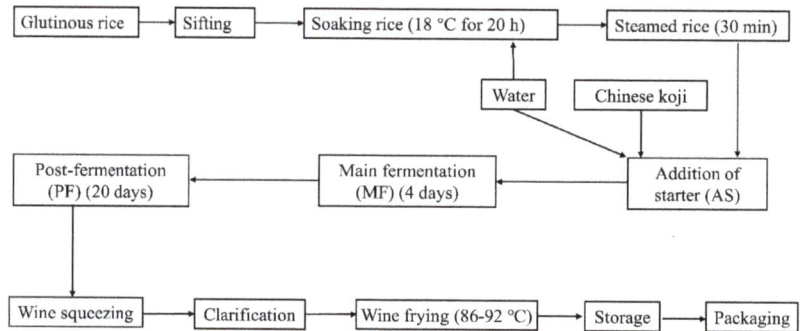

Figure 1. Diagram of the Chinese rice wine production process.

2.6. Separation of the Amine Oxidases

Cell-free extracts were obtained by using the method of Callejon [22]. The bacterial cells from a 1 L culture were collected by centrifugation at 10,000 rpm, 20 min at 4 °C and washed twice with 50 mM sodium phosphate buffer (PBS), pH 7.4. The samples were resuspended in PBS buffer containing 1 mM of phenyl methylsulfonyl fluoride (PMSF) as protease inhibitor. Cell-free extracts were obtained by disrupting the bacterial cells with 1 g of 106 μM diameter glass beads in a Mikro-dismenbrator® Sartorius: 10 cycles of 40 s, alternating 5 cycles of disruption with a cooling step of 5 min in ice. The samples were centrifuged at 13,000 rpm for 15 min (PrismR, Labnet, USA), and supernatants were saved at −20 °C until use. The protein content was determined by using the bicinchoninic acid assay kit (BCA, Solarbio, Beijing, China). Monoamine oxidase (MAO) assay kit and diamine oxidase (DAO) assay kit (Jiancheng Institute, Nanjing, China) were both used to determine the amine oxidase activity. The MAO assay kit was based on the ability of MAO to form H_2O_2 substrate, which could be determined by a fluorimetric method. The DAO assay kit was based on the oxidation of PUT to pyrroline plus NH_3 and H_2O_2, which can be determined by the fluorimetric method.

The cell-free extracts were further ultracentrifuged at 47,000 rpm for 1 h, and the supernatant was precipitated by 75% saturation of ammonium sulfate precipitation [22]. The protein was redissolved with 50 mM PBS and were loaded onto a Sephadex G-100 column (1.6 cm × 70 cm) followed by a linear gradient elution with a flow rate of 1 mL/min. The protein fraction was collected and measured at 280 nm by using a HD-93-1 spectrophotometer (Purkinje General Instrument Co. Ltd., Beijing, China). There fractions were collected (P1, P2 and P3, Supplement Figure S1), and were then concentrated and freeze-dried. The degradation ability of the fractions was further evaluated by incubation with 50 mg/L eight biogenic amines at pH 4.0, 33 °C for 2 h.

2.7. Identification of the Amine Oxidases

The fractions separated from the cell-free extracts were digested with trypsin (Promega, Madison, WI, USA) overnight at 37 °C and were identified by LC-MS/MS using the Easy nLC-1000 nano ultra-high-pressure system (Thermo Fisher Scientific, San Jose, CA, USA) coupling with a Q Exactive mass spectrometer (Thermo Fisher Scientific, San Jose, CA, USA). The peptide mixture was loaded onto a Zorbax 300SB-C18 peptide traps (Agilent Technologies, Wilmington, DE, USA) in buffer A (0.1% Formic acid) and separated with a linear gradient of 4%–50% buffer B (80% acetonitrile and 0.1% formic acid) for 50 min, 50%–100% B for 4 min, and held at 100% B for 6 min at a flow rate of 250 nL/min. The mass spectrometer was operated in positive ion mode. MS data was acquired using a data-dependent top10 method dynamically choosing the most abundant precursor ions from the survey scan for high-energy collisional dissociation (HCD) fragmentation and was searched by using MASCOT engine and Proteome Discoverer 1.3 against the local uniport_lactobocilluspiantarum database.

2.8. Enzymatic Properties of the Amine Oxidases

Effects of temperatures (15, 20, 25, 28, 30, 35, 40, 80 °C at pH 4.0 for 2 h), pH (3.0–5.0) at 30 °C for 2 h, and metal ions (0.2 mol/L, copper ion, ferrous ion, zinc ion, calcium ion and magnesium ion) at 30 °C for 2 h (pH 4.0) on the amine oxidase degradation activity were further investigated.

2.9. Statistical Analysis

All samples were prepared in three independent and each was analyzed in triplicate by the analysis of variance (ANOVA). The results were considered significant at $p \leq 0.05$ by the Duncan test.

3. Result

3.1. Strains Screening and Identification

A total of 61 strains were isolated from the five major stages (soaking rice, steamed rice, addition of starter, main fermentation and post-fermentation, Figure 1) of CRW fermentation. After screening their potentials to degrade/eliminate the contents of BAs, about 30% of strains were able to degrade BAs even though most of them degraded BAs to less than 10% extents (results not known). Only one strain drew attentions for more than 40% degradation efficiency of the BAs (Table 1). 16S rDNA sequencing identified that the strain had 100% similarity in 16S rDNA sequences to *Lactobacillus plantarum* CAU 3823 (GenBank accession no. MF424991.1). In the details, *Lactobacillus plantarum* CAU 3823 was a *L. plantarum* that exhibited the greatest potential for BAs degradation, as 56% degradation, for TRY, 41% for PHE, 42% for PUT, 43% for CAD, 40% for TYR, 45% for HIS, 44% for SPD and 43% for SPM, which should be considered in the further analysis.

Table 1. Percentage (%) of degradation of the biogenic amines by *Lactobacillus plantarum* CAU 3823 from Chinese rice wine [a].

Strains	Tryptamine	Phenylethylamine	Putrescine	Cadaverine	Tyramine	HISTAMINE	Spermidine	Spermine
Lactobacillus plantarum CAU 3823	55.95 ± 6.59	40.85 ± 9.87	41.82 ± 7.97	42.79 ± 7.76	40.12 ± 8.09	44.72 ± 7.56	43.51 ± 8.39	42.56 ± 8.41

[a] 10^7 cfu/mL of *Lactobacillus plantarum* CAU 3823 was incubated in the Man Rogosa Sharpe agar (MRS) liquid medium contaminated with 50 mg/L of each amine at pH 5.5 for 48 h.

3.2. The Bacterial Growth Ability

The growth ability of *L. plantarum* CAU 3823 at different temperatures (28 °C, 33 °C and 37 °C) was shown in Figure 2. *L. plantarum* CAU 3823 was able to grow at different temperatures, showing $OD_{600} > 1$ at main fermentation temperature (33 °C) for 9–25 h and post-fermentation temperature (28 °C) for 12~25 h. The maximum OD_{600} value of 1.4 was found at different temperatures at 25 h of growth, suggesting the good growth trends indicated that *L. plantarum* CAU 3823 could be used in industry producing CRW fermentation.

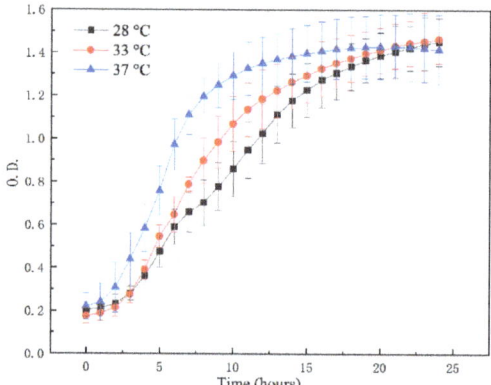

Figure 2. The growth ability of *L. plantarum* CAU 3823 at different temperatures (28 °C, 33 °C and 37 °C). Growth curves are representative of all determinations.

3.3. Changes in the BAs Induced by L. plantarum in Pilot Scale Fermentation

To investigate the capability to degrade BAs of *L. plantarum* CAU 3823 to the BAs in pilot scale fermentation of CRW, RP-HPLC was applied to quantify the contents of BAs in CRW incubation with various levels (10^5, 10^6 and 10^7 cfu/mL) of *L. plantarum* CAU 3823 as extra starter during fermentation, and the results are shown in Figure 3. Compared to control group, the total contents of BAs in CRW with *L. plantarum* CAU 3823 were significantly lower ($p < 0.05$) during the entire fermentation period (Figure 3A). The degradation percentages of BAs were 32%, 54% and 58%, respectively, at low, middle and high level of *L. plantarum* CAU 3823 at the main fermentation stage, suggesting the dose dependent manner. Total content of BAs was significantly reduced to 34%, 60% and 61% at low, middle and high levels of *L. plantarum* CAU 3823, respectively, at 5th day of post-fermentation, and similar degradation efficiency was obtained in the 10th day of post-fermentation and 20th day of post-fermentation, respectively.

The degrading abilities of *L. plantarum* CAU 3823 to TRY, PUT, HIS, CAD, PHE, SPD and SPM were also studied in Figure 3B–H, respectively. A marked decrease in the contents of BAs was observed during fermentation with the increasing of the strain content. As the most content of BAs detected in Chinese rice wine, TRY was degraded by *L. plantarum* CAU 3823 with the degradation rate of 39% at low level, 56% at middle level and 58% at high level strain at main fermentation; 41% at low level, 60% at middle level and 62% at high level strain at post-fermentation 5d; 51% at low level, 63% at middle level and 66% at high level strain at post-fermentation 10d; and 49% at low level, 57% at middle level and 61% at high level strain at post-fermentation 20d (Figure 3B). Similar degradation efficiency to PUT, HIS, CAD, PHE, SPD and SPM was also found as follows: PUT with 13% reduction at low level, 39% at middle level and 43% at high level strain; HIS with 4% at low level, 42% at middle level and 55% at high level; PHE with 45% at low level, 74% at middle level and 82% at high level; CAD with 38% at low level, 55% at middle level and 55% at high level; SPD with 23% at low level, 46% at middle level and 89% at high level; SPM with 25% at low level, 50% at middle level and 75%, respectively, at high level at the end of post-fermentation. Overall, more than 40% contents of BAs could be degraded incubation with *L. plantarum* CAU 3823 at the middle and high levels than the one at low level during fermentation.

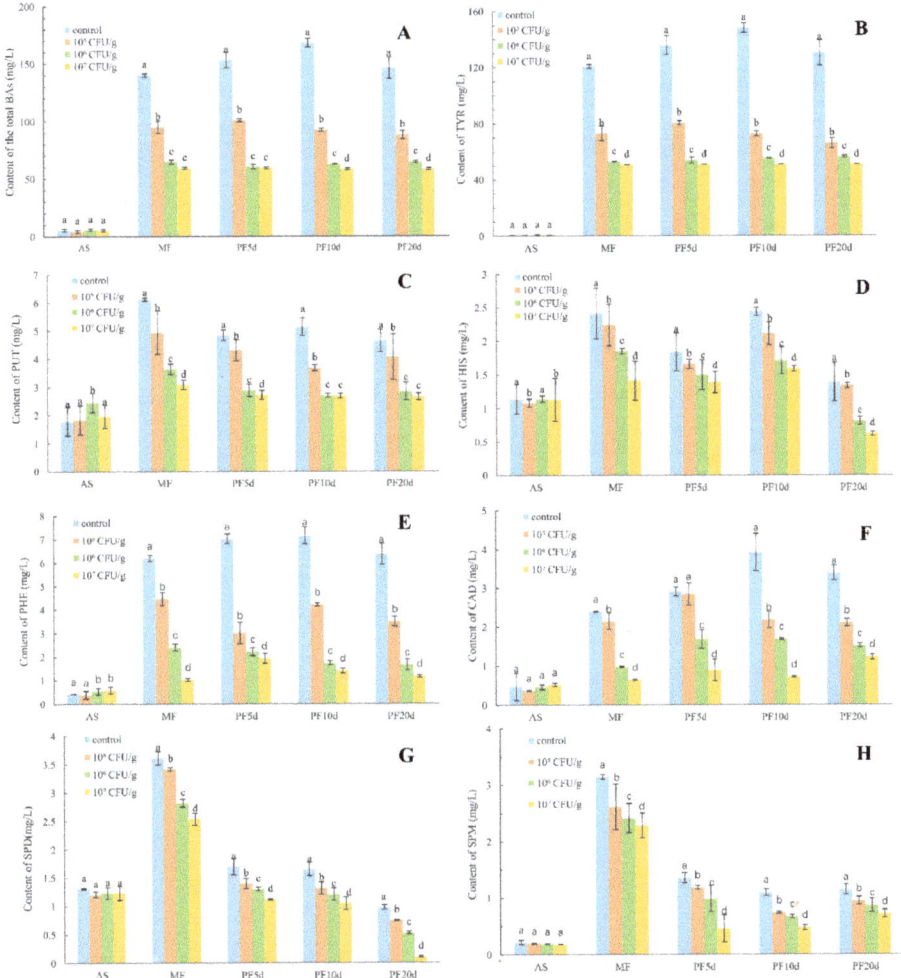

Figure 3. The contents of the total biogenic amines (BAs, **A**), tyramine (TYR, **B**), putrescine (PUT, **C**), Histamine (HIS, **D**) phenylethylamine (PHE, **E**), cadaverine (CAD, **F**), spermidine (SPD, **G**) and spermine (SPM, **H**) in Chinese rice wine adding different level of *L. plantarum* CAU 3823 at the post-fermentation and main fermentation stage during different fermentation stages (addition of starter (AS); main fermentation (MF); post-fermentation 5d (PF5d); post-fermentation 10d (PF10d); post-fermentation 20d (PF20d)).

3.4. Total Acid and pH in Pilot Scale Fermentation

As shown in Table 2, the changes in total acid and pH value of Chinese rice wine when different levels of *L. plantarum* CAU 3823 were added during fermentation were investigated, to evaluate the effect of this strain on the quality of CRW. At the initial stage of starter addition, there was no difference ($P > 0.05$) in lactic acid content and pH value among the four CRW samples. The total acid content of the CRW showed a slightly increase from 6.53 at low level to 6.86 g/L at middle level strain incubated with *L. plantarum* CAU 3823 at the end of post-fermentation, compared to the control group of 5.94 g/L. However, the total acid of CRW of 9.14 g/L incubated with high level of *L. plantarum* CAU 3823 indicated the over-acidification.

Table 2. Changes in the total acid and pH in the Chinese rice wine adding different level of *L. plantarum* CAU 3823 at the post-fermentation and main fermentation stage during different fermentation stages (addition of starter; main fermentation; post-fermentation 5d; post-fermentation 10d; post-fermentation 20d).

	Addition the Selected Strain (cfu/mL)	The Addition of Starter	Main Fermentation	Post-Fermentation 5d	Post-Fermentation 10d	Post-Fermentation 20d
Total acid (g/L)	Control	6.03 ± 0.22 [a]	3.81 ± 0.15 [a]	4.91 ± 0.07 [a]	5.55 ± 0.33 [a]	5.94 ± 0.20 [a]
	10^5 (low level)	6.17 ± 0.13 [a]	4.93 ± 0.13 [b]	5.41 ± 0.19 [b]	5.92 ± 0.19 [a]	6.53 ± 0.13 [b]
	10^6 (middle level)	5.92 ± 0.19 [a]	6.01 ± 0.14 [c]	6.51 ± 0.14 [c]	6.74 ± 0.44 [b]	6.86 ± 0.13 [d]
	10^7 (high level)	6.03 ± 0.15 [a]	6.04 ± 0.10 [c]	7.06 ± 0.09 [c]	8.01 ± 0.23 [c]	9.14 ± 0.45 [c]
pH	Control	6.33 ± 0.19 [a]	4.04 ± 0.12 [a]	4.19 ± 0.05 [a]	4.21 ± 0.03 [b]	4.14 ± 0.12 [a]
	10^5 (low level)	6.37 ± 0.28 [a]	4.00 ± 0.14 [a]	4.36 ± 0.12 [a]	4.12 ± 0.07 [a]	3.99 ± 0.16 [a]
	10^6 (middle level)	6.45 ± 0.22 [a]	3.84 ± 0.16 [a]	4.34 ± 0.08 [a]	4.45 ± 0.13 [b]	3.87 ± 0.12 [a]
	10^7 (high level)	6.43 ± 0.23 [a]	3.71 ± 0.04 [b]	4.24 ± 0.12 [a]	4.32 ± 0.12 [b]	3.63 ± 0.03 [b]

Presented data (mean ± standard deviation) are the mean values of three independent samples and each analyzed in triplicate. Values in a column with different superscripts differ significantly ($p < 0.05$).

3.5. Alcohol Content, Total Sugar, Non-Sugar Solid and Amino Acid Nitrogen in Pilot Scale Fermentation

The effects of *L. plantarum* CAU 3823 on the alcohol content, total sugar, non-sugar solid and amino acid nitrogen in the Chinese rice wine were analyzed after production process. As presented in Table 3, there was no notable change in alcohol, amino acid nitrogen and total sugar contents among the CRWs incubated with low and middle level of *L. plantarum* CAU 3823. The non-sugar solid was markedly higher ($p < 0.05$) when CRW was fermented involving with the selected strain.

Table 3. The alcohol content, amino acid nitrogen, total sugar and non-sugar solid in the Chinese rice wine after production process.

Addition the Selected Strain (cfu/mL)	Alcohol Content (% vol)	Amino Acid Nitrogen (g/L)	Total Sugar (g/L)	Non-Sugar Solid (g/L)
Control	11.52 ± 0.23 [a]	1.44 ± 0.11 [a]	31.98 ± 1.37 [a]	39.81 ± 0.33 [a]
10^5 (low level)	11.49 ± 0.35 [a]	1.28 ± 0.35 [a]	15.35 ± 2.34 [b]	62.34 ± 0.32 [c]
10^6 (middle level)	10.33 ± 0.41 [b]	0.82 ± 0.13 [b]	11.98 ± 3.25 [b]	71.52 ± 0.18 [d]
10^7 (high level)	9.29 ± 0.25 [c]	0.59 ± 0.02 [c]	10.97 ± 2.23 [b]	51.16 ± 0.25 [b]

Presented data (mean ± standard deviation) are the mean values of three independent samples and each analyzed in triplicate. Values in a column with different superscripts differ significantly ($p < 0.05$).

3.6. Sensory Evaluation

The sensory characteristics of CRW adding with different levels of the isolated strain were described by the 30 sensory panelists. As presented in Figure 4, CRW with high level of strain exhibited the lowest score (appearance 6, aroma 7, taste 6, mouthfeel 6 and harmony 6.2) among the four CRW samples. No significant difference was observed between the CRW incubated with middle level and low level strain compared to the control CRW ($p > 0.05$), indicating *L. plantarum* CAU 3823 with low and middle level would not have an influence on the sensory behaviors of the Chinese rice wine.

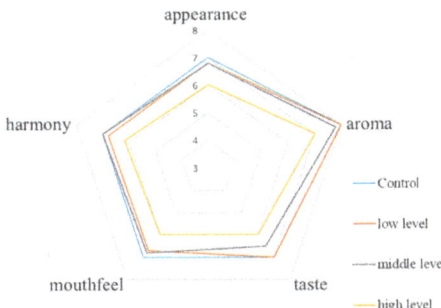

Figure 4. Average radar map of the Chinese rice wine including different level of biogenic amine-reduced *Lactobacillus plantarum* based on sensory scores.

3.7. Purification and Identification of the Amine Oxidases

To gain a deeper insight into the amine-degrading activity exhibited by *L. plantarum* CAU 3823, LC-MS/MS experiments were designed to show whether the amine oxidases existed in the strain. Cell-free extracts were obtained at a protein concentration of 5.5 mg/mL (Table 4). The MAO activity was 36.9 U/mg and the DAO activity was 128 U/L at 37 °C, pH = 7 in the cell-free extracts (Table 4). Three fractions were collected from a Sephadex G-100 column (Supplement Figure S1), and little DAO activity was detected in all three fractions, but only fraction 1 showed a good MAO activity of 19.8 U/mg compared to fraction 2 of 2.4 U/mg, and no amine oxidase activity was determined in fraction 3, which might be due to the low protein concentration.

To further investigate the amine degradation ability, the BA degradation rate (%) was calculated by incubating the three fractions with the eight BAs at pH 4.0, 33 °C for 2 h (Table 5). The BAs contents in fraction 1 significantly declined with the degradation rate of 41.9% for TYR, 41.1% for HIS, 40.3% for PUT, 44.3% for PHE, 41.1% for CAD, 41% for SPD, 43.5% for SPM and 47.9% for TRY. However, there were slight or little changes observed in the BA contents in the Fractions 2 and 3.

The fraction 1 was further identified by using LC-MSMS. Ten proteins including 9 amine oxidase proteins were identified in fraction 1, and hereinto, 8 amine oxidase proteins were monoamine oxidases, including 4 amine oxidase [flavin-containing] A (accession: P58027, P21396, Q5NU32 and A0A011QTL0), 2 amine oxidase [flavin-containing] B (accession: Q5RE98 and A0QU10), 1 monoamine oxidase [flavin-containing] (accession: A0A375EQX7) and 1 monoamine oxidase (accession: U2EF11) (Supplement Table S1). The MWs of the amine oxidases were closer and range from 46 to 60 kDa.

Table 4. The protein concentration, monoamine oxidase activity and diamine oxidase activity of the cell-free extracts (37 °C, pH = 7).

	Protein Concentration (mg/mL)	Monoamine Oxidase Activity (U/mg)	Diamine Oxidase Activity ($\times 10^{-4}$ U/mg)
Cell-free extracts	5.5	36.9 ± 5.2	1.3 ± 0.1
Fraction 1	3.1	19.8 ± 2.6	ND
Fraction 2	1.6	2.4 ± 1.2	ND
Fraction 3	0.5	ND	ND

ND = Not determined.

Table 5. Degradation percentages (%) of the eight biogenic amines in the three fractions by Sephadex separation incubation with 50 mg/L of the eight biogenic amines at pH 4.0, 33 °C for 2 h.

	Tryptamine	Phenylethylamine	Putrescine	Cadaverine	Histamine	Tyramine	Spermidine	Spermine
Fraction 1	47.9	44.3	40.3	41.1	41.1	41.9	41	43.5
Fraction 2	ND	0.3	0.7	ND	1.2	3.8	ND	ND
Fraction 3	ND	ND	ND	ND	ND	ND	ND	ND

ND = Not determined.

3.8. Amine Oxidases Assays

As shown in Figure 5, the purified amine oxidases mixture (fraction 1) retained its activity in a wide temperature range from 15 to 80 °C and was shown to maintain the 50% MAO activity after on heat treatment at 80 °C for 2 h. The optimal temperature for the amine oxidase activity was 28 °C and the MAO activity was 36.9 U/mg (Figure 5A). The MAO activities increased from 22.3 U/mg to 35.9 U/mg accompanied by the pH value from 3.0 to 5.0 while the amine oxidases were incubated at 30 °C for 2 h (Figure 5B). All the ions could inhibit the MAO activity, as 73%, 31%, 58%, 64% and 79% activity retained when adding 0.2 mol/L Zn^{2+}, Cu^{2+}, Fe^{2+}, Ca^{2+} and Mg^{2+}, respectively (Figure 5C).

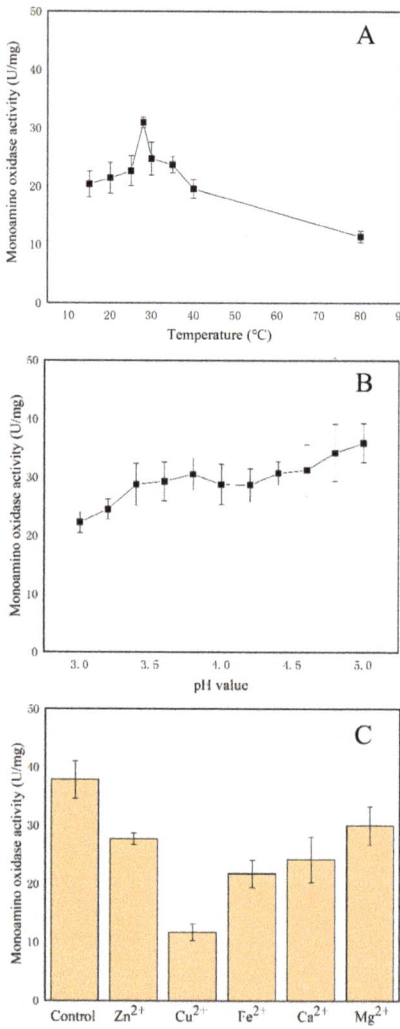

Figure 5. The monoamine oxidase (MAO) activity in the amine oxidase mixture at different temperatures (**A**) at pH 4.0 for 2 h; different pH (**B**) at 30 °C for 2 h and different metal ions (**C**) at 30 °C for 2 h (pH 4.0).

4. Discussion

Biogenic amines are considered as potential health risks since high amounts of them can lead to a series of health problems. The intake of foods with high level of BAs could induce the release of adrenaline and noradrenaline, provoking gastric acid secretion, increased cardiac output, migraine, tachycardia, increased blood sugar levels, and higher blood pressure [23]. Several researches supported the view that the BAs were formed in winemaking mainly by lactic acid bacteria carrying specific metabolic pathways that convert precursor amino acids into BAs [24]. In contrast, there is a lack of studies concerning BAs degradation by food sourced micro-organisms in wine, especially in Chinese rice wine.

In this paper, a *L. plantarum* CAU 3823, isolated from Chinese rice wine, can degrade more than 40% of the BAs, especially the five major BAs of TYR, PUT, HIS, PHE and CAD in Chinese rice wine. A similar research in grade wine showed that only one strain, *L. casei* IFI-CA 52, showed a strong ability to degrade the BAs (54% HIS, 55% TRY and 65% PUT) isolated from wine/ grape cell cultures of 85 strains [18]. However, the histamine-degrading ability of *L. casei* IFI-CA 52 was only 17% when addition of 12% ethanol, suggesting that the ability of *L. casei* IFI-CA 52 to reduce amine concentrations in wines would be rare. Regrettably, the ability of this strain to degrade other BAs was not analyzed. Moreover, a pilot scale fermentation, rather than addition of ethanol, would be a better choice to simulate accurately the complicated wine matrix.

In our experiment, pilot scale fermentation tests had proved that *L. plantarum* CAU 3823 was competent to be used as an extra starter in CRW industrial producing. Chinese koji was added at the beginning of brewing, which could bring in lots of bacteria, thus the BAs accumulated significantly at the beginning [13]. The BAs concentration showed a notably increase in the common CRW (the control group) from the starter addition stage to 10-days post-fermentation, indicating the proliferation of bacteria [13]. The concentration of BAs decreased at the end of post-fermentation, which might be due to the bacteria growth inhibition as the total acid increased during fermentation. According to our results, *L. plantarum* CAU 3823 could degrade the BAs in the CRW brewing process, and the formation of biogenic amines was further degraded by increasing the dose of strain. In this study, HIS, TYR, PUT and CAD were degraded significantly during the pilot scale fermentation, especially TYR, which indicated *L. plantarum* CAU 3823 could provide a more safety traditional fermented beverage for consumers.

Identification of functional microorganisms in CRW to reduce the formation of BAs has received more interest. Liu, Yu [13] utilized an in vivo screening process based on the next-generation sequencing technology to find BA-decreasing microorganism in CRW, and three *Lactobacillus* strains were detected that would not form biogenic amines, but only *L. plantarum* JN01 could grow under 15% ethanol, and the wine could form an unpleasant rancidity taste and more than 8 g/L total acid when the *L. plantarum* JN01 was more than 0.01 gDCW/t. Indeed, high level of functional bacteria could bring about unsatisfactory changes in CRW. A similar trend found in the current study showed that the total acid increased, and alcohol content decreased when 10^7 cfu/mL (high level) of *L. plantarum* CAU 3823 was added into the fermentation mash. Although the sensory scores were also decreased, the whole CRW was within the acceptable range for consumers at high level of the strain. Therefore, *L. plantarum* CAU 3823 could be the best choice to date to decrease BAs in CRW.

As a traditional alcoholic beverage, total sugar, alcoholic degree, pH value, total acid, amino acid nitrogen and non-sugar solid would play important roles in the flavor, taste and nutrition of Chinese rice wine [22]. Although high level (10^7 cfu/mL) of *L. plantarum* CAU 3823 could degrade the BAs maximally, undesirable influence on the acceptability was also noteworthy. Low level (10^5 cfu/mL) and middle level (10^6 cfu/mL) of *L. plantarum* CAU 3823 could eliminate the negative effect on the qualities of the wine, and what's more important, similar sensory characteristics were obtained in CRW. Thus, to degrade the content of BAs in CRW to the highest extent, middle level (10^6 cfu/mL) of the *L. plantarum* could be chosen in the CRW fermentation process.

Non-sugar solids, a major nutrition indicator to evaluate the quality grade of CRW, are mainly composed of dextrin, glycerin, non-volatile acid, protein and hydrolysates [25]. Interestingly, the content of non-sugar solids was increased remarkably when *L. plantarum* CAU 3823 was used, especially at middle level (10^6 cfu/mL), which provided a novel insight that the *L. plantarum* CAU 3823 could produce more non-sugar solids in CRW and thus have potential nutritional values.

BA can be converted into products via oxidation by microorganisms which can be used as a carbon and/or energy source or as a nitrogen source [26]. Limited studies attributed these transformations to amine oxidase activity derived from microorganisms. Yagodina [27] reported that flavoprotein oxidases existing in some microorganisms could catalyze the oxidation of BAs. Sekiguchi [28] found a histamine oxidase in the actinobacteria *Arthrobacter crystallopoietes* KAIT-B-007 isolated from soil. In this study, the amine oxidases from *L. plantarum* CAU 3823 were purified and characterized. Nine amine oxidase proteins, a mixture from *L. plantarum* CAU 3823, contributed the most of amine-degrading ability of *L. plantarum* CAU 3823. Eight MAOs were identified and thus confirmed a good monoamine oxidase activity shown in fraction 1. Amine oxidases can be divided into two subfamilies based on the cofactor they contain. MAO (EC 1.4.3.4) are a family of enzymes containing flavin that catalyze the oxidation of monoamines, employing oxygen to clip off their amine group [29]. The amine oxidases containing copper as cofactor (EC 1.4.3.6) are homodimers, which contain three subclass, namely, diamine oxidase, primary-amine oxidase and diamine oxidase [30]. Amine oxidase [flavin-containing] A and B can catalyze the oxidative deamination of biogenic amines [31]. Amine oxidase [flavin-containing] B that in humans was encoded by the MAOB gene could preferentially degrade PHE [32], which confirmed 44.3% PHE degradation in fraction 1. An "aromatic cage" has been found to play a steric role in substrate binding and in flavin accessibility and helps to increase the substrate amine nucleophilicity [33], which might enhance BA degradation. It is noted that no diamine oxidase was identified although cell-free extracts showed diamine oxidase activity.

To provide a seemingly feasible solution to degrade the BAs in foodstuffs, the biochemical character assays of the amine oxidases mixture from *L. plantarum* CAU 3823 were designed. The enzymes were very thermostable, as the activity remained stable at 80 °C, and were fully stable over the pH range of 3–5. Similar results were reported that a putrescine oxidase from *Rhodococcus erythropolis* NCIMB 11540 could be stable at 50 °C for 2 h [34] and a thermostable histamine oxidase was found in *Arthrobacter crystallopoietes* KAIT-B-007 [29]. These results indicated that the amine oxidases could be stable to use in fermented food processing.

5. Conclusions

In this paper, *Lactobacillus plantarum* CAU 3823 was a *L. plantarum* originating from Chinese rice wine which could effectively degrade the BAs. Middle level (10^6 cfu/mL) of *L. plantarum* could be an optimal choice to decrease the BAs maximally while keeping the CRW character and quality in the pilot scale fermentation. Nine amine oxidase proteins were identified from *L. plantarum* using Sephadex separation followed by LC-MS/MS analysis. The enzymes were very thermostable and fully stable at pH 3–5. All the ions can inhibit the amine oxidase to an extent. *L. plantarum* seemed to be an interesting species displaying BAS degradation, both in culture media conditions and in CRW fermentation, suggesting its suitability as a commercial malolactic starter. This paper provided an efficient method to decrease the biogenic amine contents in the traditional fermented food made by multiple microbes like wine, rice wine, sausages, vinegar, cheese, kimchi and so on.

Supplementary Materials: The following are available online at http://www.mdpi.com/2304-8158/8/8/312/s1. Figure S1: The three fractions separated by a Sephadex G-100 column, Table S1: A group of proteins by Sephadex separation followed by LC-MS/MS analysis in fraction 1.

Author Contributions: T.N. and Y.M. conceived and designed the experiments; T.N. and Y.G. performed the experiments; T.N. and Y.G. analyzed the data; T.N. and X.L. wrote the paper.

Funding: This work was supported by the National Key Research and Development Program of China (No. 2018YFC1604303-04).

Conflicts of Interest: The authors declare no conflicts of interest.

References

1. Kim, J.Y.; Kim, D.; Park, P.; Kang, H.-I.; Ryu, E.K.; Kim, S.M. Effects of storage temperature and time on the biogenic amine content and microflora in Korean turbid rice wine, Makgeolli. *Food Chem.* **2011**, *128*, 87–92. [CrossRef] [PubMed]
2. Guo, X.; Guan, X.; Wang, Y.; Li, L.; Wu, D.; Chen, Y.; Pei, H.; Xiao, D. Reduction of biogenic amines production by eliminating the PEP4 gene in Saccharomyces cerevisiae during fermentation of Chinese rice wine. *Food Chem.* **2015**, *178*, 208–211. [CrossRef] [PubMed]
3. Alvarez, M.A.; Moreno-Arribas, M.V. The problem of biogenic amines in fermented foods and the use of potential biogenic amine-degrading microorganisms as a solution. *Trends Food Sci. Technol.* **2014**, *39*, 146–155. [CrossRef]
4. Xia, X.; Zhang, Q.; Zhang, B.; Zhang, W.; Wang, W. Insights into the Biogenic Amine Metabolic Landscape during Industrial Semidry Chinese Rice Wine Fermentation. *J. Agric. Food Chem.* **2016**, *64*, 7385–7393. [CrossRef] [PubMed]
5. Ancín-Azpilicueta, C.; González-Marco, A.; Jiménez-Moreno, N. Current Knowledge about the Presence of Amines in Wine. *Crit. Rev. Food Sci. Nutr.* **2008**, *48*, 257–275. [CrossRef] [PubMed]
6. Guo, Y.Y.; Yang, Y.P.; Peng, Q.; Han, Y. Biogenic amines in wine: A review. *Int. J. Food Sci. Technol.* **2015**, *50*, 1523–1532. [CrossRef]
7. Liu, S.P.; Yu, J.X.; Wei, X.L.; Ji, Z.W.; Zhou, Z.L.; Meng, X.Y.; Mao, J. Sequencing-based screening of functional microorganism to decrease the formation of biogenic amines in Chinese rice wine. *Food Control* **2016**, *64*, 98–104. [CrossRef]
8. Torlois, S.; Joyeux, A.; Moreno-Arribas, V.; Lonvaud-Funel, A.; Bertrand, A. Isolation, properties and behaviour of tyramine-producing lactic acid bacteria from wine. *J. Appl. Microbiol.* **2000**, *88*, 584–593.
9. Moreno-Arribas, M.; Polo, M.; Jorganes, F.; Muñoz, R. Screening of biogenic amine production by lactic acid bacteria isolated from grape must and wine. *Int. J. Food Microbiol.* **2003**, *84*, 117–123. [CrossRef]
10. Zhang, F.; Xue, J.; Wang, D.; Wang, Y.; Zou, H.; Zhu, B. Dynamic changes of the content of biogenic amines in Chinese rice wine during the brewing process. *J. Inst. Brew.* **2013**, *119*, 294–302. [CrossRef]
11. Chen, S.; Xu, Y. The Influence of Yeast Strains on the Volatile Flavour Compounds of Chinese Rice Wine. *J. Inst. Brew.* **2010**, *116*, 190–196. [CrossRef]
12. Yongmei, L.; Xin, L.; Xiaohong, C.; Mei, J.; Chao, L.; Mingsheng, D. A survey of biogenic amines in Chinese rice wines. *Food Chem.* **2007**, *100*, 1424–1428. [CrossRef]
13. Callejon, S.; Sendra, R.; Ferrer, S.; Pardo, I. Identification of a novel enzymatic activity from lactic acid bacteria able to degrade biogenic amines in wine. *Appl. Microbiol. Biotechnol.* **2014**, *98*, 185–198. [CrossRef] [PubMed]
14. Capozzi, V.; Russo, P.; Ladero, V.; Fernandez, M.; Fiocco, D.; Alvarez, M.A.; Grieco, F.; Spano, G. Biogenic Amines Degradation by Lactobacillus plantarum: Toward a Potential Application in Wine. *Front. Microbiol.* **2012**, *3*, 122. [CrossRef] [PubMed]
15. Leuschner, R.; Hammes, W. Tyramine degradation by micrococci during ripening of fermented sausage. *Meat Sci.* **1998**, *49*, 289–296. [CrossRef]
16. Dapkevicius, M.L.; Nout, M.; Rombouts, F.M.; Houben, J.H.; Wymenga, W. Biogenic amine formation and degradation by potential fish silage starter microorganisms. *Int. J. Food Microbiol.* **2000**, *57*, 107–114. [CrossRef]
17. Landete, J.; Ferrer, S.; Pardo, I. Biogenic amine production by lactic acid bacteria, acetic bacteria and yeast isolated from wine. *Food Control* **2007**, *18*, 1569–1574. [CrossRef]
18. García-Ruiz, A.; González-Rompinelli, E.M.; Bartolomé, B.; Moreno-Arribas, M.V. Potential of wine-associated lactic acid bacteria to degrade biogenic amines. *Int. J. Food Microbiol.* **2011**, *148*, 115–120. [CrossRef]
19. Cui, Y.; Qu, X.; Li, H.; He, S.; Liang, H.; Zhang, H.; Ma, Y. Isolation of halophilic lactic acid bacteria from traditional Chinese fermented soybean paste and assessment of the isolates for industrial potential. *Eur. Food Res. Technol.* **2012**, *234*, 797–806. [CrossRef]
20. Yu, H.; Ying, Y.; Fu, X.; Lu, H. Quality Determination of Chinese Rice Wine Based on Fourier Transform near Infrared Spectroscopy. *J. Near Infrared Spectrosc.* **2006**, *14*, 37–44. [CrossRef]

21. Shen, F.; Ying, Y.; Li, B.; Zheng, Y.; Hu, J. Prediction of sugars and acids in Chinese rice wine by mid-infrared spectroscopy. *Food Res. Int.* **2011**, *44*, 1521–1527. [CrossRef]
22. Callejon, S.; Sendra, R.; Ferrer, S.; Pardo, I. Ability of Kocuria varians LTH 1540 To Degrade Putrescine: Identification and Characterization of a Novel Amine Oxidase. *J. Agric. Food Chem.* **2015**, *63*, 4170–4178. [CrossRef] [PubMed]
23. Caston, J.; Eaton, C.; Gheorghiu, B.; Ware, L. Tyramine induced hypertensive episodes and panic attacks in hereditary deficient monoamine oxidase patients. *J. S. C. Med. Assoc. 1975* **2002**, *98*, 187.
24. Beneduce, L.; Romano, A.; Capozzi, V.; Lucas, P.; Barnavon, L.; Bach, B.; Vuchot, P.; Grieco, F.; Spano, G. Biogenic amine in wines. *Ann. Microbiol.* **2010**, *60*, 573–578. [CrossRef]
25. Ouyang, Q.; Zhao, J.; Chen, Q. Measurement of non-sugar solids content in Chinese rice wine using near infrared spectroscopy combined with an efficient characteristic variables selection algorithm. *Spectrochim. Acta Part A Mol. Biomol. Spectrosc.* **2015**, *151*, 280–285. [CrossRef] [PubMed]
26. Levering, P.R.; Van Dijken, J.P.; Veenhuis, M.; Harder, W.; Dijken, J.P. Arthrobacter P1, a fast growing versatile methylotroph with amine oxidase as a key enzyme in the metabolism of methylated amines. *Arch. Microbiol.* **1981**, *129*, 72–80. [CrossRef] [PubMed]
27. Yagodina, O.V.; Nikol'Skaya, E.B.; Khovanskikh, A.E.; Kormilitsyn, B.N. Amine Oxidases of Microorganisms. *Zhurnal Evoliutsionnoĭ Biokhimii I Fiziol.* **2002**, *29*, 864–869.
28. Sekiguchi, Y.; Makita, H.; Yamamura, A.; Matsumoto, K. A thermostable histamine oxidase from Arthrobacter crystallopoietes KAIT-B-007. *J. Biosci. Bioeng.* **2004**, *97*, 104–110. [CrossRef]
29. Tipton, K.F.; Boyce, S.; O'Sullivan, J.; Davey, G.P.; Healy, J. Monoamine Oxidases: Certainties and Uncertainties. *Curr. Med. Chem.* **2004**, *11*, 1965–1982. [CrossRef]
30. Cona, A.; Rea, G.; Angelini, R.; Federico, R.; Tavladoraki, P. Functions of amine oxidases in plant development and defence. *Trends Plant Sci.* **2006**, *11*, 80–88. [CrossRef]
31. Grimsby, J.; Chen, K.; Wang, L.J.; Lan, N.C.; Shih, J.C. Human monoamine oxidase A and B genes exhibit identical exon-intron organization. *Proc. Natl. Acad. Sci. USA* **1991**, *88*, 3637–3641. [CrossRef] [PubMed]
32. Yang, H.Y.; Neff, N.H. Beta-phenylethylamine: A specific substrate for type B monoamine oxidase of brain. *J. Pharmacol. Exp. Ther.* **1973**, *187*, 365–371.
33. Li, M.; Binda, C.; Mattevi, A.; Edmondson, D.E. Functional Role of the "Aromatic Cage" in Human Monoamine Oxidase B: Structures and Catalytic Properties of Tyr435 Mutant Proteins. *Biochemistry* **2006**, *45*, 4775–4784. [CrossRef] [PubMed]
34. Van Hellemond, E.W.; Van Dijk, M.; Heuts, D.P.H.M.; Janssen, D.B.; Fraaije, M.W. Discovery and characterization of a putrescine oxidase from Rhodococcus erythropolis NCIMB 11540. *Appl. Microbiol. Biotechnol.* **2008**, *78*, 455–463. [CrossRef] [PubMed]

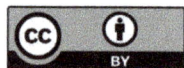

© 2019 by the authors. Licensee MDPI, Basel, Switzerland. This article is an open access article distributed under the terms and conditions of the Creative Commons Attribution (CC BY) license (http://creativecommons.org/licenses/by/4.0/).

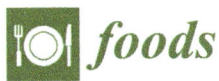

Article

The Role of *Enterococcus faecium* as a Key Producer and Fermentation Condition as an Influencing Factor in Tyramine Accumulation in *Cheonggukjang*

Young Kyoung Park [1], Young Hun Jin [1], Jun-Hee Lee [1], Bo Young Byun [1], Junsu Lee [1], KwangCheol Casey Jeong [2,3] and Jae-Hyung Mah [1,*]

1. Department of Food and Biotechnology, Korea University, 2511 Sejong-ro, Sejong 30019, Korea; eskimo@korea.ac.kr (Y.K.P.); younghoonjin3090@korea.ac.kr (Y.H.J.); bory92@korea.ac.kr (J.-H.L.); by-love23@hanmail.net (B.Y.B.); jpang@korea.ac.kr (J.L.)
2. Department of Animal Sciences, University of Florida, Gainesville, FL 32611, USA; kcjeong@ufl.edu
3. Emerging Pathogens Institute, University of Florida, Gainesville, FL 32611, USA
* Correspondence: nextbio@korea.ac.kr; Tel.: +82-44-860-1431

Received: 10 June 2020; Accepted: 8 July 2020; Published: 11 July 2020

Abstract: The study evaluated the role of *Enterococcus faecium* in tyramine production and its response to fermentation temperature in a traditional Korean fermented soybean paste, *Cheonggukjang*. Tyramine content was detected in retail *Cheonggukjang* products at high concentrations exceeding the recommended limit up to a factor of 14. All retail *Cheonggukjang* products contained *Enterococcus* spp. at concentrations of at least 6 Log CFU/g. Upon isolation of *Enterococcus* strains, approximately 93% (157 strains) produced tyramine at over 100 µg/mL. The strains that produced the highest concentrations of tyramine (301.14–315.29 µg/mL) were identified as *E. faecium* through 16S rRNA sequencing. The results indicate that *E. faecium* is one of the major contributing factors to high tyramine content in *Cheonggukjang*. During fermentation, tyramine content in *Cheonggukjang* groups co-inoculated with *E. faecium* strains was highest at 45 °C, followed by 37 °C and 25 °C. The tyramine content of most *Cheonggukjang* groups continually increased as fermentation progressed, except groups fermented at 25 °C. At 45 °C, the tyramine content occasionally exceeded the recommended limit within 3 days of fermentation. The results suggest that lowering fermentation temperature and shortening duration may reduce the tyramine content of *Cheonggukjang*, thereby reducing the safety risks that may arise when consuming food with high tyramine concentrations.

Keywords: *Cheonggukjang*; *Enterococcus faecium*; tyramine; biogenic amines; fermentation temperature; fermentation duration; tyrosine decarboxylase gene (*tdc*)

1. Introduction

Cheonggukjang is a traditional Korean soybean paste produced by fermenting soybeans with *Bacillus subtilis*. Traditional methods of *Cheonggukjang* production utilize rice straw added to steamed soybeans for a short fermentation period of approximately 2–3 days, while starter cultures are used instead of rice straw for modern methods of production [1,2]. Fermentation of *Cheonggukjang* is a process involving microbial enzymatic proteolysis resulting in uniquely characteristic savory aromatic and flavor properties [3]. Consumption of *Cheonggukjang* has been reported to be associated with numerous benefits such as antioxidative, antihypertensive, thrombolytic, and antimicrobial properties [4,5]. However, despite the beneficial properties of *Cheonggukjang*, potentially hazardous biogenic amines (BAs) may be produced during fermentation of the proteinous food rich in precursor amino acids.

The majority of BAs are formed through the reductive amination of ketones and aldehydes, as well as the decarboxylation of amino acids by microbially produced enzymes [6]. Though BAs are essential for the regulation of protein synthesis, nucleic acid functions, and membrane stabilization in living cells, consumption of food products with high concentrations of BAs may result in toxicological effects [7–10]. The excessive intake of food products such as mackerel, pacific saury, sardines, and tuna may result in "scombroid poisoning" owing to potentially high concentrations of toxic histamine that may cause symptoms similar to an allergic reaction including diarrhea, dyspnea, headache, hives, and hypotension [10–13]. Overconsumption of foods with high concentrations of tyramine may potentially result in a "cheese crisis" with various symptoms including heart failure, hemorrhages, hypertensive crisis, high blood pressure, and severe headaches [9,10,14,15]. Such a high content of tyramine produced by microbial tyrosine decarboxylase activity has occasionally been found in tyrosine-rich foods such as cheese [16,17] and soybean-based fermented products [18–20]. Therefore, Ten Brink, et al. [21] suggested BA toxicity limits of 30 mg/kg for β-phenylethylamine, 100 mg/kg for histamine, and 100–800 mg/kg for tyramine in foods.

Previous studies by Ko, et al. [18], Jeon, et al. [19], and Seo, et al. [20] on the BA content of *Cheonggukjang* have shown that tyramine in particular has been detected in high concentrations up to 1913.51, 251.66, and 905.0 mg/kg, respectively. Ibe, et al. [22] suggested that *Enterococcus faecium* may be largely responsible for the BA content of *Miso* (a Japanese fermented soybean paste). Notably, numerous studies have reported that *Enterococcus* spp. possess the tyrosine decarboxylase gene (*tdc*) [23,24]. Moreover, in particular Kang and Park [25] and Kang, et al. [26] confirmed the presence of *E. faecium* in *Cheonggukjang*, while a previous study by Jeon, et al. [19] showed that *Enterococcus* spp. isolated from *Cheonggukjang* exhibited tyramine production at concentrations of at least 351.59 µg/mL. Taken together, the previous reports imply that *E. faecium* may also be responsible for the BA content of *Cheonggukjang*. Meanwhile, the growth of *Enterococcus* spp. has been reported to occur at temperatures ranging from 10 °C up to 45 °C that overlap with *Cheonggukjang* fermentation temperatures ranging from 25 to 50 °C [27–30]. The corresponding range in temperature may be beneficial for *E. faecium* growth and tyramine production during the fermentation of contaminated *Cheonggukjang* products. Furthermore, a previous study reported that tyramine content increases in fermented soybeans as fermentation progresses [19]. According to Bhardwaj, et al. [31], the production of tyramine by *E. faecium* strains may be affected by incubation conditions such as temperature and time. Therefore, the current study assessed the safety risk of BAs (particularly tyramine) in *Cheonggukjang*, clarified the microorganism responsible for tyramine accumulation, and evaluated the effect of fermentation temperature/duration on *E. faecium* growth and subsequent tyramine production in the food.

2. Materials and Methods

2.1. Cheonggukjang Products

Six representative, but different *Cheonggukjang* products were purchased from various retail markets in the Republic of Korea and stored at 4 °C until further experimentation. Within a day of storage, the BA content of *Cheonggukjang* products was measured, followed by physicochemical and microbial analyses.

2.2. Physicochemical Analyses

To investigate the influencing factors such as pH, salinity, and water activity on BA content in *Cheonggukjang*, the physicochemical properties of *Cheonggukjang* samples (retail *Cheonggukjang* products purchased and *Cheonggukjang* groups fermented in this study) were measured as described below. Samples weighing 10 g using an analytical balance (Ohaus Adventurer™, Ohaus Corporation, Parsippany, NJ, USA) were homogenized with 90 mL of distilled water using a stomacher (Laboratory Blender Stomacher 400, Seward, Ltd., Worthing, UK). The pH of the homogenates was measured using a pH meter (Orion 3-star pH Benchtop Thermo Scientific, Waltham, MA, USA), while salinity was measured using the procedure described by the Association of Official Analytical Chemists

(AOAC; Official Method 960.29) [32]. The water activity of the samples was measured using an electric hygrometer (AquaLab Pre, Meter Group, Inc., Pullman, WA, USA).

2.3. Microbial Analyses

The analysis of the microbial community in *Cheonggukjang* samples was conducted using Plate Count Agar (PCA; Difco, Becton Dickinson, Sparks, MD, USA); de Man, Rogosa, and Sharpe (MRS; Conda, Madrid, Spain) agar; and m-Enterococcus Agar (m-EA; MB Cell, Seoul, Korea) for the enumeration of total mesophilic viable bacteria, lactic acid bacteria, and *Enterococcus* spp., respectively. Samples weighing 10 g were homogenized with 90 mL of sterile 0.1% peptone saline using a stomacher. The homogenates were 10-fold serially diluted with 0.1% peptone saline up to 10^{-5}, and 100 µL of each dilution was spread on PCA, MRS agar, and m-EA in duplicates. Incubation conditions were set according to the manufacturer's instructions: PCA at 37 °C for 24 h and m-EA at 37 °C for 48 h under aerobic condition; MRS agar at 37 °C for 48 h under anaerobic condition. Anaerobic condition was achieved using an anaerobic chamber (Coy Lab. Products, Inc., Grass Lake, MI, USA) containing an atmosphere of 95% nitrogen and 5% hydrogen. After incubation, the bacterial concentrations of the *Cheonggukjang* samples were calculated by enumerating the colony-forming units (CFU) on the plates of respective media with approximately 10 to 300 colonies [33] and adjusting for the dilution.

2.4. Isolation and Identification of Enterococcus Strains from Retail Cheonggukjang Products

A total of 169 *Enterococcus* strains were isolated from retail *Cheonggukjang* products according to the method described by Mareková, et al. [34], with minor modifications. Upon enumeration of colonies on m-EA, individual colonies were streaked on MRS agar and incubated at 37 °C for 48 h under anaerobic condition. Single colonies were streaked again on MRS agar and incubated under the same conditions. The pure single colonies were inoculated in MRS broth, incubated at 37 °C for 48 h, and stored at −70 °C using glycerol (20%, *v/v*).

The identities (at species level) of the individual *Enterococcus* strains that displayed the highest tyramine production were further investigated through sequence analysis of 16S rRNA gene amplified with the universal bacterial primer pair 518F (5′-CCAGCAGCCGCGGTAATACG-3′) and 805R (5′-GACTACCAGGGTATCTAAT-3′) (Solgent Co., Daejeon, Korea). The identities of sequences were determined using the basic local alignment search tool (BLAST) of the National Center for Biotechnology Information (NCBI; http://www.ncbi.nlm.nih.gov/BLAST/).

2.5. Preparation of Cheonggukjang

To investigate the effect of fermentation temperature on tyramine production by *E. faecium*, several temperatures were set for in situ *Cheonggukjang* fermentation experiments. The temperature for *Cheonggukjang* fermentation (intermediate-temperature group) was determined based upon previous studies in which 37 °C was reported as the temperature commonly used for *Cheonggukjang* production [19,35,36]. In addition, the temperatures of 25 °C and 45 °C used by other studies for *Cheonggukjang* fermentation were utilized for the low and high temperature groups, respectively [29,30].

White soybeans (*Glycine* max Merrill) were purchased from a retail market in the Republic of Korea. The soybeans were soaked in distilled water at 4 °C for 12 h, and subsequently drained for 1 h. Approximately 200 g of soybeans were adjusted to a final salinity of 2.40% according to the salinity of *Cheonggukjang* outlined in the 9th revision of the Korean food composition table [37] and subsequently steamed at 125 °C for 30 min using an autoclave. The steamed soybeans were cooled to 50 °C and inoculated with bacterial inocula in M/15 Sörensen's phosphate buffer (pH 7) to final concentrations of approximately 6 Log CFU/g of *B. subtilis* KCTC 3135 (also designated as ATCC 6051; type strain) and 4 Log CFU/g of *E. faecium* KCCM 12118 (ATCC 19434; type strain) or *E. faecium* CJE 216 (strain isolated from *Cheonggukjang* and selected owing to both strong tyramine production and *tdc* gene expression). The control group (without any *E. faecium* strains) was inoculated with only *B. subtilis* KCTC 3135 to a final concentration of 6 Log CFU/g. The sizes of inocula were selected with consideration of the cell count of each microorganism in *Cheonggukjang* products determined in our previous study [19]. The inoculated steamed soybeans were then fermented at 25 °C, 37 °C, or 45 °C for 3 days. Approximately 20 g of the fermented soybeans were collected daily during fermentation to measure the BA content as well as physicochemical and microbial properties. Fermented soybeans sampled during fermentation were stored at −70 °C for further testing, as required.

2.6. BA Analyses in Cheonggukjang Samples and Bacterial Cultures

2.6.1. BA Extraction from *Cheonggukjang* Samples and Bacterial Cultures

Quantification of the BA content of *Cheonggukjang* was conducted as previously described by Ben-Gigirey, et al. [38]. Five grams of *Cheonggukjang* with 20 mL of 0.4 M perchloric acid (Sigma-Aldrich, St. Louis, MO, USA) were homogenized by vortex (Vortex-Genie, Scientific industries, Bohemia, NY, USA) and stored at 4 °C for 2 h. The mixture was then centrifuged at 3000× g for 10 min at 4 °C (1736R, Labogene, Seoul, Korea), and the supernatant was collected. Upon resuspension of the pellet with 20 mL of 0.4 M perchloric acid, the mixture was stored at 4 °C for 2 h and centrifuged again at 3000× g at 4 °C for 10 min. The supernatant was combined with the previously collected supernatant and adjusted to a final volume of 50 mL with 0.4 M perchloric acid. Then, the extract was filtered through Whatman paper No. 1 (Whatman International Ltd., Maidstone, UK).

The bacterial production of BAs was measured using the procedures described by Eerola, et al. [39], modified by Ben-Gigirey, et al. [38,40], and further modified in the present study to culture *Enterococcus* spp. based on Marcobal, et al. [41]. A loopful (10 µL) of glycerol stock of each enterococcal strain was inoculated in 5 mL of MRS broth supplemented with 0.5% of each amino acid, including L-histidine monohydrochloride monohydrate, L-tyrosine disodium salt hydrate, L-ornithine monohydrochloride, L-lysine monohydrochloride (pH 5.8), and 0.0005% pyridoxal-HCl (all from Sigma-Aldrich) and incubated at 37 °C for 48 h. Approximately 100 µL of the broth culture was then transferred to another tube containing 5 mL of the same medium. Upon incubation at 37 °C for 48 h, the broth culture was filtered using a sterile syringe with a 0.2 µm membrane (Millipore Co., Bedford, MA, USA). Then, 9 mL of 0.4 M perchloric acid were added to 1 mL of the filtered broth culture and mixed by a vortex mixer. The mixture was reacted in a cold chamber at 4 °C for 2 h and centrifuged at 3000× g at 4 °C for 10 min. The extract was filtered through Whatman paper No. 1.

2.6.2. Preparation of Standard Solutions for High Performance Liquid Chromatography (HPLC) Analysis

Standard solutions with concentrations of 0, 10, 50, 100, and 1000 ppm were prepared for tryptamine, β-phenylethylamine hydrochloride, putrescine dihydrochloride, cadaverine dihydrochloride, histamine dihydrochloride, tyramine hydrochloride, spermidine trihydrochloride, and spermine tetrahydrochloride (all from Sigma-Aldrich). Internal standard solution with the same concentrations was prepared using 1,7-diaminoheptane (Sigma-Aldrich).

2.6.3. Derivatization of Extracts and Standards

Derivatization of BAs was conducted according to the method described by Eerola, et al. [39]. One milliliter of extract or standard solution prepared as aforementioned was mixed with 200 µL of 2 M sodium hydroxide and 300 µL of saturated sodium bicarbonate (all from Sigma-Aldrich). Two milliliters of dansyl chloride (Sigma-Aldrich) solution (10 mg/mL) in acetone were added to the mixture and incubated at 40 °C for 45 min. The residual dansyl chloride was removed by adding 100 µL of 25% ammonium hydroxide and incubating for 30 min at 25 °C. Using acetonitrile, the mixture was adjusted to a final volume of 5 mL and centrifuged at 3000× g for 5 min. After filtration using 0.2 µm pore-size filters (Millipore), the filtered supernatant was kept at 4 °C until further analysis using HPLC.

2.6.4. Chromatographic Separations

Chromatographic separation of BAs was conducted according to the method previously developed by Eerola, et al. [39] and modified by Ben-Gigirey, et al. [40]. An HPLC unit (YL9100, YL Instruments Co., Ltd., Anyang, Korea) equipped with a UV/vis detector (YL Instruments) and Autochro-3000 data system (YL Instruments) was used. For chromatographic separation, a Nova-Pak C_{18} 4 μm column (150 mm × 4.6 mm, Waters, Milford, MA, USA) held at 40 °C was utilized. The mobile phases were 0.1 M ammonium acetate dissolved in deionized water (solvent A; Sigma-Aldrich) and acetonitrile (solvent B; SK chemicals, Ulsan, Korea) adjusted to a flow rate of 1 mL/min with a linear gradient starting from 50% of solvent B reaching 90% by 19 min. A 10 μL sample was injected and monitored at 254 nm. The limits of detection were approximately 0.1 μg/mL for all BAs in standard solutions and bacterial cultures, and about 0.1 mg/kg for all BAs in food matrices [42].

2.7. Gene Expression Analyses in Bacterial Cultures and Cheonggukjang

2.7.1. RNA Extraction and Reverse Transcription

Expression analysis of tyrosine decarboxylase gene (*tdc*) involved RNA extraction from bacterial cultures (for in vitro experiments) and *Cheonggukjang* samples (viz., *Cheonggukjang* groups prepared through fermentation; for in situ fermentation experiments) with a Ribo-Ex Total RNA isolation solution (Geneall, Seoul, Korea). The extraction was conducted according to the manufacturer's instructions with minor modifications as follows. To prepare bacterial culture for in vitro gene expression analysis, a loopful (10 μL) of glycerol stock of each enterococcal strain was inoculated in 5 mL of MRS broth supplemented with 0.5% L-histidine monohydrochloride monohydrate, L-tyrosine disodium salt hydrate, L-ornithine monohydrochloride, L-lysine monohydrochloride (pH 5.8), and 0.0005% pyridoxal-HCl (all from Sigma-Aldrich) and incubated at 37 °C for 48 h. Approximately 100 μL of the broth culture was then transferred to another tube containing 5 mL of the same medium and incubated under the same conditions. As for *Cheonggukjang* samples, 10 g of *Cheonggukjang* were gently mixed with 40 mL of phosphate buffer in a sterile bag, and the liquid part was collected. Subsequently, 3 mL of the bacterial culture or all liquid part of the mixture were immediately transferred into a 50 mL conical tube and centrifuged at 10,000× g at 4 °C for 5 min. After removing the supernatant, the pellet was suspended with 7 mL of phosphate buffer and centrifuged under the same conditions. Then, the pellet was homogenized with 800 μL of Ribo-Ex reagent in a bacterial lysing tube (Lysing Matrix B; MP Biomedicals, Santa Ana, CA, USA) using a Precellys 24 homogenizer (Bertin Technologies, Montigny, France) with two cycles for 30 s at 6800 rpm, pausing for 90 s between cycles. Approximately 200 μL of chloroform were added to the lysate, vortexed, and centrifuged at 10,000× g for 1 min. Approximately 400 μL of the supernatant were mixed with 600 μL of chilled absolute ethanol. The mixture was reacted at −70 °C for 15 min and purified with a Nucleospin RNA kit (Macherey-Nagel, Düren, Germany) according to the manufacturer's instructions. The quality of the extracted RNA was evaluated using a NanoDrop 1000 spectrophotometer (Thermo Fisher, Waltham, MA, USA).

ReverTra Ace qPCR RT Master Mix with gDNA Remover kit (Toyobo, Osaka, Japan) containing reverse transcriptase, RNase inhibitor, oligo (dT) primers, random primers, and deoxynucleoside triphosphates (dNTPs) was used to synthesize cDNA from 1 μL of extracted RNA according to the manufacturer's instructions. Reverse transcription was conducted under the following conditions: 37 °C for 15 min, 50 °C for 5 min, and 98 °C for 5 min. After the reaction, the resulting cDNA was stored at −70 °C until quantitative PCR analysis.

2.7.2. Quantitative PCR Analysis

As designed by Kang, et al. [43], *q-tdc* F (5′-AGACCAAGTAATTCCAGTGCC-3′) and *q-tdc* R (5′-CACCGACTACACCTAAGATTGG-3′) primers were used for the quantitation of *tdc* gene expression by *E. faecium*. The primers for reference genes including *q-gap* F (5′-ATACGACACAACTCAAGGACG-3′) and *q-gap* R (5′-GATATCTACGCCTAGTTCGCC-3′) [34], along with *tufA*-RT F (5′-TACACGCCACTAC

GCTCAC-3′) and *tufA*-RT R (5′-AGCTCCGTCCATTTGAGCAG-3′) [44] were used for the normalization of *tdc* gene expression. The efficiency of each set of primers for reverse transcription quantitative polymerase chain reaction (RT-qPCR) was determined by the following equation: $E = 10^{(-1/S)} - 1$, where E is the amplification efficiency and S is the slope of standard curves generated through threshold cycle (Ct) values of serial dilutions of cDNA obtained from reverse-transcription of RNA from *E. faecium* KCCM 12118.

For the RT-qPCR analysis of *tdc* gene expression in bacterial cultures and *Cheonggukjang* samples, 5 µL of a 10-fold diluted cDNA were added to 15 µL of a master mix containing 10 µL of Power SYBR Green PCR Master Mix (Applied Biosystems, Foster City, CA, USA), 3 µL of RNase free water, and 1 µL of each primer (forward and reverse; 500 nM). Subsequently, thermal cycling was conducted using an Applied Biosystems 7500 Real-Time PCR system (Applied Biosystems) with the thermal cycling conditions programmed as follows: initial denaturation at 95 °C for 10 min; 40 cycles at 95 °C for 15 s (denaturation step), and 60 °C for 60 s (annealing and elongation steps, unless otherwise mentioned). Annealing and elongation conditions for primer *tufA*-RT were set at 55 °C for 60 s. Melting curve analysis was conducted using the RT-PCR system to confirm the specificity and to analyze the amplified products. Ct values were detected when the emissions from fluorescence exceeded the fixed threshold automatically determined by thermocycler software. Relative expression of *tdc* genes was further calculated by the $2^{-(\Delta\Delta ct)}$ method, normalized to the expression levels detected in *E. faecium* KCCM 12118 (refer to Figure 2) or *Cheonggukjang* groups fermented at 37 °C (refer to Figure 6), and expressed as n-fold differences to compare gene expression levels in different bacterial cultures and *Cheonggukjang* samples.

2.8. Statistical Analyses

Data were presented as means and standard deviations of duplicates or triplicates. All measurements on retail products were performed in triplicates, while the other experiments were conducted in duplicate. The significance of differences was determined by one-way analysis of variance (ANOVA) with Fisher's pairwise comparison module of the Minitab statistical software, version 17 (Minitab Inc., State College, PA, USA), and differences with probability (p) value of <0.05 were considered statistically significant.

3. Results and Discussion

3.1. Physicochemical Properties of Retail Cheonggukjang Products

Physicochemical and microbial properties as well as BA content in retail *Cheonggukjang* products were analyzed to estimate the contributing factors to BA content (particularly tyramine) in *Cheonggukjang* (Sections 3.1–3.3). Table 1 displays the physicochemical properties of *Cheonggukjang* products purchased from retail markets in the Republic of Korea. The pH ranged from 6.39 to 7.05, with an average pH of 6.84 ± 0.23 (mean ± standard deviation). The results were similar to the study conducted by Lee, et al. [45], which reported the average pH of *Cheonggukjang* to be 7.0 ± 0.8. Jeon, et al. [19] and Yoo, et al. [46] also reported the average pH of *Cheonggukjang* to be pH 6.07 ± 0.72 (range of pH 4.62–8.14) and pH 7.21 ± 0.59 (range of pH 5.89–7.95), respectively. Such differences in the pH of the *Cheonggukjang* products may be owing to different fermentation conditions [47] and/or fermentation metabolites [48]. The salinity of retail *Cheonggukjang* products ranged from 1.95 to 9.36% with an average salinity of 5.16 ± 2.78%. In comparison, Ko, et al. [18], Jeon, et al. [19], and Kang, et al. [49] reported the average salinity of *Cheonggukjang* to be 2.12 ± 1.66% (0.12–11.51%), 1.56 ± 1.19% (0.10–5.33%), and 3.51 ± 2.45 (1.64–8.39%), respectively. Though the salinity of the *Cheonggukjang* products was found to vary substantially, Ko, et al. [18] suggested that the large differences in *Cheonggukjang* salinities may be traced to the production process, as some methods utilize the addition of different amounts of salt to preserve the fermented soybean product. The water activity of retail *Cheonggukjang* products ranged from 0.919 to 0.973 with an average of 0.951 ± 0.019. In a previous study by Kim, et al. [47], the average water activity was found to be 0.962 ± 0.028 (0.857–0.991). Overall, the physicochemical properties of retail *Cheonggukjang* products analyzed in the current study were mostly similar to the values reported in previous studies. Although the results of the current study did not show any correlation between physicochemical properties and BA content (especially tyramine) based on linear regression analyses (data not shown), it is noteworthy that the ranges of the physicochemical parameters were within the specific conditions for the growth of *E. faecium*, which are as follows: pH, from 4 to 10 [50]; salinity, up to 7% [50]; water activity, above 0.940 [51].

Table 1. Physicochemical properties of retail *Cheonggukjang* products.

Products [1]	pH	Salinity (%)	Water Activity
CJ1	6.91 ± 0.03 [2]	5.54 ± 0.09	0.948 ± 0.002
CJ2	6.84 ± 0.02	7.25 ± 0.06	0.919 ± 0.001
CJ3	6.87 ± 0.02	3.16 ± 0.06	0.968 ± 0.002
CJ4	6.99 ± 0.03	1.95 ± 0.09	0.973 ± 0.002
CJ5	7.05 ± 0.05	9.36 ± 0.59	0.944 ± 0.003
CJ6	6.39 ± 0.03	3.71 ± 0.34	0.954 ± 0.003
Average	6.84 ± 0.23	5.16 ± 2.78	0.951 ± 0.019

[1] CJ: *Cheonggukjang*; [2] Mean ± standard deviation were calculated from triplicate experiments.

3.2. Microbial Properties of Retail Cheonggukjang Products

Table 2 shows the microbial properties of retail *Cheonggukjang* products. The number of total mesophilic viable bacteria ranged from 8.54 to 9.81 Log CFU/g, with an average of 9.27 ± 0.45 Log CFU/g. Comparatively, Ko, et al. [18] and Jeon, et al. [19] reported the total counts of viable mesophilic bacteria of *Cheonggukjang* products to be 7.50 ± 1.01 Log CFU/g (5.30–9.98 Log CFU/g) and 9.65 ± 0.77 Log CFU/g (8.23–11.66 Log CFU/g), respectively. The wide range of total mesophilic viable bacteria may result from an insufficient standardization of *Cheonggukjang* manufacturing processes such as different fermentation materials and conditions [18,47]. *Enterococcus* spp. were detected at concentrations of 6.64–7.99 Log CFU/g, with an average of 7.17 ± 0.49 Log CFU/g. The number of lactic acid bacteria was found to be approximately 6.66–8.12 Log CFU/g, with an average of 7.09 ± 0.58 Log CFU/g (Table 2). For comparison, a study by Kang and Park [25] showed that *Enterococcus* spp. were detected in all 31 *Cheonggukjang* products at concentrations of 3.51–8.46 Log CFU/g, with an average of 5.95 ± 1.60 Log CFU/g. In the report, approximately 58% and 16.8% of the isolated *Enterococcus* strains were identified as *E. faecium* and *E. faecalis*, respectively. The presence of *E. faecium* in *Cheonggukjang* was also reported by Kang, et al. [26]. The reported results on the presence of *Enterococcus* spp. at high concentrations in *Cheonggukjang* concurred with the findings of the current study. As *E. faecium* has been reported as a pathogenic and/or tyramine-producing bacterium detected in some foods including Chinese and Japanese fermented soybean products, previous studies have mentioned that preventative measures are necessary to avoid contamination during the manufacturing of fermented foods [52–55]. The traditional *Cheonggukjang* production process may also be susceptible to contamination by harmful microbes owing to the reliance on rice straw containing *B. subtilis* for fermentation [56]. In fact, according to Heu, et al. [57], rice straw contains a variety of bacteria, including mesophiles, thermophiles, coliforms, and actinomycetes, as well as fungi. Moreover, as sterilization processes are not utilized in the manufacturing of *Cheonggukjang*, occasional contamination by tyramine-producing bacteria such as *E. faecium* may be present in the final product. The results of the current and previous studies suggest that further research appears to be necessary for the development of methods to inhibit *E. faecium* growth during the manufacturing of *Cheonggukjang* as well as other fermented soybean products described above.

Table 2. Microbial properties of retail *Cheonggukjang* products.

Products [1]	Total Mesophilic Viable Bacteria (Log CFU/g)	*Enterococcus* spp. (Log CFU/g)	Lactic Acid Bacteria (Log CFU/g)
CJ1	9.45 ± 0.06 [2]	7.32 ± 0.03	7.45 ± 0.10
CJ2	9.04 ± 0.09	6.78 ± 0.14	6.66 ± 0.10
CJ3	9.81 ± 0.25	6.64 ± 0.01	6.70 ± 0.15
CJ4	9.57 ± 0.15	7.27 ± 0.03	6.96 ± 0.09
CJ5	8.54 ± 0.48	7.00 ± 0.08	6.67 ± 0.18
CJ6	9.20 ± 0.44	7.99 ± 0.04	8.12 ± 0.01
Average	9.27 ± 0.45	7.17 ± 0.49	7.09 ± 0.58

[1] CJ: *Cheonggukjang*; [2] Mean ± standard deviation were calculated from triplicate experiments; CFU: colony-forming units.

3.3. BA Content of Retail Cheonggukjang Products

Cheonggukjang contains abundant BA precursor amino acids such as lysine, histidine, tyrosine, and phenylalanine [58]. The high amino acid content may pose a risk for conversion into BAs during *Cheonggukjang* fermentation. In the present study, tryptamine, β-phenylethylamine, putrescine, cadaverine, histamine, tyramine, spermidine, and spermine contents in retail *Cheonggukjang* products were detected at concentrations of 70.63 ± 44.74 mg/kg, 36.22 ± 29.55 mg/kg, 10.80 ± 5.07 mg/kg, 18.57 ± 9.08 mg/kg, 8.37 ± 2.40 mg/kg, 457.42 ± 573.15 mg/kg, 121.92 ± 19.69 mg/kg, and 187.20 ± 110.27 mg/kg, respectively (Table 3). A previous study suggested toxicity limits of 30 mg/kg for β-phenylethylamine, 100 mg/kg for histamine, and 100–800 mg/kg for tyramine in foods [21]. Therefore, the evaluation of the BA content of the *Cheonggukjang* products was continued with regard to the aforementioned BA intake limits with the exception of tyramine (at 100 mg/kg). Evaluation of β-phenylethylamine content in two *Cheonggukjang* products revealed that concentrations exceeded the recommended limit of 30 mg/kg, with one product exceeding the limit by a factor of approximately 3. Though the histamine content of all *Cheonggukjang* products was found to be below the recommended limit of 100 mg/kg, the tyramine content of three products exceeded the 100 mg/kg limit by factors of 2, 9, and 14, respectively. Other studies have reported similarly high concentrations of tyramine in *Cheonggukjang*. Ko, et al. [18] and Seo, et al. [20] reported the highest concentrations of tyramine in *Cheonggukjang* products, exceeding the recommended limit by factors of 19 and 9, respectively. Furthermore, Cho, et al. [59], Han, et al. [60], and Jeon, et al. [19] reported that *Cheonggukjang* products contained high concentrations of tyramine, which exceeded the recommended limit by up to factors of 5, 5, and 3, respectively. Altogether, as β-phenylethylamine and tyramine content of several *Cheonggukjang* products exceeded the recommended limits, overconsumption of such fermented soybean products may occasionally result in adverse effects on the body. Moreover, *Cheonggukjang* was found to contain other BAs enhancing the toxicity of β-phenylethylamine and tyramine. Therefore, further research remains necessary for precautionary measures and remedial methods to reduce the BA content of *Cheonggukjang* to ensure the safety of the fermented soybean food.

Table 3. Biogenic amine (BA) content of retail *Cheonggukjang* products.

Products [1]	BA Content (mg/kg) [2]							
	TRP	PHE	PUT	CAD	HIS	TYR	SPD	SPM
CJ1	115.06 ± 19.72 [A,3]	31.66 ± 3.82 [B]	8.54 ± 3.45 [BC]	22.66 ± 0.82 [C]	8.60 ± 0.88 [B]	222.25 ± 15.1 [C]	137.88 ± 1.76 [A]	292.99 ± 27.86 [A]
CJ2	86.02 ± 3.12 [B]	16.06 ± 2.24 [B]	12.18 ± 0.73 [B]	29.95 ± 0.82 [A]	12.69 ± 0.28 [A]	57.14 ± 8.06 [D]	99.99 ± 4.25 [C]	206.32 ± 23.82 [B]
CJ3	118.27 ± 5.97 [A]	27.22 ± 2.00 [B]	18.33 ± 4.93 [A]	26.58 ± 1.65 [B]	6.50 ± 1.00 [C]	80.83 ± 3.91 [D]	96.82 ± 4.09 [C]	201.63 ± 5.77 [B]
CJ4	54.87 ± 3.18 [C]	22.20 ± 7.06 [B]	11.36 ± 2.28 [B]	8.28 ± 0.54 [F]	5.86 ± 0.37 [C]	898.41 ± 79.43 [B]	125.61 ± 4.64 [B]	91.09 ± 24.03 [C]
CJ5	47.85 ± 4.04 [C]	24.48 ± 1.97 [B]	11.61 ± 4.21 [B]	13.57 ± 0.21 [D]	8.65 ± 0.51 [B]	61.98 ± 6.30 [D]	125.98 ± 7.60 [B]	305.05 ± 17.35 [A]
CJ6	1.70 ± 2.94 [D]	95.58 ± 46.97 [A]	2.81 ± 1.77 [C]	10.19 ± 0.50 [E]	7.84 ± 0.33 [B]	1424.04 ± 62.43 [A]	145.18 ± 7.64 [A]	26.20 ± 8.51 [D]
Average	70.63 ± 44.74	36.22 ± 29.55	10.80 ± 5.07	18.57 ± 9.08	8.37 ± 2.40	457.42 ± 573.15	121.92 ± 19.69	187.20 ± 110.27

[1] CJ: *Cheonggukjang*; [2] TRP: tryptamine, PHE: β-phenylethylamine, PUT: putrescine, CAD: cadaverine, HIS: histamine, TYR: tyramine, SPD: spermidine, SPM: spermine; [3] Mean ± standard deviation were calculated from triplicate experiments. Mean values in the same column followed by different letters (A–F) are significantly different ($p < 0.05$).

3.4. In Vitro BA Production by Enterococcus Strains Isolated from Retail Cheonggukjang Products

Microbial decarboxylation of free amino acids is one of the main causing factors in the production of BAs, and various microorganisms, including *Bacillus*, *Clostridium*, Enterobacteriaceae, enterococci, *Lactobacillus*, and *Pseudomonas*, are capable of producing the decarboxylases responsible for the conversion of amino acids into BAs [21,61,62]. Considering previous studies in which *Enterococcus* spp. have been suggested to be responsible for tyramine accumulation in Chinese and Japanese fermented soybean products [52,53], the current study analyzed the BA production capabilities of 169 enterococcal strains isolated from retail *Cheonggukjang* products using an MRS broth-based assay medium. As shown in Figure 1, the production of tryptamine, β-phenylethylamine, putrescine, cadaverine, spermidine, and spermine was observed at concentrations lower than 10 μg/mL. Histamine production by 168 of the 169 strains was detected at quantities lower than 2 μg/mL; however, only one strain was capable of producing histamine at 96.06 μg/mL. Though tyramine production ranged from ND (not detected) to 315.29 μg/mL, 157 strains (about 93%) produced over 100 μg/mL. Through 16S rRNA sequencing, the seven strains (CJE 101, CJE 115, CJE 119, CJE 128, CJE 130, CJE 210, and CJE 216) that produced the highest levels of tyramine (301.14–315.29 μg/mL; refer to Figure 2) among the enterococcal strains were all identified as *E. faecium*. Novella-Rodríguez, et al. [63] suggested that the presence of Enterobacteriaceae or enterococci may result in the production of BAs in contaminated food products. Marcobal, et al. [64] demonstrated that *E. faecium* possesses a gene that codes an enzyme capable of L-tyrosine decarboxylation. According to Ibe, et al. [22], high levels of tyramine in *Miso* (a Japanese fermented soybean paste) products may partially result from tyramine production by *E. faecium*. Jeon, et al. [19] reported that *Enterococcus* spp. exhibited strong production of tyramine ranging from 0.41 μg/mL to 351.59 μg/mL in assay media. The author also found tyramine-producing *Bacillus* spp. (up to 123.08 μg/mL) and suggested that the species is one of the major tyramine producers in *Cheonggukjang* along with *Enterococcus* species based on the in situ fermentation experiment. Consequently, the present results suggest that *Enterococcus* spp. (particularly *E. faecium*) may be largely responsible for high tyramine concentrations in *Cheonggukjang*.

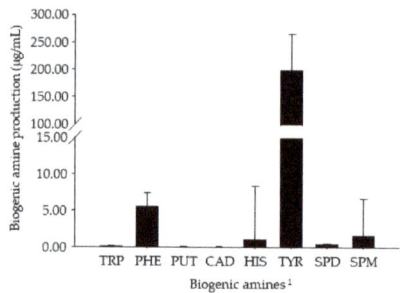

Figure 1. Biogenic amine (BA) production by *Enterococcus* strains (n = 169) isolated from retail *Cheonggukjang* products. Error bars indicate standard deviations calculated from duplicate experiments.
[1] TRP: tryptamine, PHE: β-phenylethylamine, PUT: putrescine, CAD: cadaverine, HIS: histamine, TYR: tyramine, SPD: spermidine, SPM: spermine.

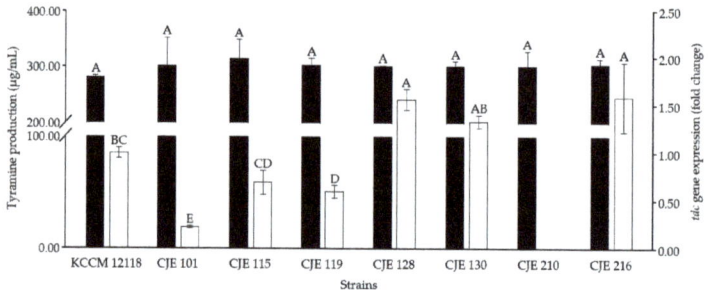

Figure 2. Comparison of tyramine production and *tdc* expression by *E. faecium* strains. ■: tyramine production, □: *tdc* gene expression. The expression levels observed in *E. faecium* strains isolated from retail *Cheonggukjang* products were normalized to that detected in *E. faecium* KCCM 12118 (type strain). The *tdc* gene expression was not detected in *E. faecium* strain CJE 210. Mean values followed by different letters are significantly different ($p < 0.05$). Error bars indicate standard deviations calculated from duplicate experiments.

3.5. Selection of Tyramine-Producing E. faecium Strain for Cheonggukjang Fermentation Based on Tyrosine Decarboxylase Gene Expression In Vitro

In the current study, the efficiency of primer sets *q-tdc* (for the quantitation of *tdc* gene expression) along with *q-gap* and *tufA*-RT (for the normalization of *tdc* gene expression) was calculated to be 100.71%, 94.84%, and 95.03%, respectively. An amplification efficiency between 90 and 110% indicates that the results of gene expression obtained using RT-qPCR are reproducible [65].

The aforementioned primer sets were used to detect *tdc* gene expression by the seven *E. faecium* strains (CJE 101, CJE 115, CJE 119, CJE 128, CJE 130, CJE 210, and CJE 216) with the highest tyramine production in vitro as described in the previous section (note that the primer sets were also used for in situ gene expression analysis). Among the strains, *E. faecium* strain CJE 216 showed the highest expression level of *tdc* gene (Figure 2). Considering the highest *tdc* gene expression as well as tyramine production in vitro, the CJE 216 strain was selected as an inoculant for fermentation experiments in the next section.

3.6. Tyramine Production by E. faecium during Cheonggukjang Fermentation at Various Temperatures

3.6.1. Changes in Physicochemical and Microbial Properties during *Cheonggukjang* Fermentation at Various Temperatures

As the results of the previous sections indicated that *E. faecium* was most likely one of the major contributing factors to high levels of tyramine in *Cheonggukjang*, in situ fermentation experiments were performed to empirically investigate the influence of *E. faecium* on tyramine content in *Cheonggukjang*. For the in situ fermentation experiments, three experimental groups of *Cheonggukjang* were used: control group inoculated with only *B. subtilis* KCTC 3135, and other two groups co-inoculated with the *B. subtilis* strain and each *E. faecium* strain (*E. faecium* KCCM 12118 or *E. faecium* CJE 216). Each group was further divided into three groups based on fermentation temperatures of 25 °C, 37 °C, and 45 °C (low-, intermediate-, and high-temperature groups, respectively). As shown in Figure 3, the changes in the physicochemical and microbial properties of *Cheonggukjang* were measured at 24-hour intervals for 3 days of fermentation. The pH of all *Cheonggukjang* groups was lowest on day 2, with progressively lower pH depending on the fermentation temperature, independent of which inoculum was used. The pH on day 2 of *Cheonggukjang* fermentation at 25 °C, 37 °C, and 45 °C ranged from pH 6.34 to 6.36, pH 5.90 to 6.09, and pH 5.49 to 5.88, respectively (Figure 3a). Loizzo, et al. [66] suggested that decarboxylases are produced by bacteria owing to a mechanism to neutralize acidic environments that restrict the growth of the bacteria. A previous study reported that low pH between 4.0 and 5.5 may result in the production of BAs [67]. Therefore, in this study, as the *Cheonggukjang* groups fermented at 45 °C (high-temperature group) resulted in a lower pH than other groups fermented at 37 °C and 25 °C (intermediate- and low-temperature groups, respectively), regardless of inoculum, the BA content was expected to be detected at the highest concentration among all *Cheonggukjang* groups. As for water activity, all *Cheonggukjang* groups remained within 0.95–0.97 during fermentation (Figure 3b).

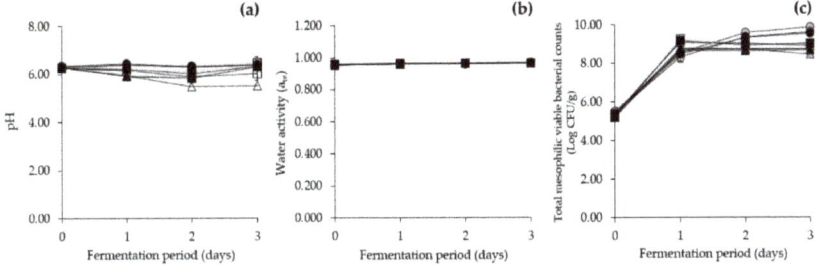

Figure 3. Physicochemical and microbial properties during *Cheonggukjang* fermentation at various temperatures. (**a**) pH, (**b**) water activity, (**c**) total mesophilic viable bacterial counts. •: 25 °C, ■: 37 °C, ▲: 45 °C (inoculated with only *B. subtilis* KCTC 3135); •: 25 °C, ■: 37 °C, ▲: 45 °C (inoculated with *B. subtilis* KCTC 3135 and *E. faecium* KCCM 12118); ○: 25 °C, □: 37 °C, △: 45 °C (inoculated with *B. subtilis* KCTC 3135 and *E. faecium* CJE 216). Error bars indicate standard deviations calculated from duplicate experiments.

The counts of total mesophilic viable bacteria, most probably attributed to *B. subtilis* inoculated, showed that microbial concentrations started from approximately 6 Log CFU/g on day 0 and remained at approximately 8–9 Log CFU/g throughout *Cheonggukjang* fermentation at all three temperatures, regardless of the presence or absence of *E. faecium* inoculum (Figure 3c). The total mesophilic viable bacteria in *Cheonggukjang* increased as fermentation temperature decreased; however, on day 1, those in the groups fermented at 25 °C and 45 °C showed growth up to 8 Log CFU/g, while those in the groups fermented at 37 °C exhibited the highest counts at 9 Log CFU/g. The results concurred with a previous finding that 37 °C is the optimal in situ growth temperature for *B. subtilis* during *Cheonggukjang* fermentation [29]. Similarly, Mann, et al. [68] reported the optimal in vitro growth temperature for *B. subtilis* strains isolated from *Cheonggukjang* to be 37 °C.

The enterococcal count in *Cheonggukjang* co-inoculated with *E. faecium* KCCM 12118 at approximately 4 Log CFU/g (and *B. subtilis* KCTC 3135 at 6 Log CFU/g as well) increased by 1.63 Log CFU/g, 3.52 Log CFU/g, and 4.06 Log CFU/g after 3 days of fermentation at 25 °C, 37 °C, and 45 °C, respectively (Figure 4). In *Cheonggukjang* co-inoculated with *E. faecium* CJE 216 at 4 Log CFU/g (and *B. subtilis* KCTC 3135), enterococcal count increased at all fermentation temperatures of 25 °C,

37 °C, and 45 °C by 3.48 Log CFU/g, 4.78 Log CFU/g, and 4.80 Log CFU/g, respectively, by day 3. *Enterococcus* spp. were not detected in the control group for the duration of the fermentation period. The results displayed progressively higher enterococcal counts that increased alongside rising fermentation temperatures with the highest enterococcal counts in *Cheonggukjang* fermented at 45 °C (high-temperature group). The findings were comparable to a previous study by Morandi, et al. [69], which showed that lower fermentation temperatures weakened *E. faecium* growth as the reported generation time at 25 °C was nearly two times longer than at 37 °C. *E. faecium* has been reported to display active growth within the temperature range of 37–53 °C, with an optimal growth temperature of 42.7 °C [50,70]. The current and previous studies, therefore, indicate that the use of high fermentation temperatures such as 45 °C may enhance *E. faecium* growth, thereby increasing the potential for high tyramine production during *Cheonggukjang* fermentation.

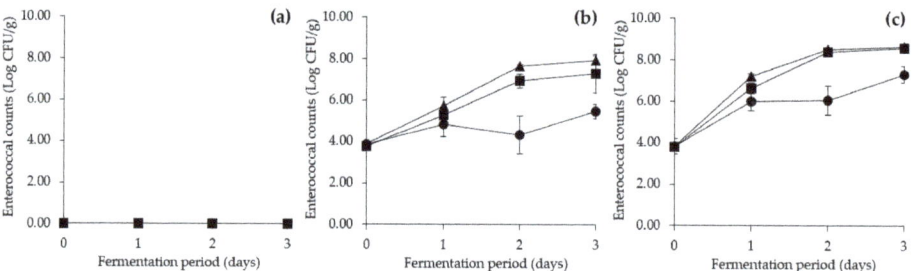

Figure 4. Effect of fermentation temperature on enterococcal counts in *Cheonggukjang* inoculated with (**a**) *B. subtilis* KCTC 3135, (**b**) *B. subtilis* KCTC 3135 and *E. faecium* KCCM 12118, and (**c**) *B. subtilis* KCTC 3135 and *E. faecium* CJE 216. ●: 25 °C, ■: 37 °C, ▲: 45 °C. Error bars indicate standard deviations calculated from duplicate experiments.

3.6.2. Effect of Fermentation Temperature on Tyramine Content in *Cheonggukjang*

The tyramine content of *Cheonggukjang* co-inoculated with either *E. faecium* KCCM 12118 or *E. faecium* CJE 216, along with *B. subtilis* KCTC 3135, was measured during fermentation, as seen in Figure 5. The tyramine content of the control group without *E. faecium* was detected at concentrations that did not exceed 10 mg/kg in all fermentation conditions (Figure 5a). In contrast, other groups with *E. faecium* contained higher levels of tyramine, which indicated that *E. faecium* was capable of and responsible for producing tyramine in *Cheonggukjang*. In *Cheonggukjang* groups co-inoculated with *E. faecium* KCCM 12118, initial tyramine content increased by 0.78 mg/kg, 33.36 mg/kg, and 101.17 mg/kg at 3 days of fermentation at 25 °C, 37 °C, and 45 °C, respectively (Figure 5b). As for *Cheonggukjang* groups co-inoculated with *E. faecium* CJE 216, initial tyramine content increased by 1.59 mg/kg, 74.11 mg/kg, and 85.14 mg/kg at 25 °C, 37 °C, and 45 °C, respectively, by day 3 of fermentation (Figure 5c). All *Cheonggukjang* groups fermented at 25 °C contained the lowest tyramine concentrations at less than 10 mg/kg during the entire fermentation duration. However, at 45 °C, the *Cheonggukjang* group co-inoculated with *E. faecium* KCCM 12118 displayed an exceptionally high tyramine content detected at 105.13 ± 5.68 mg/kg, exceeding the recommended limit, as expected owing to the acidic pH described in Section 3.6.1. Both *E. faecium* strains appeared to continuously produce tyramine during *Cheonggukjang* fermentation at 37 °C and 45 °C (Figure 5b,c). The results of the current study are in agreement with findings reported by Kalhotka, et al. [71], which showed a stronger in vitro tyramine production by *E. faecium* incubated at 37 °C than at 25 °C. According to Morandi, et al. [69], *E. faecium* metabolic activity was detected to be higher at 37 °C than at 25 °C during milk fermentation. The previous studies have indicated that lower temperatures may reduce both metabolic activity and tyramine production of *E. faecium*. BA content during fermentation at higher temperatures may even reach dangerously high levels as reported by Kang, et al. [43]. In the same report, tyramine concentrations in *E. faecium*-inoculated *Cheonggukjang* fermented at 45 °C for

48 h increased (up to 698.67 mg/kg) during the fermentation period, and consequently exceeded the recommended limit for consumption. Jeon, et al. [19] also reported strong tyramine production by *Enterococcus* spp. during soybean fermentation at 37 °C. The report demonstrated that tyramine concentrations continued to increase as fermentation progressed. Given the results, safety precautions regarding the limitation of fermentation duration and temperature appear to be necessary as extended periods of fermentation as well as high fermentation temperatures may increase tyramine content in *Cheonggukjang* beyond the recommended safe limit for consumption. Besides, the results showing a lower tyramine content in *Cheonggukjang* during fermentation at lower temperatures coincide with the results in the previous section that displayed a reduction in enterococcal count alongside a decrease in fermentation temperature. Taken together, the present study indicates that lower fermentation temperatures inhibit enterococcal growth, thereby limiting acid production and maintaining low levels of tyramine in *Cheonggukjang*. Therefore, utilizing lower temperatures for *Cheonggukjang* fermentation may reduce the risks associated with *Enterococcus* growth and tyramine accumulation.

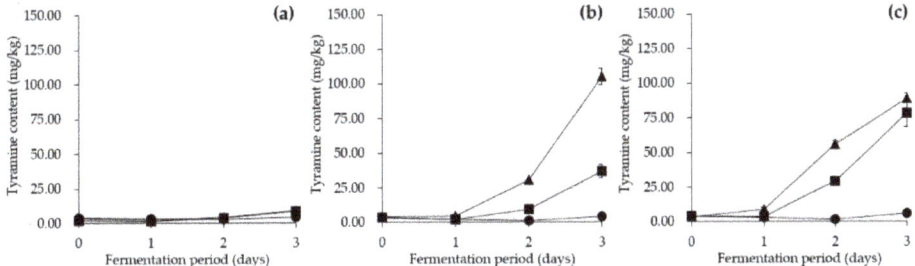

Figure 5. Effect of fermentation temperature on tyramine content in *Cheonggukjang* inoculated with (a) *B. subtilis* KCTC 3135, (b) *B. subtilis* KCTC 3135 and *E. faecium* KCCM 12118, and (c) *B. subtilis* KCTC 3135 and *E. faecium* CJE 216. ●: 25 °C, ■: 37 °C, ▲: 45 °C. Error bars indicate standard deviations calculated from duplicate experiments.

3.6.3. Effect of Fermentation Temperature on *tdc* Gene Expression by *E. faecium* Strains in *Cheonggukjang*

The changes in *tdc* gene expression by tyramine-producing *E. faecium* strains were detected and quantified during fermentation of *Cheonggukjang* at 25 °C, 37 °C, and 45 °C. As *Cheonggukjang* is mostly fermented at 37 °C, the *tdc* gene expression detected in *Cheonggukjang* groups fermented at 45 °C was normalized to that detected in the corresponding groups fermented at 37 °C according to the *E. faecium* strains used as inoculants. In *Cheonggukjang* fermented at 25 °C, tyramine content continuously remained at concentrations lower than 10 mg/kg, and *tdc* gene expression by *E. faecium* KCCM 12118 and *E. faecium* CJE 216 was not detected in all *Cheonggukjang* groups. In contrast, the highest *tdc* gene expression by *E. faecium* KCCM 12118 was detected in *Cheonggukjang* fermented at 45 °C and was upregulated in the range of 1.90- to 7.15-fold throughout *Cheonggukjang* fermentation, compared with that in *Cheonggukjang* fermented at 37 °C (Figure 6a–c, left). As for *Cheonggukjang* fermented at 45 °C with *E. faecium* CJE 216, downregulation of *tdc* gene expression was observed at 0.82-fold on day 1, and the expression was then upregulated in the range of 1.90- to 3.39-fold thereafter (Figure 6a–c, right). Consequently, both tyramine content and *tdc* gene expression were highest in *Cheonggukjang* groups fermented at 45 °C (viz., high-temperature group). Nonetheless, the variation in detected *tdc* gene expression levels during fermentation did not necessarily reflect the tyramine content observed for *Cheonggukjang*. After one day of fermentation, the *Cheonggukjang* group with *E. faecium* CJE 216 fermented at 37 °C contained a lower tyramine content than at 45 °C; however, *tdc* gene expression was slightly higher at 37 °C as described right above. The results showed that there may be differences between gene expression level and enzyme activity (and products thereof). Glanemann, et al. [72] reported that, in vitro, the mRNA response levels do not necessarily reflect the protein response levels or enzyme activity. As previously suggested by Ladero, et al. [73], while the correlation between BA content and gene expression is not always linear, RT-qPCR remains a reliable method to detect and quantify BA-producing bacteria in food products. Similarly, in our preliminary tests conducted under different incubation conditions, tyramine production by *E. faecium* strains in an assay medium appeared to be insignificantly related to *tdc* gene expression level (data not shown). Therefore, utilizing HPLC analysis appears to be essential for the quantification of BA content and/or bacterial BA production in food samples [31,73,74]. When utilized in conjunction, the complementary methods, that is, HPLC and RT-qPCR, sufficiently allow for the quantitative analysis of both the BA content and tyramine-producing bacteria (including enterococci) in food products [24,31]. In the present study, the results derived from both techniques indicated that the fermentation of *Cheonggukjang* at high temperatures results in increased *tdc* gene expression and tyramine production. Therefore, low-temperature fermentation appears to be necessary to minimize both *tdc* gene expression and tyramine production by *Enterococcus* spp. and thereby ensure the safety of fermented soybean products.

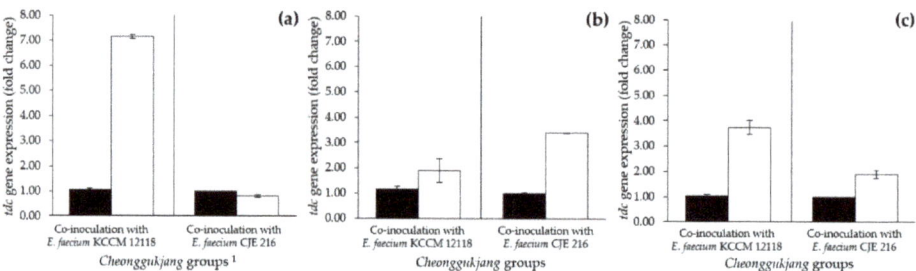

Figure 6. Effect of fermentation temperature on *tdc* expression by *E. faecium* strains in *Cheonggukjang* on (**a**) day 1, (**b**) day 2, and (**c**) day 3 of fermentation. ■: 37 °C, □: 45 °C. [1] *Cheonggukjang* groups were co-inoculated with *B. subtilis* (KCTC 3135) and *E. faecium* (KCCM 12118 or CJE 216) strains. The expression levels observed in groups fermented at 45 °C were normalized to those detected in the corresponding groups fermented at 37 °C. Expression of *tdc* gene was not detected in *Cheonggukjang* fermented at 25 °C. Error bars indicate standard deviations calculated from duplicate experiments.

4. Conclusions

The current study assessed the safety risk of tyramine in *Cheonggukjang*, diagnosed the microbial causative agent (i.e., *E. faecium*) responsible for high tyramine levels, and evaluated the impact of fermentation temperature on enterococcal growth (as well as acid production and *tdc* gene expression) and tyramine production. Of the retail *Cheonggukjang* examined, half of the products contained tyramine content that exceeded the recommended limit for safe consumption by up to a factor of approximately 14. *E. faecium* strains isolated from the retail *Cheonggukjang* products were highly capable of producing tyramine in assay media, which indicated that the species is principally, or at least partly, responsible for tyramine accumulation in the food.

During in situ fermentation at different temperatures, the tyramine content of *Cheonggukjang* groups co-inoculated with *B. subtilis* (used as an inoculant to ferment soybeans) and *E. faecium* (either isolated in this study or designated previously as the type strain) strains was highest at 45 °C, followed by 37 °C and 25 °C. On the other hand, the control group inoculated with only *B. subtilis* strain (without any *E. faecium* inoculants) had the lowest tyramine content at all fermentation temperatures, which supported the notion that *E. faecium* may be a key producer of tyramine in *Cheonggukjang*. Another implication of the results was that a lower fermentation temperature leads to a lower tyramine content below the recommended limit in *Cheonggukjang*, even though the tyramine content continually increases during fermentation. Therefore, low temperatures and a short fermentation duration may reduce the accumulation of tyramine caused by *E. faecium* growth in *Cheonggukjang*, thereby reducing the safety risks associated with consuming food with high BA concentrations.

Author Contributions: Conceptualization, Y.K.P. and J.-H.M.; Investigation, Y.K.P., Y.H.J., J.-H.L., B.Y.B., and J.L.; Formal analysis, J.L.; Writing—original draft, Y.K.P.; Writing—review and editing, Y.K.P., Y.H.J., K.C.J., and J.-H.M.; Supervision: J.-H.M. All authors have read and agreed to the published version of the manuscript.

Funding: This work was supported by the National Research Foundation of Korea (NRF) grant funded by the Korea government (MSIT) (no. 2020R1I1A3052118).

Acknowledgments: The authors thank Jae Hoan Lee and Alixander Mattay Pawluk of Department of Food and Biotechnology at Korea University for technical assistance and English editing, respectively.

Conflicts of Interest: The authors declare no conflict of interest.

References

1. Jang, C.H.; Lim, J.K.; Kim, J.H.; Park, C.S.; Kwon, D.Y.; Kim, Y.-S.; Shin, D.H.; Kim, J.-S. Change of isoflavone content during manufacturing of *cheonggukjang*, a traditional Korean fermented soyfood. *Food Sci. Biotechnol.* **2006**, *15*, 643–646.
2. Kim, K.-J.; Ryu, M.-K.; Kim, S.-S. *Chungkook-jang Koji* fermentation with rice straw. *Korean J. Food Sci. Technol.* **1982**, *14*, 301–308.
3. Hong, S.W.; Kim, J.Y.; Lee, B.K.; Chung, K.S. The bacterial biological response modifier enriched *Chungkookjang* fermentation. *Korean J. Food Sci. Technol.* **2006**, *38*, 548–553.
4. Lee, J.-O.; Ha, S.-D.; Kim, A.-J.; Yuh, C.-S.; Bang, I.-S.; Park, S.-H. Industrial application and physiological functions of *Chongkukjang*. *Food Sci. Ind.* **2005**, *38*, 69–78.
5. Hwang, J.-S.; Kim, S.-J.; Kim, H.-B. Antioxidant and blood-pressure reduction effects of fermented soybean, Chungkookjang. *Korean J. Microbiol.* **2009**, *45*, 54–57.
6. Askar, A.; Treptow, H. *Biogene Amine in Lebensmitteln: Vorkommen, Bedeutung und Bestimmung*, 1st ed.; Eugen Ulmer: Stuttgart, Germany, 1986; pp. 21–74.
7. Silla Santos, M.H. Biogenic amines: Their importance in foods. *Int. J. Food Microbiol.* **1996**, *29*, 213–231. [CrossRef]
8. Shalaby, A.R. Significance of biogenic amines to food safety and human health. *Food Res. Int.* **1996**, *29*, 675–690. [CrossRef]
9. Ladero, V.; Calles-Enriquez, M.; Fernández, M.; Alvarez, M.A. Toxicological effects of dietary biogenic amines. *Curr. Nutr. Food Sci.* **2010**, *6*, 145–156. [CrossRef]
10. EFSA Panel on Biological Hazards (BIOHAZ). Scientific opinion on risk based control of biogenic amine formation in fermented foods. *EFSA J.* **2011**, *9*, 2393. [CrossRef]
11. Taylor, S.L.; Eitnmiller, R.R. Histamine food poisoning: Toxicology and clinical aspects. *Crit. Rev. Toxicol.* **1986**, *17*, 91–128. [CrossRef]
12. Kovacova-Hanuskova, E.; Buday, T.; Gavliakova, S.; Plevkova, J. Histamine, histamine intoxication and intolerance. *Allergol. Immunopathol.* **2015**, *43*, 498–506. [CrossRef] [PubMed]
13. Maintz, L.; Novak, N. Histamine and histamine intolerance. *Am. J. Clin. Nutr.* **2007**, *85*, 1185–1196. [CrossRef] [PubMed]
14. Smith, T.A. Amines in food. *Food Chem.* **1981**, *6*, 169–200. [CrossRef]
15. Stratton, J.E.; Hutkins, R.W.; Taylor, S.L. Biogenic amines in cheese and other fermented foods: A review. *J. Food Prot.* **1991**, *54*, 460–470. [CrossRef]
16. Linares, D.M.; Martín, M.; Ladero, V.; Alvarez, M.A.; Fernández, M. Biogenic amines in dairy products. *Crit. Rev. Food Sci. Nutr.* **2011**, *51*, 691–703. [CrossRef]
17. Schirone, M.; Tofalo, T.; Fasoli, G.; Perpetuini, G.; Corsetti, A.; Manetta, A.C.; Ciarrocchi, A.; Suzzi, G. High content of biogenic amines in Pecorino cheeses. *Food Microbiol.* **2013**, *34*, 137–144. [CrossRef]
18. Ko, Y.-J.; Son, Y.-H.; Kim, E.-J.; Seol, H.-G.; Lee, G.-R.; Kim, D.-H.; Ryu, C.-H. Quality properties of commercial *Chungkukjang* in Korea. *J. Agric. Life Sci.* **2012**, *46*, 177–187.
19. Jeon, A.R.; Lee, J.H.; Mah, J.-H. Biogenic amine formation and bacterial contribution in *Cheonggukjang*, a Korean traditional fermented soybean food. *LWT Food Sci. Technol.* **2018**, *92*, 282–289. [CrossRef]
20. Seo, M.-J.; Lee, C.-D.; Lee, J.-N.; Yang, H.-J.; Jeong, D.-Y.; Lee, G.-H. Analysis of biogenic amines and inorganic elements in *Cheonggukjang*. *Korean J. Food Preserv.* **2019**, *26*, 101–108. [CrossRef]
21. Ten Brink, B.; Damink, C.; Joosten, H.M.L.J.; Huis in 't Veld, J.H.J. Occurrence and formation of biologically active amines in foods. *Int. J. Food Microbiol.* **1990**, *11*, 73–84. [CrossRef]

22. Ibe, A.; Nishima, T.; Kasai, N. Bacteriological properties of and amine-production conditions for tyramine-and histamine-producing bacterial strains isolated from soybean paste (miso) starting materials. *Jpn. J. Toxicol. Environ. Health* **1992**, *38*, 403–409. [CrossRef]
23. Torriani, S.; Gatto, V.; Sembeni, S.; Tofalo, R.; Suzzi, G.; Belletti, N.; Gardini, F.; Bover-Cid, S. Rapid detection and quantification of tyrosine decarboxylase gene (*tdc*) and its expression in gram-positive bacteria associated with fermented foods using PCR-based methods. *J. Food Prot.* **2008**, *71*, 93–101. [CrossRef] [PubMed]
24. Ladero, V.; Fernández, M.; Cuesta, I.; Alvarez, M.A. Quantitative detection and identification of tyramine-producing enterococci and lactobacilli in cheese by multiplex qPCR. *Food Microbiol.* **2010**, *27*, 933–939. [CrossRef] [PubMed]
25. Kang, T.-M.; Park, J.-H. Isolation and antibiotic susceptibility of *Enterococcus* spp. from fermented soy paste. *J. Korean Soc. Food Sci. Nutr.* **2012**, *41*, 714–720. [CrossRef]
26. Kang, H.-R.; Lee, Y.-L.; Hwang, H.-J. Potential for application as a starter culture of tyramine-reducing strain. *J. Korean Soc. Food Sci. Nutr.* **2017**, *46*, 1561–1567. [CrossRef]
27. Svec, P.; Devriese, L.A. Enterococcus. In *Bergey's Manual of Systematics of Archaea and Bacteria*, 2nd ed.; De Vos, P., Garrity, G.M., Jones, D., Krieg, N.R., Ludwig, W., Rainey, F.A., Schleifer, K.-H., Whitman, W.B., Eds.; Springer: New York, NY, USA, 2015; Volume 3, pp. 594–607.
28. Food Information Statistics System. Available online: http://www.atfis.or.kr/article/M001050000/view.do?articleId=2452&page=5&searchKey=&searchString=&searchCategory= (accessed on 29 May 2020).
29. Kim, I.-J.; Kim, H.-K.; Chung, J.-H.; Jeong, Y.-K.; Ryu, C.-H. Study of functional *Chungkukjang* contain fibrinolytic enzyme. *Korean J. Life Sci.* **2002**, *12*, 357–362.
30. Lee, N.-R.; Go, T.-H.; Lee, S.-M.; Hong, C.-O.; Park, K.-M.; Park, G.-T.; Hwang, D.-Y.; Son, H.-J. Characteristics of Chungkookjang prepared by *Bacillus amyloliquefaciens* with different soybeans and fermentation temperatures. *Korean J. Microbiol.* **2013**, *49*, 71–77. [CrossRef]
31. Bhardwaj, A.; Gupta, H.; Iyer, R.; Kumar, N.; Malik, R.K. Tyramine-producing enterococci are equally detected on tyramine production medium, by quantification of tyramine by HPLC, or by *tdc* gene-targeted PCR. *Dairy Sci. Technol.* **2009**, *89*, 601–611. [CrossRef]
32. AOAC. *Official Methods of Analysis of AOAC International*, 18th ed.; AOAC International: Gaithersburg, MD, USA, 2005.
33. ISO 7218:2007. *Microbiology of Food and Animal Feeding Stuffs—General Requirements and Guidance for Microbiological Examinations*; ISO: Geneva, Switzerland, 2007.
34. Mareková, M.; Lauková, A.; DeVuyst, L.; Skaugen, M.; Nes, I.F. Partial characterization of bacteriocins produced by environmental strain *Enterococcus faecium* EK13. *J. Appl. Microbiol.* **2003**, *94*, 523–530. [CrossRef]
35. Ryu, M.S.; Yang, H.-J.; Kim, J.W.; Jeong, S.-J.; Jeong, S.-Y.; Eom, J.-S.; Jeong, D.-Y. Potential probiotics activity of *Bacillus* spp. from traditional soybean pastes and fermentation characteristics of *Cheonggukjang*. *Korean J. Food Preserv.* **2017**, *24*, 1168–1179. [CrossRef]
36. Lee, J.S.; Lee, M.H.; Kim, J.M. Changes in quality characteristics of *cheonggukjang* added with quinoa during fermentation period. *Korean J. Food Nutr.* **2018**, *31*, 24–32.
37. National Institute of Agricultural Sciences. Available online: https://koreanfood.rda.go.kr:2360/eng/fctFoodSrchEng/engMain (accessed on 7 May 2020).
38. Ben-Gigirey, B.; Vieites Baptista De Sousa, J.M.; Villa, T.G.; Barros-Velazquez, J. Changes in biogenic amines and microbiological analysis in albacore (*Thunnus alalunga*) muscle during frozen storage. *J. Food Prot.* **1998**, *61*, 608–615. [CrossRef] [PubMed]
39. Eerola, S.; Hinkkanen, R.; Lindfors, E.; Hirvi, T. Liquid chromatographic determination of biogenic amines in dry sausages. *J. AOAC Int.* **1993**, *76*, 575–577. [CrossRef]
40. Ben-Gigirey, B.; Vieites Baptista De Sousa, J.M.; Villa, T.G.; Barros-Velazquez, J. Histamine and cadaverine production by bacteria isolated from fresh and frozen albacore (*Thunnus alalunga*). *J. Food Prot.* **1999**, *62*, 933–939. [CrossRef] [PubMed]
41. Marcobal, Á.; Martín-Álvarez, P.J.; Moreno-Arribas, M.V.; Muñoz, R. A multifactorial design for studying factors influencing growth and tyramine production of the lactic acid bacteria *Lactobacillus brevis* CECT 4669 and *Enterococcus faecium* BIFI-58. *Res. Microbiol.* **2006**, *157*, 417–424. [CrossRef] [PubMed]
42. Yoon, H.; Park, J.H.; Choi, A.; Hwang, H.-J.; Mah, J.-H. Validation of an HPLC analytical method for determination of biogenic amines in agricultural products and monitoring of biogenic amines in Korean fermented agricultural products. *Toxicol. Res.* **2015**, *31*, 299–305. [CrossRef]

43. Kang, H.-R.; Kim, H.-S.; Mah, J.-H.; Kim, Y.-W.; Hwang, H.-J. Tyramine reduction by tyrosine decarboxylase inhibitor in *Enterococcus faecium* for tyramine controlled *cheonggukjang*. *Food Sci. Biotechnol.* **2018**, *27*, 87–93. [CrossRef]
44. Top, J.; Paganelli, F.L.; Zhang, X.; van Schaik, W.; Leavis, H.L.; Van Luit-Asbroek, M.; van der Poll, T.; Leendertse, M.; Bonten, M.J.M.; Willems, R.J.L. The *Enterococcus faecium* enterococcal biofilm regulator, EbrB, regulates the *esp* operon and is implicated in biofilm formation and intestinal colonization. *PLoS ONE* **2013**, *8*, e65224. [CrossRef]
45. Lee, E.S.; Kim, Y.S.; Ryu, M.S.; Jeong, D.Y.; Uhm, T.B.; Cho, S.H. Characterization of *Bacillus licheniformis* SCK A08 with antagonistic property against *Bacillus cereus* and degrading capacity of biogenic amines. *J. Food Hyg. Saf.* **2014**, *29*, 40–46. [CrossRef]
46. Yoo, S.-M.; Choe, J.-S.; Park, H.-J.; Hong, S.-P.; Chang, C.-M.; Kim, J.-S. Physicochemical properties of traditional *Chonggugjang* produced in different regions. *Appl. Biol. Chem.* **1998**, *41*, 377–383.
47. Kim, J.-W.; Kim, Y.-S.; Jeong, P.-H.; Kim, H.-E.; Shin, D.-H. Physicochemical characteristics of traditional fermented soybean products manufactured in folk villages of Sunchang region. *J. Food Hyg. Saf.* **2006**, *21*, 223–230.
48. Jeong, W.J.; Lee, A.R.; Chun, J.; Cha, J.; Song, Y.-S.; Kim, J.H. Properties of *cheonggukjang* fermented with *Bacillus* strains with high fibrinolytic activities. *J. Food Sci. Nutr.* **2009**, *14*, 252–259. [CrossRef]
49. Kang, S.J.; Kim, S.S.; Chung, H.Y. Comparison of physicochemical characteristics and consumer perception of *Cheongkukjang*. *J. Korean Soc. Food Sci. Nutr.* **2014**, *43*, 1104–1111. [CrossRef]
50. Oh, S.-J.; Mah, J.-H.; Kim, J.-H.; Kim, Y.-W.; Hwang, H.-J. Reduction of tyramine by addition of *Schizandra chinensis* Baillon in Cheonggukjang. *J. Med. Food* **2012**, *15*, 1109–1115. [CrossRef] [PubMed]
51. International Commission on Microbiological Specifications for Foods International Association of Microbiological Societies. Reduced water activity. In *Microbial Ecology of Foods*, 1st ed.; Silliker, J.H., Elliot, R.P., Baird-Parker, A.C., Bryan, F.L., Christian, J.H.B., Clark, D.S., Olson, J.C., Roberts, T.A., Eds.; Academic Press: New York, NY, USA, 1980; Volume 1, pp. 70–91.
52. Li, L.; Ruan, L.; Ji, A.; Wen, Z.; Chen, S.; Wang, L.; Wei, X. Biogenic amines analysis and microbial contribution in traditional fermented food of Douchi. *Sci. Rep.* **2018**, *8*, 1–10. [CrossRef] [PubMed]
53. Takebe, Y.; Takizaki, M.; Tanaka, H.; Ohta, H.; Niidome, T.; Morimura, S. Evaluation of the biogenic amine-production ability of lactic acid bacteria isolated from tofu-misozuke. *Food Sci. Technol. Res.* **2016**, *22*, 673–678. [CrossRef]
54. Giraffa, G. Enterococci from foods. *FEMS Microbiol. Rev.* **2002**, *26*, 163–171. [CrossRef]
55. Giraffa, G.; Carminati, D.; Neviani, E. Enterococci isolated from dairy products: A review of risks and potential technological use. *J. Food Prot.* **1997**, *60*, 732–738. [CrossRef]
56. Bandara, N.; Chung, S.-J.; Jeong, D.-Y.; Kim, K.-P. The use of the pathogen-specific bacteriophage BCP8-2 to develop a rice straw-derived *Bacillus cereus*-free starter culture. *Korean J. Food Sci. Technol.* **2014**, *46*, 115–120. [CrossRef]
57. Heu, J.-S.; Lee, I.-J.; Yoon, M.-H.; Choi, W.-Y. Adhesive microbial populations of rice straws and their effects on Chungkukjang fermentation. *Korean J. Agric. Sci.* **1999**, *26*, 77–83.
58. Seok, Y.-R.; Kim, Y.-H.; Kim, S.; Woo, H.-S.; Kim, T.-W.; Lee, S.-H.; Choi, C. Change of protein and amino acid composition during *Chungkook-Jang* fermentation using *Bacillus licheniformis* CN-115. *Korean J. Agic. Sci.* **1994**, *37*, 65–71.
59. Cho, T.-Y.; Han, G.-H.; Bahn, K.-N.; Son, Y.-W.; Jang, M.-R.; Lee, C.-H.; Kim, S.-H.; Kim, D.-B.; Kim, S.-B. Evaluation of biogenic amines in Korean commercial fermented foods. *Korean J. Food Sci. Technol.* **2006**, *38*, 730–737.
60. Han, G.-H.; Cho, T.-Y.; Yoo, M.-S.; Kim, C.-S.; Kim, J.-M.; Kim, H.-A.; Kim, M.-O.; Kim, S.-C.; Lee, S.-A.; Ko, Y.-S.; et al. Biogenic amines formation and content in fermented soybean paste (*cheonggukjang*). *Korean J. Food Sci. Technol.* **2007**, *39*, 541–545.
61. Rice, S.L.; Eitenmiller, R.R.; Koehler, P.E. Biologically active amines in food: A review. *J. Milk Food Technol.* **1976**, *39*, 353–358. [CrossRef]
62. Rodriguez-Jerez, J.J.; Giaccone, V.; Colavita, G.; Parisi, E. *Bacillus macerans*—A new potent histamine producing micro-organism isolated from Italian cheese. *Food Microbiol.* **1994**, *11*, 409–415. [CrossRef]

63. Novella-Rodríguez, S.; Veciana-Nogues, M.T.; Roig-Sagues, A.X.; Trujillo-Mesa, A.J.; Vidal-Carou, M.C. Evaluation of biogenic amines and microbial counts throughout the ripening of goat cheeses from pasteurized and raw milk. *J. Dairy Res.* **2004**, *71*, 245–252. [CrossRef] [PubMed]
64. Marcobal, A.; de las Rivas, B.; Moreno-Arribas, M.V.; Munoz, R. Evidence for horizontal gene transfer as origin of putrescine production in *Oenococcus oeni* RM83. *Appl. Environ. Microbiol.* **2006**, *72*, 7954–7958. [CrossRef] [PubMed]
65. Condori, J.; Nopo-Olazabal, C.; Medrano, G.; Medina-Bolivar, F. Selection of reference genes for qPCR in hairy root cultures of peanut. *BMC Res. Notes* **2011**, *4*, 392. [CrossRef] [PubMed]
66. Loizzo, M.R.; Menichini, F.; Picci, N.; Puoci, F.; Spizzirri, U.G.; Restuccia, D. Technological aspects and analytical determination of biogenic amines in cheese. *Trends Food Sci. Technol.* **2013**, *30*, 38–55. [CrossRef]
67. Cosansu, S. Determination of biogenic amines in a fermented beverage, boza. *J. Food Agric. Environ.* **2009**, *7*, 54–58.
68. Mann, S.-Y.; Kim, E.-A.; Lee, G.-Y.; Kim, R.-U.; Hwang, D.-Y.; Son, H.-J.; Kim, D.-S. Isolation and identification of GABA-producing microorganism from *Chungkookjang*. *J. Life Sci.* **2013**, *23*, 102–109. [CrossRef]
69. Morandi, S.; Brasca, M.; Alfieri, P.; Lodi, R.; Tamburini, A. Influence of pH and temperature on the growth of *Enterococcus faecium* and *Enterococcus faecalis*. *Le Lait* **2005**, *85*, 181–192. [CrossRef]
70. Van den Berghe, E.; De Winter, T.; De Vuyst, L. Enterocin A production by *Enterococcus faecium* FAIR-E 406 is characterised by a temperature-and pH-dependent switch-off mechanism when growth is limited due to nutrient depletion. *Int. J. Food Microbiol.* **2006**, *107*, 159–170. [CrossRef] [PubMed]
71. Kalhotka, L.; Manga, I.; Přichystalová, J.; Hůlová, M.; Vyletělová, M.; Šustová, K. Decarboxylase activity test of the genus *Enterococcus* isolated from goat milk and cheese. *Acta Vet. BRNO* **2012**, *81*, 145–151. [CrossRef]
72. Glanemann, C.; Loos, A.; Gorret, N.; Willis, L.B.; O'brien, X.M.; Lessard, P.A.; Sinskey, A.J. Disparity between changes in mRNA abundance and enzyme activity in *Corynebacterium glutamicum*: Implications for DNA microarray analysis. *Appl. Microbiol. Biotechnol.* **2003**, *61*, 61–68. [CrossRef] [PubMed]
73. Ladero, V.; Linares, D.M.; Fernández, M.; Alvarez, M.A. Real time quantitative PCR detection of histamine-producing lactic acid bacteria in cheese: Relation with histamine content. *Food Res. Int.* **2008**, *41*, 1015–1019. [CrossRef]
74. Spano, G.; Russo, P.; Lonvaud-Funel, A.; Lucas, P.; Alexandre, H.; Grandvalet, C.; Coton, E.; Coton, M.; Barnavon, L.; Bach, B.; et al. Biogenic amines in fermented foods. *Eur. J. Clin. Nutr.* **2010**, *64*, S95–S100. [CrossRef]

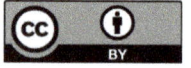

© 2020 by the authors. Licensee MDPI, Basel, Switzerland. This article is an open access article distributed under the terms and conditions of the Creative Commons Attribution (CC BY) license (http://creativecommons.org/licenses/by/4.0/).

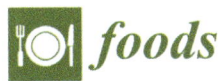

Article

Biogenic Amines, Phenolic, and Aroma-Related Compounds of Unroasted and Roasted Cocoa Beans with Different Origin

Umile Gianfranco Spizzirri [1], Francesca Ieri [2,*], Margherita Campo [2], Donatella Paolino [3], Donatella Restuccia [1] and Annalisa Romani [2]

1. Department of Pharmacy, Health and Nutritional Sciences, University of Calabria, I-87036 Rende (CS), Italy
2. Department of Statistic, Informatics and Applications "G. Parenti" (DiSIA)—University of Florence, Phytolab Laboratory, via Ugo Schiff 6, 50019 Sesto Fiorentino (FI), Italy
3. Department of Experimental and Clinical Medicine, University of Catanzaro "Magna Græcia", 88100 Catanzaro, Italy
* Correspondence: francesca.ieri@unifi.it; Tel.: +39-055-457-3676

Received: 27 June 2019; Accepted: 30 July 2019; Published: 1 August 2019

Abstract: Biogenic amines (BAs), polyphenols, and aroma compounds were determined by chromatographic techniques in cocoa beans of different geographical origin, also considering the effect of roasting (95, 110, and 125 °C). In all samples, methylxantines (2.22–12.3 mg kg^{-1}) were the most abundant followed by procyanidins (0.69–9.39 mg kg^{-1}) and epicatechin (0.16–3.12 mg kg^{-1}), all reduced by heat treatments. Volatile organic compounds and BAs showed variable levels and distributions. Although showing the highest BAs total content (28.8 mg kg^{-1}), Criollo variety presented a good aroma profile, suggesting a possible processing without roasting. Heat treatments influenced the aroma compounds especially for Nicaragua sample, increasing more than two-fold desirable aldehydes and pyrazines formed during the Maillard cascade and the Strecker degradation. As the temperature increased, the concentration of BAs already present in raw samples increased as well, although never reaching hazardous levels.

Keywords: cocoa nibs; roasting; bioactive amines; polyphenols; volatile organic compounds; geographical areas

1. Introduction

Cocoa beans represent the basic raw material in the production of chocolate and cocoa-based products. During processing, cocoa beans undergo important manipulations, including fermentation and roasting, which drastically influence the quality of the final product. During fermentation, cocoa beans are exposed to the action of various microorganisms and enzymes, while in the roasting process, high temperatures determine important modifications on the cocoa bean's composition [1].

Cocoa is a food rich in polyphenols, mainly flavonoids, procyanidins, and flavan-3-ols. The preservation or enhancement of cocoa procyanidins is of great importance since these compounds, despite their poor bioavailability, have been related to the health beneficial effects of cocoa, particularly in cardiovascular diseases [2]. Polyphenol and xanthine content in cocoa seeds changes during ripening and during the processing phases [3]. Microbial activity during fermentation and the drying process contribute to settling the amounts of theobromine and caffeine and their relative abundances, polyphenol amounts, in particular of catechin and epicatechin, and the amounts of organic acids, sugars, mannitol, ethanol, and alkaloids, thus influencing the quality and the biological properties of the finished product [4]. At the beginning of fermentation, during the first three days, the highest contents of total phenolic compounds and total anthocyanins prevailed in cocoa beans. Finally, at the end of cocoa beans fermentation, the lowest contents of total phenolic compounds, and total anthocyanins, were observed [5].

In addition, roasting temperature has been seen to have effects on the flavanols amounts causing losses and structural modifications, particularly epimerization of both monomers and polymers. At high roasting temperatures, a progressive loss of (−)-epicatechin and (+)-catechin and an increase in (−)-catechin were observed as a result of heat-related epimerization from (−)-epicatechin; additionally, a temperature-related epimerization of procyanidin dimers has been reported [6,7]. These structural modifications could have negative effects on the biological properties of the product, being (−)-epicatechin the most bioavailable isomer and (−)-catechin the one with the lowest bioavailability. Roasting processes may also cause reduction of the content of hydroxycynnamic compounds, clovamide in particular [8], with a possible further reduction of the antioxidant activity.

The secret of the flavor of chocolate, so highly appreciated worldwide, resides mainly in its volatile aromatic fraction. Its complex composition depends on the cocoa bean genotype and is the consequence of several processes [9,10]. To date, descriptive studies have identified >600 volatile compounds in cocoa and chocolate products [11,12], mainly pyrazines, esters, amines and amides, acids, and hydrocarbons. Besides cocoa flavor precursors, also toxic molecules, such as biogenic amines (BAs), can be produced during processing. BAs are a class of organic, basic, nitrogenous compounds with low molecular weight, are usually part of bioactive molecules of cocoa beans and derivatives. They mainly derived by decarboxylation of corresponding amino acids, due to the action of suitable enzymes widely distributed in spoilage bacteria and other microorganisms, as well as in naturally occurring and/or artificially added bacteria involved in food fermentation [5,13]. Although several amines (i.e., natural polyamines) are present in living cells and contribute to promoting many human physiological functions, these compounds can represent a serious health hazard for humans, when present in food in significant amounts or ingested in the presence of potentiating factors, such as amine oxidase-inhibiting drugs, alcohol, and gastrointestinal diseases. Then, their attendance in foodstuffs is often undesirable, because often associated with several of pathological syndromes, such as headaches, respiratory distress, heart palpitations, hypo- or hypertension and several allergenic disorders [14]. In particular, tyramine, β-phenylethylamine, and histamine have been considered as the initiators of hypertension and dietary-induced migraines, while the neurotransmitter serotonin is essential in the regulation of appetite, body temperature, and sleep [15].

Generally speaking, a variety of factors determining cocoa and cocoa derivatives quality are strongly related to the cocoa beans processing, from the opening of the fruit until the end of industrial processes [16]. In addition, qualitative characteristics of the cocoa beans are a consequence of the differences in the farming practices regarding growing, fermenting, and drying the cocoa beans, with significant differences sometimes found in samples from the same country [16,17].

Recently, it has been reported that in cocoa beans the amino acid oxidative decarboxylation can be also obtained during food processing suggesting a new chemical, heat-induced formation of BAs [18]. It follows that, in addition to the amino acid catabolism produced by microorganisms, amino acids can also be degraded chemically as a consequence of thermal treatment of foods [19]. These reactions are responsible for the formation of taste and flavor compounds, reducing, at the same time, the concentration of essential amino acids and contributing to the accumulation of compounds that may be dangerous for consumers, such as BAs [20]. It follows that two main reasons can be underlined accounting for the analysis of BAs in foods: first their potential toxicity; second the possibility of using them as food quality markers as their concentration can be related with the hygienic-sanitary quality of the process and with the freshness of the raw materials and the processed products. As BAs have been widely exploited as important indicators of safety and quality in a variety of foods, many papers appeared in recent years reporting their quantitative determination in many fermented and non-fermented foods, including cocoa and its derivatives [13].

In this work, the quantitative determination of biogenic amines, xanthine, and polyphenol molecules was performed by liquid chromatography (LC) techniques on cocoa beans from different origin. The aroma profile of cocoa nibs was investigated by headspace solid-phase micro-extraction (HS-SPME) combined with gas chromatography-mass spectrometry (GC-MS). Additionally, the same compounds were monitored after roasting process at different temperatures to establish a possible correlation between heating and different biomolecules profiles.

2. Materials and Methods

2.1. Samples

Seven cocoa beans samples from different world areas and years were considered as reported in Table 1. All fruits studied in this work were considered as well fermented. Approximately 500 g portions of Coviriali and O'Payo cocoa beans of uniform size were random selected from 50 kg of each nib variety peeled and roasted in a forced airflow-drying oven ROASTER CENTOVENTI vertiflow® system (Selmi Chocoloate Machinery, Cuneo, Italy) at Meraviglie S.r.l. (Verona, Italy). Applied in these studies, heat treatment parameters were chosen to obtain a range of roasted beans with acceptable physico-chemical and sensory properties. The parameters of thermal processing were optimized to avoid over-roasting, varying time of roasting as soon as bean cracking occurs, as follows: temperatures of 95, 110, and 125 °C for 60, 30, and 20 min respectively. Samples from all bean types were prepared using differentiated methods according to the analyses carried out as reported in the subsections of the experimental section.

Table 1. List of samples. ^{nr}not roasted; ^{r1}95 °C; ^{r2}110 °C; ^{r3}125 °C.

ID	Sample	Year	Variety	Country	Region
1^{nr}	CAMINO VERDE	2015	Nacional Forastero	Ecuador	Guayas
2^{nr}	MADAGASCAR	2015	Trinitario	Madagascar	Sambirano
3^{nr}	COVIRIALI	2015	Forastero	Peru	Junín
$4^{nr}, 4^{r1}, 4^{r2}, 4^{r3}$	COVIRIALI	2016	Forastero	Peru	Junín
5^{nr}	CHENI	2016	Forastero	Peru	Satipo
$6^{nr}, 6^{r1}, 6^{r2}$	O'PAYO	2016	Trinitario	Nicaragua	North Caribbean Coast Autonomous Region
7^{nr}	CRIOLLO	2016	Criollo	Indonesia	Bali

2.2. Chemicals

BAs spermine (SPM, tetrahydrochloride), spermidine (SPD, trihydrochloride), putrescine (PUT, dihydrochloride), histamine (HIM, dihydrochloride), tyramine (TYR, hydrochloride), β-phenylethylamine (PHE, hydrochloride), cadaverine (CAD, hydrochloride), as well as dansyl chloride, ammonia (30%), perchloric acid, and LC solvents (acetonitrile and methanol LC grade) were purchased from Sigma-Aldrich (Milford, MA, USA). Ultrapure water was obtained from Milli-Q System (Millipore Corp., Milford, MA, USA). Filters (0.45 and 0.20 µm) were purchased from Sigma-Aldrich. SPE C18 cartridges (0.5 g) were obtained from Supelco Inc. (Bellefonte, PA, USA). All GC chemicals were from Sigma-Aldrich (Milford, MA, USA). The HPLC grade standards (±)-catechin hydrate, theobromine, caffeic acid, quercetin-3-glucoside were purchased from Sigma-Aldrich (Milford, MA, USA).

2.3. Samples Preparation for the Analysis of Polyphenols and Xanthines

The peeled cocoa beans were crushed in a mortar, then 1.0 g accurately weighed of crushed material was extracted in 10.0 mL of a solution EtOH:H_2O 70:30 at pH 3.2 by addition of HCOOH, at room temperature, for 24 h under stirring. The solid material was removed by filtration under vacuum and the extracts analyzed by high performance liquid chromatography coupled with diode array detection and electrospray ionization mass spectrometer (HPLC-DAD-ESI-MS) and by high performance liquid chromatography coupled with diode array detection and fluorescence detector (HPLC-DAD-FLD).

2.4. Chromatographic Conditions Xanthine and Polyphenol Determination

The method used for the quali-quantitative analysis, and described below, was optimized according to literature data and previous studies of this research group about polyphenolic compounds and xanthines, and modifying them based on the specific results [8,21–23]. The analyses were performed using a HP-1200 Liquid Chromatograph with a DAD and a fluorescence detector and a HP-1100 MSD API Electrospray (Agilent Technologies, Palo Alto, CA, USA) operating in negative and positive ionization mode. Gas temperature was 350 °C, flow rate 10.0 L/min, nebulizer pressure 30 psi, quadrupole temperature 300 °C, capillary voltage 3500 V, and fragmentor 120 eV.

For the chromatographic separation a Luna C18 250 × 4.60 mm, 5 μm (Phenomenex, Torrance, CA, USA) column was used operating at 26 °C. A multistep linear solvent gradient starting from 95% H_2O at pH 3.2 by addition of HCOOH (A), up to 100% CH_3CN (B) was performed with a flow rate of 0.8 mL min^{-1} over a 63 min period. In detail, the applied gradient started with 95% A; from 95% A to 85% A in 20 min; isocratic elution 85% A until 30 min; from 85% A to 75% A in 9 min; isocratic elution 75% A until 47 min; from 75% A to 15% A in 2 min; isocratic elution 15% A until 53 min; from 15% A to 0% A in 2 min; 0% A until 60 min; from 0% A to the initial conditions in 3 min. Figure 1 reports on the chromatographic profile of raw O'Payo bean extract (2016) by DAD at 280 nm (A) and 330 nm (B) and FLD ex. 280 nm; em. 315 nm (C).

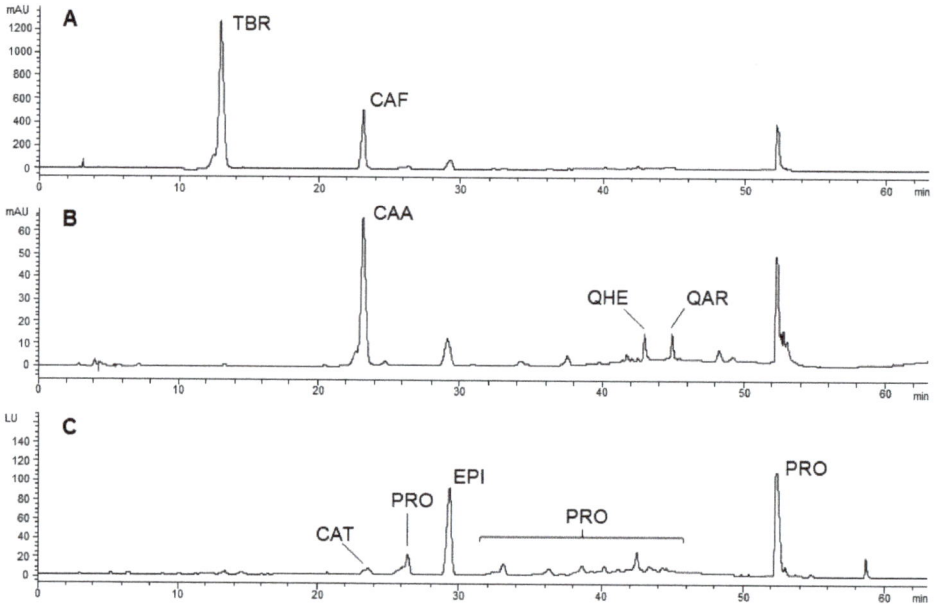

Figure 1. Chromatographic profile of raw O'Payo bean extract (2016): diode array detection (DAD) 280 nm (**A**) and 330 nm (**B**); fluorescence detector (FLD) ex. 280 nm; em. 315 nm (**C**). TBR—Theobromine; CAF—Caffeine; PRO—Procyanidins; CAA—Caffeoyl aspartic acid; QHE—Quercetin hexoside; QAR—Quercetin arabinoside; CAT—Catechin; EPI—Epicatechin.

2.5. Calibration

Quantitation of xanthines, flavonols, hydroxycinnamic derivatives, and procyaninides was performed by HPLC-DAD using five-point regression curves built with the available standards. Curves with an $r^2 > 0.9998$ were considered. Calibration was performed at the wavelength of the maximum UV-Vis absorbance, applying the correction of molecular weight. In particular, the extinction coefficient of each quantified compound being comparable to that of the specific standard used for its calibration, the weights in mg were calculated by multiplying the weight obtained from the calibration by a correction factor given by the ratio between the molecular weight of the compound and the molecular weight of the standard used for its calibration. In particular, xanthines were calibrated at 280 nm using theobromine as reference; procyanidins were calibrated at 280 nm using catechin hydrate as reference; hydroxycinnamic derivatives were calibrated at 330 nm using caffeic acid as reference; flavanols were calibrated at 350 nm using quercetin as reference. The quantitation of catechin and epicatechin was performed by HPLC-FLD, using a five point calibration curve ($r^2 = 0.9999$) built with standard solutions of catechin hydrate. The fluorescence detector was set as follows: excitation wavelength 280 nm; emission wavelength 315 nm [24].

2.6. HS-SPME-GC-MS Analyses

Headspace solid-phase micro-extraction combined with gas chromatography–mass spectrometry (HS-SPME-GC-MS) was selected as the most suitable technique to recover and analyze the Volatile Organic Compounds (VOCs) in peeled cocoa beans samples. Samples were ground and homogenous powders were obtained. A total of 1 g of the powdered sample, was placed into a 20-mL screw cap vial fitted with PTFE/silicone septa. An Internal Standard (IS) in suitable amount was added to each sample (IS: ethylacetate-D8; 1-Butanol-D10; ethyl hexanoate-D11; 5-methyl-hexanol; acetic acid-D3; Hexanoic acid-D11; 3,4-Dimethylphenol;). The Internal Standard was used for normalizing the analyte responses over the area of the IS, to minimize the instrumental error during the time of analysis.

After some trials aimed at optimizing amounts of sample, exposure time, and temperature, SPME conditions were set as follows: after 5 min of equilibration at 60 °C, VOCs were absorbed exposing a 1-cm divinilbenzene/carboxen/polydimethylsiloxane SPME fiber (DVB/CAR/PDMS by Supelco) for 15 min into the vial headspace under orbital shaking (500 rpm) and then immediately desorbed at 280 °C in a gas chromatograph injection port operating in split less mode. The chromatographic analysis was performed in a GC system coupled to quadrupole mass spectrometry using an Agilent 7890a GC equipped with a 5975C MSD (Agilent Technologies, Palo Alto, CA, USA). The separation of analytes was achieved by an Agilent DB InnoWAX column (length 50 m, id 0.20 µm, df 0.40 µm). Chromatographic conditions were: initial temperature 40 °C, then 10 °C min^{-1} up to 260 °C, hold for 6.6 min. Compounds were tentatively identified by comparing calculated Kovats retention index and mass spectra of each peak with those reported in mass spectral databases, namely the standard NIST08/Wiley98 libraries. Quadrupole MS operated in full-scan mode from which the specific ions of the analyte were extracted. Only the compounds with higher intensity were identified in order to select major compounds over a complex mixture of VOCs. Each sample was analyzed in triplicate.

2.7. Amine Standard Solutions and Calibration

A calibration curve was built starting from 1.0 mg mL^{-1} standard solution of each amine in purified water and preparing 12 BAs standard mixtures to a final volume of 25 mL employing HClO$_4$ 0.6 mol L^{-1}. Amine final concentrations were 0.1, 0.5, 0.8, 2.0, 4.0, 5.0, 10.0, 16.0, 25.0, 50.0, 75.0, and 100.0 µg mL^{-1}. The comparison between the retention times of peaks of samples and standard solutions allowed the identification of each BA. Standard concentration against peak area allowed to build a calibration plot, and six independent replicates for each concentration level were performed. Moreover, the matrix effect was evaluated by comparison of external calibration plots, depicting concentration of standard solutions versus peak area, with standard addition method plots, depicting peak area versus concentration of standard solutions added to the sample. No significant matrix effect was recorded because of the slopes of the two plots were not significantly different. Quantitative determination was then accomplished by direct interpolation in the external calibration plot of each BA. Chromatogram of a standard mixture of BAs is displayed in Figure 2A.

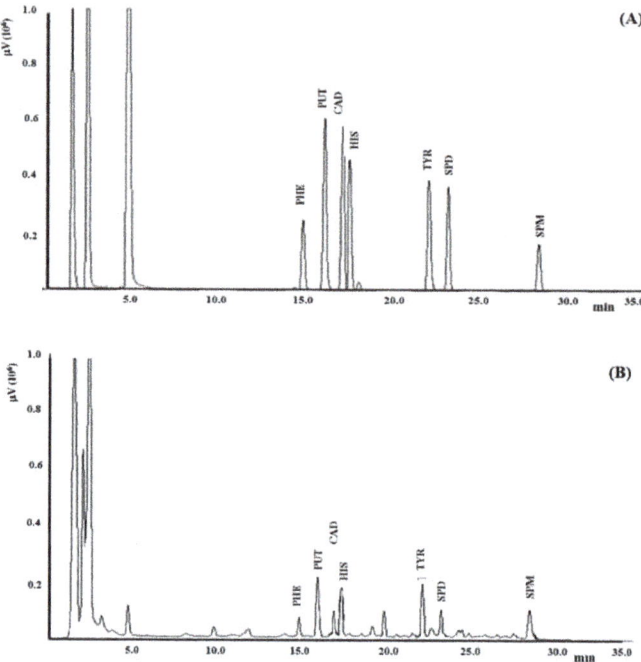

Figure 2. LC-UV chromatogram of biogenic amines (BAs) standard mixture at concentration of 100 µg mL^{-1} (**A**) and sample 1 (**B**). The chromatogram was obtained employing gradient conditions as specified in the Materials and Methods section.

2.8. BAs Extraction and Purification

The extraction of BAs from peeled cocoa beans samples was performed by adding 20 mL of HClO$_4$ 0.6 mol L^{-1} to about 5.0 g of grounded sample, in a 50.0 mL test tube. The mixture was homogenized (vortex at 40 Hz for 40 min), centrifuged (10,000× g for 20 min), filtered (syringe filter 0.20 µm), collected in a plastic vial and purified by SPE on a C$_{18}$ sorbent (conditioning: 2.0 mL of H$_2$O and 2.0 mL (two times) of CH$_3$OH; loading: 5.0 mL of the basified sample; washing: 2.0 mL of NH$_4$OH at pH 11.0; eluting: 2.0 mL (two times) of CH$_3$OH). Nitrogen gas was employed to dry eluting solution providing a solid residue that was re-dissolved in a plastic test tube with 1.3 mL of extraction solvent.

To perform recovery experiments sample 1 was spiked, before the extraction procedure, with an aliquot of standard mixture of BAs. Specifically, 5.0 g of peeled cocoa beans were spiked with 1.0 mL of 25.0 mg L^{-1} BAs standard solution. Method validation was obtained in terms of recovery percentages, linearity, intra- and inter-day repeatability, limits of quantification and limits of detection (LOQs and LODs), to confirm analytical suitability [25].

Dansylation reaction was performed by adding at 1.0 mL of standard solution (or acid sample extract spiked with BAs or acid sample extract) 200 µL of NaOH 2.0 mol L^{-1}, 300 µL of saturated NaHCO$_3$ solution and 2.0 mL of dansyl-chloride solution (10.0 mg mL^{-1} in acetone prepared just before use). After 30 min, dansyl-chloride in excess was removed with 100 µL of NH$_4$OH 25% (v/v) and the suspension filtered by a 0.45 µm syringe filters. Finally, 20 µL was injected for LC-UV analysis. Figure 2B shows a chromatogram of sample 1.

2.9. Chromatographic Conditions for BAs Quantification

Jasco PU-2080 instrument equipped with a Rheodyne 7725 injector with a 20 mL sample loop and a gradient pump (PU-2089 plus, Jasco Inc., Easton, MD, USA) was employed to obtain the chromatograms. The system was interfaced with an UV detector operating at λ = 254 nm (UV-2075, Jasco Inc., Easton, MD, USA). Data were collected and analyzed with an integrator Jasco-Borwin1. A reverse-phase C18 column (250 mm × 4.6 I.D., 5 mm) (Supelco Inc., Bellefonte, PA, USA) equipped with a C18 guard-pak (10 mm × 4.6 I.D., 5 mm) were used (Supelco Inc., Bellefonte, PA, USA) for separation of BAs. Two solvent reservoirs containing (A) purified water and (B) acetonitrile were used to separate all the BAs with a gradient elution which began with 3 min of isocratic program A-B 50:50 (v/v) reaching after 20 min A-B 10:90 (v/v). Then 3 min of isocratic elution was carried out and 4 min further where necessary to restore again the starting conditions (A-B 50:50, v/v). A constant flow at 1.2 mL min^{-1} was employed.

2.10. Statistical Analyses

All analyses were performed in triplicate and data were expressed as mean ± relative standard deviations (RSD). Studies of the correlation coefficient and linear regression, calculation of average, assessment of repeatability, standard deviation, and RSD were performed using Microsoft Excel 2010 software. Significance was performed using a one-way analysis of variance (ANOVA) test, employing Duncan's multiple range test at significance level $p < 0.05$.

3. Results and Discussion

3.1. Polyphenol Content in Cocoa Beans

To identify the phenolic compounds and xanthines, UV-Vis absorption spectra, mass spectra and literature data were used and combined for tentative identification of the analytes. In the present study, catechin and epicatechin were quantified through calibration by using a FLD detector, whereas oligomeric and polymeric procyanidins were quantified through DAD calibration. FLD calibration was used for catechin and epicatechin because of its higher sensibility and specificity, needed for catechin in particular, that often partially coelutes with caffeine, and is always present in low amounts with respect to this latter (average amount of catechin with respect to caffeine: 5.2% in the analyzed samples). In these conditions, the fact that both catechin and caffeine have also very similar wavelengths of maximum UV-Vis absorption hinders a correct quantification of the flavanol by using a DAD detector. Conversely, unlike caffeine, catechin and epicatechin emit a very intense fluorescence signal in the experimental conditions (excitation wavelength 280 nm; emission wavelength 315 nm), easily detectable and measurable also in presence of methylxanthines [24,26]. On the other hand, for the calibration of the other procyanidins a DAD detector is needed, because fluorescence detection is insensitive to procyanidins containing a gallic acid ester and/or gallocatechins as monomeric units [23]. In this case, the use of a fluorescence detector could lead to an underestimation of the total procyanidin content.

In Table 2 polyphenol distributions and total amounts in fermented, not-roasted cocoa beans of different origin are reported. Xanthines, theobromine in particular, are the most abundant compounds and their amounts decrease with increasing roasting temperature, after an initial slight increase by roasting at 95 °C, probably due to a further loss of water after the drying process.

Among the raw samples analyzed, the highest in polyphenols were 1^{nr} (Camino verde 2015), 3^{nr} (Coviriali 2015) and 6^{nr} (O'Payo 2016), respectively with 10.67, 10.53, and 12.96 mg g^{-1} total polyphenols. In all samples, it is possible to observe a clear predominance of epicatechin with respect to catechin; the highest [epicatechin]:[catechin] ratio (27.9) was found for the raw sample from Madagascar (2015), but its low content in polyphenols (1.44 mg g^{-1}) suggests a lower quality with respect to the other samples under study. The other two samples harvested in 2015 (Camino verde and Coviriali) appear not to contain catechin, so it was impossible to evaluate the ratio even though the epicatechin amount appears to be high in particular for the Camino verde sample (2.84 mg g^{-1}). The lowest [epicatechin]/[catechin] ratio was found for the raw samples Cheni and Criollo (5.0 for both the samples).

Table 2. HPLC/DAD quantitative analysis of methylxantines and polyphenols in cocoa nibs. Results in mg g^{-1} vegetal material. Data obtained from triplicate analysis with relative standard deviation (SD) 2–5%.

	1^{nr}	2^{nr}	3^{nr}	5^{nr}	7^{nr}	4^{nr}	4^{r1}	4^{r2}	4^{r3}	6^{nr}	6^{r1}	6^{r2}
Theobromine	8.65 ^{f}	1.95 ^{a}	7.81 ^{de}	7.69 ^{d}	7.61 ^{d}	8.49 ^{f}	8.52 ^{f}	7.68 ^{d}	7.14 ^{c}	8.08 ^{e}	10.08 ^{g}	6.68 ^{b}
Caffeine	2.01 ^{c}	0.27 ^{a}	1.89 ^{c}	1.70 ^{b}	0.96 ^{c}	3.81 ^{e}	2.81 ^{d}	2.18 ^{c}	1.60 ^{b}	2.60 ^{d}	2.04 ^{c}	2.03 ^{c}
Catechin	nd ^{a}	0.01 ^{b}	nd ^{a}	0.17 ^{g}	0.06 ^{c}	0.20 ^{h}	0.15 ^{f}	0.10 ^{d}	0.14 ^{f}	0.24 ^{i}	0.12 ^{e}	0.12 ^{e}
Epicatechin	2.84 ^{i}	0.16 ^{a}	0.84 ^{e}	0.87 ^{e}	0.32 ^{b}	1.98 ^{g}	1.08 ^{f}	0.58 ^{c}	0.73 ^{d}	3.12 ^{j}	2.22 ^{h}	0.69 ^{d}
Procyanidins	7.58 ^{h}	1.00 ^{b}	9.39 ^{j}	8.15 ^{i}	0.62 ^{a}	2.47 ^{f}	1.29 ^{d}	1.17 ^{c}	1.01 ^{b}	9.17 ^{j}	5.17 ^{g}	1.92 ^{e}
Quercetin hexoside	0.03 ^{c}	0.02 ^{b}	0.03 ^{c}	0.05 ^{d}	0.02 ^{b}	<LOQ ^{a}	0.07 ^{e}	0.05 ^{d}	0.05 ^{d}	0.03 ^{c}	0.05 ^{d}	0.02 ^{b}
Quercetin arabinoside	0.04 ^{e}	0.03 ^{d}	0.04 ^{e}	0.05 ^{f}	0.02 ^{c}	<LOQ ^{a}	0.09 ^{h}	0.06 ^{g}	0.06 ^{g}	0.05 ^{f}	0.10 ^{i}	0.01 ^{b}
Caffeoyl aspartic acid	0.12 ^{b}	0.13 ^{b}	0.24 ^{c}	<LOQ ^{a}	0.24 ^{c}	0.51 ^{h}	0.43 ^{g}	0.76 ^{i}	0.38 ^{f}	0.34 ^{e}	0.29 ^{d}	0.28 ^{d}
Hydroxycinnamic der.	0.06 ^{b}	0.09 ^{c}	nd ^{a}	nd ^{a}	nd ^{a}	nd ^{a}	nd ^{a}	nd ^{a}	nd ^{a}	nd ^{a}	nd ^{a}	nd ^{a}
N-caffeoyl-L-DOPA	<LOQ ^{a}	<LOQ ^{a}	<LOQ ^{a}	<LOQ ^{a}	<LOQ ^{a}	<LOQ ^{a}	<LOQ ^{a}	<LOQ ^{a}	<LOQ ^{a}	<LOQ ^{a}	<LOQ ^{a}	<LOQ ^{a}
Epicatechin:catechin ratio		27.9		5.0	5.0	9.7	7.0	6.0	5.3	12.9	18.7	5.9
Total xanthines	10.66 ^{d}	2.22 ^{a}	9.71 ^{c}	9.39 ^{c}	8.58 ^{b}	12.30 ^{f}	11.33 ^{e}	9.86 ^{c}	8.74 ^{b}	10.68 ^{d}	12.12 ^{f}	8.71 ^{b}
Total polyphenols	10.67 ^{i}	1.44 ^{b}	10.55 ^{i}	9.29 ^{h}	1.28 ^{a}	5.16 ^{f}	3.11 ^{d}	2.72 ^{d}	2.37 ^{c}	12.96 ^{j}	7.95 ^{g}	3.04 ^{e}

Different letters express significant differences ($p < 0.05$). ^{nr}not roasted; ^{r1}95 °C; ^{r2}110 °C; ^{r3}125 °C. nd means not detected and <LOQ means under limit of quantification.

For Coviriali 2016 and O'Payo 2016 beans it was possible to compare the polyphenols contents after roasting at 110 °C, confirming that the total amounts of polyphenols significantly decrease with respect to the raw samples; Coviriali beans were roasted also at a higher temperature (125 °C) with a further decreasing of total polyphenols. According to previously reported data [27,28], also [epicatechin]/[catechin] ratios follow the same trend depending on the roasting process at high temperature. Procyanidins, quantified as catechin equivalents, are the most abundant polyphenols in all samples and their amounts also appear to be negatively influenced by the roasting process [28]. Two flavonolic compounds were found, quercetin hexoside and quercetin arabinoside, in low amounts and apparently not depending on the roasting temperature. The only hydroxycynnamic derivative present in the extracts was caffeoyl aspartic acid [3].

The characteristics of cocoa beans and derived food products, such as hydrophilic and volatile secondary metabolites profile, organoleptic properties, antioxidant activity etc., depend not only on fermentation and processing methods, but also on several variables related to genetics, geographical regions of cultivation, agronomical practices, and climatic conditions [29,30]. In particular, concerning phenolic compounds, the low amount of total polyphenols (1.28 mg g^{-1}) found for Criollo variety is reliable based on literature data that identify this variety as the one with the lowest content of polyphenols [31,32]. The Forastero variety includes also Nacional Forastero that is the Forastero variety cultivated in northern Ecuador [31]. The analyzed Forastero samples were harvested in 2015 (Nacional Forastero from Ecuador, sample 1^{nr}, and Forastero from Junìn region, Peru, sample 3^{nr}) and 2016 (Forastero from Junìn region, sample 4^{nr}, and Forastero from Satipo region, Peru, sample 5^{nr}). For Forastero beans harvested in 2015, no significant difference was found between their contents of total polyphenols; interestingly, catechin was not detected in either of the two samples. Conversely, statistically significant differences were found between epicatechin and procyanidins contents. For Forastero beans harvested in 2016, total polyphenols are higher in the sample from Satipo region than in the one from Junìn region, but it must be taken into consideration that the total polyphenols content varies also according to climate variations, thus possibly from one year to another, as it can be seen for the two Junìn region samples of 2015 and 2016 (10.55 and 5.16 mg/g total polyphenols respectively). Moreover, a small difference was found between their contents of catechin, whereas the difference between epicatechin amounts is more evident. The differences between polyphenolic compositions are evident for the two samples of Trinitario variety from Sambirano region, Madagascar (sample 2^{nr}) and Bali, Indonesia (sample 6^{nr}). Sample 6^{nr}, not roasted, is the highest in polyphenols among all the samples analyzed in the present study (12.96 mg/g total polyphenols), and its polyphenols content consists mainly of procyanidins (9.17 mg/g). Sample 2^{nr} shows a consistently lower total polyphenols content (1.44 mg/g), of which 1.00 mg/g procyanidins remaining the most represented polyphenolic subclass. Monomeric flavanols are also higher in the sample from Indonesia, but the epicatechin/catechin ratio is better for the other sample (12.9 vs. 27.9). Again, it must be noted that the samples 2^{nr} and 6^{nr} differ not only concerning their geographical origins but also regarding the years of production (2015 and 2016).

3.2. VOCs in Cocoa Beans

After a successful fermentation process, it is necessary to reduce the water content of the cocoa seeds to between 5% and 8% and this is achieved by drying [33]. The drying process is not only important in preserving the cocoa seeds but also plays a very crucial role in the development of cocoa flavor and the overall quality of the raw cocoa seeds. Cocoa is dried to minimize the formation of molds and to reduce the acid level and astringency of the beans. Then the roasting of the cocoa seeds takes place in the consumer countries. Among the cacao beans analyzed, the 7^{nr} sample (Criollo) beans will be used by a chocolate maker that produces raw chocolate, so beans will be not roasted and never reach temperatures of more than 42 °C. Especially for this product, the quality of cocoa beans is a very big determinant of the final taste of the chocolate. Cocoa flavor resides in volatile fraction, which is composed of a complex mixture of up to 600 compounds with new research continuously increasing this number [12].

HS-SPME coupled to GC-MS has proven a valuable tool for analysis of volatile and semi-volatile compounds from cocoa and chocolate products. The technique is very sensitive to experimental conditions and in this study, the DVB/CAR-PDMS fiber was found to afford the most efficient extraction of both volatile and semi-volatile compounds from the analyte's headspace according to literature [34].

The HS-SPME-GC-MS analysis of raw cocoa seeds allowed the extraction of a complex mixture of VOCs and the compounds with higher intensity were selected and reported in Table 3. The key VOCs considered in this work belonged to the class of alcohols, aldehydes, esters, acids, ketones, pyrazines, and terpenes and they have all been previously reported in other works [12,34].

The main VOCs were associated with the aroma of vinegar (acetic acid) and with the aroma of roasted and nutty (tetramethyl-pyrazine). High level of acetic acid could influence in a negative way the final aroma of chocolate, moreover pyrazines were considered important contributors to the desirable chocolate aroma [12] and changed during roasting [35]. Additionally, the aldehydes 2-methylbutanal and 3-methylbutanal are reported to have a strong influence on the chocolate flavor [12]. Phenylethyl alcohol and 3-Methylbutyl acetate were considered key aroma compounds and were associated to the odor of floral, rose and sweet, fruity, banana, respectively. There were significant differences among the types of beans, in particular for the abovementioned VOCs (Table 3). The 2^{nr} (Madagascar) sample showed highest level of acetic acid and tetramethyl-pyrazine, instead of 1^{nr} (Camino Verde) showing the lowest values. O'Payo beans (sample 6^{nr}) showed highest levels of the aldehydes with chocolate and almond aroma, 2-methylbutanal, 3-methylbutanal and benzaldehyde. Cheni beans (sample 5^{nr}) showed highest level of banana flavor (3-Methylbutyl acetate) and Coviriali beans (sample 4^{nr}) the highest value of rose aroma (Phenylethyl alcohol).

The 7^{nr} sample (Criollo) showed a large number of VOCs, not reported in Table 3, as 2-Heptanol for the class of alcohols, as 2-Pentanol acetate for esters and as 2-Heptanone for ketones. The high variety of VOCs, the low level of acetic acid and the good quantity of pyrazines and aldehydes confirmed the high quality of this variety and the possible use without roasting to produce raw chocolate.

Forastero, Criollo, Trinitario, and Nacional, the variety grown in Ecuador, exhibit differences in flavor characteristics that can be attributed to original variety but also growing conditions and geographical origin [36]. The extent to which other factors such as climate and soil chemical compositions influence the formation of flavor precursors and their relationships with final flavor quality remains unclear [36]. Some authors have studied the influence of cocoa's origin on the composition in volatile compounds and profile comparison allowed beans, liquor, and chocolate from various geographical origins to be distinguished [29,37].

Trinitario samples from Madagascar (2^{nr}) and Nicaragua (6^{nr}) exhibited high differences in many of key VOCs considered and also Forastero samples from different areas of Peru, 4^{nr} and 5^{nr}, showed significant differences in volatile composition.

Cocoa beans underwent the roasting process by means of a dry heat treatment, changing chocolate flavor. Flavor precursors developed during fermentation interact in the roasting process. Aldehydes and pyrazines are among the major compounds formed during roasting. They are formed through the heat induced Maillard reaction and Strecker degradation of amino acids and sugars [35]. The roasting process not only generated and increased the concentration of some flavor compounds through pyrolysis of sugars, but also reduced the amount of minor compounds affecting the final quality of chocolate [38]. The degree of chemical changes depends on the temperature applied during the process [38]. The HS-SPME-GC-MS analysis of roasted beans confirmed changes in VOCs during roasting as the decrease of acetic acid, especially in samples 4 where a higher level was present, and the increase of pyrazines in both samples (Table 3). Additionally, 3-methylbutanal increased with roasting, especially at 95 and 110 °C, while at 125 °C there was a return to initial values, due to the prevalence of the volatilization phenomenon compared to the production one. The loss of minor compounds that influence the chocolate's aroma as phenylethyl alcohol and benzaldehyde was observed by increasing the roasting temperature, in particular at 125 °C.

Table 3. Key aroma volatiles in raw samples and in roasted samples together with their odor descriptors, normalized peak area from Q (quantitation)-ion, and Internal Standard (IS). Data obtained from triplicate analysis with SD < 5%.

Odor Descriptor	Compound Name	1[nr]	2[nr]	4[nr]	5[nr]	6[nr]	7[nr]	4[r1]	4[r2]	4[r3]	6[r1]	6[r2]
	Alcohols											
Fruity, creamy, buttery	2,3-Butanediol	0.03 [b]	0.36 [c]	0.63 [e]	1.31 [f]	3.96 [h]	nd [a]	0.44 [d]	0.45 [d]	0.37 [c]	3.22 [g]	7.76 [i]
floral, rose	Phenylethyl alcohol	34.98 [e]	16.39 [b]	72.20 [i]	5.20 [a]	42.72 [f]	23.03 [c]	77.84 [j]	128.69 [k]	48.64 [h]	45.33 [g]	27.08 [d]
	Aldehydes											
Aldehydic, chocolate	2-methyl-Butanal	nd [a]	nd [a]	nd [a]	0.003 [b]	0.01 [c]	0.003 [b]	nd [a]	nd [a]	nd [a]	0.01 [c]	0.01 [c]
aldehydic, chocolate	3-methyl-Butanal	0.02 [b]	0.01 [a]	0.02 [b]	0.01 [a]	0.05 [e]	0.03 [c]	0.03 [c]	0.04 [d]	0.02 [b]	0.13 [f]	0.13 [f]
sweet, bitter, almond, cherry	Benzaldehyde	16.24 [g]	4.30 [b]	12.25 [d]	1.61 [a]	46.55 [k]	12.98 [e]	15.28 [f]	26.92 [j]	10.23 [c]	33.36 [i]	22.69 [h]
	Esters											
Sweet, fruity, banana	3-Methylbutyl acetate	3.46 [a]	15.96 [h]	7.61 [e]	23.13 [j]	6.54 [c]	17.85 [i]	9.63 [g]	9.38 [f]	4.53 [b]	7.64 [e]	6.96 [d]
floral, rose, honey, tropical	Acetic acid, 2-phenylethyl ester	3.38 [b]	5.96 [c]	22.19 [i]	2.46 [a]	10.54 [d]	13.80 [f]	17.02 [g]	41.48 [j]	18.03 [h]	11.39 [e]	10.69 [d]
	2,3-Butanediol diacetate	0.04 [b]	1.39 [i]	0.44 [f]	1.46 [k]	0.26 [c]	nd [a]	0.38 [e]	0.42 [f]	0.74 [h]	0.32 [d]	0.62 [g]
	Acids											
Acidic	2-methyl-Propanoic acid	0.17 [e]	0.07 [b]	0.16 [e]	0.26 [f]	0.38 [i]	0.30 [g]	0.09 [c]	0.06 [a]	0.15 [d]	0.36 [h]	0.32 [g]
Cheese, pungent, fruity	3-methyl-Butanoic acid	0.31 [f]	0.11 [b]	0.22 [d]	0.27 [e]	0.50 [i]	0.45 [h]	0.13 [c]	0.10 [a]	0.22 [d]	0.45 [h]	0.40 [g]
vinegar	Acetic acid	4.39 [a]	14.32 [j]	12.01 [i]	7.85 [f]	7.32 [e]	7.94 [fg]	6.18 [c]	5.23 [b]	8.06 [h]	6.50 [d]	8.01 [g]
fatty, sweat, cheese	Hexanoic acid	nd [a]	0.36 [e]	0.73 [f]	0.09 [b]	0.26 [c]	nd [a]	0.36 [e]	0.38 [e]	0.09 [b]	0.25 [c]	0.30 [d]
	4-hydroxy-Butanoic acid	0.04 [c]	0.03 [b]	0.06 [d]	0.02 [a]	0.02 [a]	0.03 [b]	0.02 [a]	0.02 [a]	0.03 [ab]	0.02 [a]	0.02 [a]
	Ketones											
Sweet, pungent, caramel	2,3-Butanedione	0.02 [a]	0.53 [h]	0.09 [d]	0.08 [c]	0.17 [g]	0.04 [b]	0.08 [c]	0.04 [b]	0.08 [cd]	0.15 [f]	0.13 [e]
buttery, milky, fatty	3-hydroxy-2-Butanone	0.20 [a]	1.76 [g]	1.40 [e]	1.52 [f]	2.39 [i]	0.45 [b]	1.38 [e]	0.92 [c]	1.31 [d]	3.22 [k]	1.91 [h]
Sweet, pungent, mimosa, almond	Acetophenone	0.68 [c]	0.58 [b]	1.04 [e]	0.08 [a]	3.46 [h]	0.61 [b]	0.83 [d]	1.01 [e]	0.69 [c]	2.69 [g]	1.27 [f]
musty, nutty, coumarin	2-acetylpyrrole	0.04 [a]	0.40 [b]	0.10 [b]	0.09 [b]	0.17 [c]	0.53 [e]	0.57 [f]	1.10 [h]	0.62 [g]	1.58 [h]	1.45 [i]
	Pyrazines											
Nutty, cocoa, roasted, peanut	Trimethyl-Pyrazine	0.36 [a]	4.63 [i]	1.64 [c]	1.83 [d]	1.57 [b]	2.29 [e]	2.37 [f]	2.62 [g]	3.28 [h]	7.67 [k]	7.60 [j]
Nutty, cocoa, peanut-like	Tetramethyl-Pyrazine	0.78 [a]	76.59 [k]	31.99 [g]	38.88 [h]	22.90 [d]	18.78 [b]	28.25 [f]	19.54 [c]	40.39 [i]	58.60 [j]	28.08 [e]
	Terpenes											
Citrus	Limonene	0.16 [e]	nd [a]	0.03 [c]	0.02 [b]	Nd [a]	0.05 [d]	0.02 [b]	0.02 [b]	0.02 [b]	nd [a]	nd [a]

Different letters express significant differences ($p < 0.05$). nd means not detected. [nr] not roasted; [r1] 95 °C; [r2] 110 °C; [r3] 125 °C.

3.3. BAs in Cocoa Beans

It can be assumed that, prior to roasting, the bacterial decarboxilation of the amino acids plays the main role in the BAs production in fresh cocoa beans. In fact, during fermentation, cocoa proteins can be hydrolyzed by microorganisms to release free amino acids, although their total amount can considerably vary [39]. Usually, low amounts of total free amino acids, mostly acidic, were detected in the unfermented seeds. It has been shown that after fermentation, acidic free amino acids decreased, while total free amino acids, as well as hydrophobic free amino acids, increased [40]. The latter aspect seems to be related to the characteristics of the aspartic endoprotease and the carboxypeptidase present in cocoa beans, as the first preferentially attacks hydrophobic amino acids of the storage proteins and the second releases single hydrophobic amino acids [40]. Considering the different optimal temperature and pH of these enzymes, proteolysis primarily depends on the fermentation conditions: duration and intensity of acidification, temperature, and aeration [39]. Once free amino acids are released, they can undergo decarboxylase activity by some bacterial enzymes to form amines [41]. Microbiota evolution during cocoa bean fermentation has been studied extensively, also owing to its importance in the formation of the precursor compounds of the cocoa flavor [42]. It was found that yeasts, filamentous fungi, lactic and acetic acid bacteria as well as members of the genus Bacillus, are typically present, all of them being able to produce BAs [43]. As a consequence of the protection mechanism of bacteria against the acid medium, decarboxylase activity is favored by low pH values during fermentation [44]. Moreover, contaminating bacteria can also decarboxylate amino acids to support a further accumulation of BAs.

In Table 4 BA distributions and total amounts in fermented, not-roasted cocoa beans of different origin are reported. Quantities of total BAs ranged from 13 mg kg^{-1} in sample 3a to 28.8 mg kg^{-1} in sample 7^{nr}, never reaching hazardous concentrations. Total BAs concentrations collected in Table 4 are in agreement with a recent study, who recorded the evolution of BAs in fresh cocoa beans over a fermentation period of seven days, reaching a maximum level of 39.6 mg kg^{-1} at the fourth day of fermentation [5]. On the contrary, considering samples of the same geographical origin, Oracz and Nebesny (2014) reported for raw cocoa beans from Ecuador and Indonesia, much lower total BAs content, not exceeding 5.0 and 6.0 mg kg^{-1}, respectively. However, only five BAs were considered in this study, neglecting natural polyamines PUT, SPM, and SPD, as well as, HIS and CAD, representing in our study the most abundant compounds [44].

As can be seen from data in Table 4 some variations are present, depending on the sample. This is not surprising, as it was already underlined that, when analyzing samples of cocoa beans from different countries, several attributes can be very different [45]. In fact, wide variations have been obtained considering cocoa beans coming from big producing countries, much more emphasized in samples obtained from smaller producing countries. Moreover, differences were not only country-dependent, but also farmer-dependent, as significant discrepancies were found in quality attributes of cocoa beans from the same country [39]. To this regard, it is noteworthy that samples 3^{nr} and 4^{nr} were collected from the same farm but harvested respectively in 2015 (sample 3^{nr}) and 2016 (sample 4^{nr}). As it can be seen, BAs profiles and concentrations did not significantly differ, implying a high degree of farming standardization.

Table 4. Biogenic amines (BAs) in fermented and roasted cocoa beans samples. Results in mg kg^{-1} vegetal material.

BAs	1^{nr}	2^{nr}	3^{nr}	4^{nr}	4^{r1}	4^{r2}	4^{r3}	5^{nr}	6^{nr}	6^{r1}	6^{r2}	7^{nr}
PHE	1.1 ± 0.1 ^{bc}	nd ^{a}	nd ^{a}	nd ^{a}	nd ^{a}	nd ^{a}	1.3 ± 0.2 ^{cd}	1.5 ± 0.1 ^{d}	1.0 ± 0.1 ^{b}	1.5 ± 0.1 ^{d}	2.1 ± 0.1 ^{e}	nd ^{a}
PUT	3.4 ± 0.2 ^{d}	1.5 ± 0.1 ^{a}	2.5 ± 0.1 ^{bc}	2.6 ± 0.1 ^{c}	4.0 ± 0.1 ^{e}	5.6 ± 0.2 ^{g}	7.3 ± 0.2 ^{h}	2.4 ± 0.1 ^{b}	1.5 ± 0.1 ^{a}	4.5 ± 0.2 ^{f}	10.9 ± 0.3 ^{i}	1.5 ± 0.1 ^{a}
CAD	1.8 ± 0.1 ^{c}	1.1 ± 0.1 ^{a}	1.3 ± 0.1 ^{b}	1.3 ± 0.1 ^{b}	1.8 ± 0.1 ^{c}	2.0 ± 0.1 ^{d}	2.1 ± 0.2 ^{d}	1.2 ± 0.1 ^{ab}	1.1 ± 0.1 ^{a}	1.9 ± 0.1 ^{cd}	2.6 ± 0.2 ^{f}	2.1 ± 0.1 ^{e}
HIS	4.1 ± 0.1 ^{c}	5.3 ± 0.2 ^{d}	3.5 ± 0.1 ^{b}	3.1 ± 0.1 ^{a}	8.1 ± 0.2 ^{f}	10.0 ± 0.3 ^{g}	10.3 ± 0.2 ^{g}	3.5 ± 0.1 ^{b}	5.6 ± 0.2 ^{de}	10.0 ± 0.2 ^{g}	12.8 ± 0.3 ^{h}	5.9 ± 0.2 ^{e}
TYR	4.9 ± 0.2 ^{d}	1.8 ± 0.1 ^{b}	nd ^{a}	nd ^{a}	nd ^{a}	6.7 ± 0.2 ^{e}	7.3 ± 0.2 ^{f}	4.9 ± 0.2 ^{d}	4.3 ± 0.1 ^{c}	10.8 ± 0.3 ^{g}	11.1 ± 0.3 ^{g}	4.8 ± 0.1 ^{d}
SPD	1.3 ± 0.1 ^{b}	nd ^{a}	nd ^{a}	nd ^{a}	nd ^{a}	nd ^{a}	nd ^{a}	1.9 ± 0.1 ^{c}	6.7 ± 0.2 ^{d}	9.1 ± 0.2 ^{f}	9.7 ± 0.2 ^{g}	7.3 ± 0.2 ^{e}
SPM	5.8 ± 0.2 ^{c}	4.5 ± 0.1 ^{b}	5.9 ± 0.2 ^{c}	6.0 ± 0.1 ^{c}	6.5 ± 0.2 ^{d}	6.5 ± 0.2 ^{d}	7.3 ± 0.2 ^{e}	3.5 ± 0.1 ^{a}	6.1 ± 0.2 ^{cd}	8.8 ± 0.2 ^{f}	9.1 ± 0.2 ^{f}	7.2 ± 0.2 ^{e}
Total	22.4 ± 0.2 ^{e}	14.2 ± 0.2 ^{b}	13.2 ± 0.4 ^{a}	12.9 ± 0.1 ^{a}	20.5 ± 0.2 ^{d}	30.9 ± 0.8 ^{h}	35.6 ± 0.5 ^{i}	18.9 ± 0.1 ^{c}	26.3 ± 0.2 ^{f}	46.6 ± 0.7 ^{j}	58.3 ± 0.3 ^{k}	28.8 ± 0.4 ^{g}

The values are expressed as means ± SD of three independent experiments. Different letters express significant differences ($p < 0.05$). nd means not detected or below limit of quantitation. ^{nr}not roasted; ^{r1}95 °C; ^{r2}110 °C; ^{r3}125 °C. PHE—β-phenylethylamine, PUT—putrescine, CAD—cadaverine, HIS—histamine, TYR—tyramine, SPD—spermidine, SPM—spermine.

Considering BAs profiles, the data obtained in this study clearly showed that BAs present in all samples at higher concentrations were SPM (3.5–7.2 mg kg^{-1}), HIS (3.1–5.3 mg kg^{-1}), PUT (1.5–3.4 mg kg^{-1}), and CAD (1.1–2.1 mg kg^{-1}), while TYR (not detected (nd)–4.9 mg kg^{-1}), SPD (nd–7.3 mg kg^{-1}) and PHE (nd–1.5 mg kg^{-1}) were present more rarely and at variable concentrations. The presence of natural polyamines in the cocoa beans is expected since they are ubiquitous in plants and all living organisms. It is also known the ability of the bacteria to produce some amines, e.g., TYR, as a protection against the acidic environment, while low levels of PHE in cocoa and derivatives seem to be associated with their aphrodisiac effects and mood lifting [46]. Guillen-Casla et al. (2012) [20] reported that TYR, PHE, serotonin, and HIS were the main amines in cocoa beans, although also PUT, dopamine, and ethanolamine have also been determined. Comparison among samples of same geographical origin (samples 1 and 7), displayed comparable (Ecuador) or higher (Indonesia) amounts of PHE, while our samples always showed much higher concentration of TYR for both raw cocoa beans [44]. In addition, do Carmo Brito et al. (2017) [5] found different results. Only tryptamine, TYR, SPD, and SPM were present during fermentation of fresh cocoa beans, while CAD and PUT where always undetectable in all the analyzed samples. SPD and SPM concentrations increased from the beginning to the end of fermentation, while TYR reached its maximum level at the fourth day of fermentation, decreasing afterward to initial contents [5].

It can be concluded that the differences already recorded for total BAs concentrations are much more evident when considering BAs profiles. This is a very common situation already underlined for many other foods supporting BAs accumulation. Considering that the aminogenesis takes origin from multiple and complex variables, all of which interact, a direct overlapping of the data arising from different studies (or from different samples of the same study, if they are not produced in the same way) is generally difficult to accomplish. Many parameters concerning either the hygienic conditions of the raw materials or the production process, as well as the preservation techniques, influence BAs levels and distributions [5,16,44].

In Table 4 the evolution of BAs concentration evaluated for sample 4^{nr} and 6^{nr} at different roasting temperatures (95, 110 and 125 °C samples 4^{r1}, 4^{r2}, 4^{r3} and 95 and 110 °C for sample 6^{r1}, 6^{r2}) is reported. As can be seen, the roasting temperature is strictly related to the amine total amount, reaching for sample 6^b the maximum level of 58.3 mg kg^{-1}, in agreement with Oracz and Nebesny (2014) [44]. They underlined that temperature and relative humidity of air during roasting influenced the BAs concentrations and profiles a lot. As can be noted from Table 4, sample 6^{nr} contained all the considered amine before roasting. Each amine concentration raised after processing, although to a different extent. In particular, PUT concentration showed the highest increasing factor (7.3) followed by TYR, CAD, HIS, PHE amounts with increasing factors between 2.1 and 2.6. SPD and SPM contents recorded the lowest enhancing, both with an increasing factor of 1.5. Although, with different profiles and distributions in comparison with Oracz and Nebesny (2014) [44], data obtained in our study confirmed the influence of the thermal processing on the increase of BAs concentrations in cocoa beans. This effect has been related to the transformation of free amino acids caused by the treatment at high temperature. In fact, it is now well established that during the Strecker degradation, the thermal decarboxylation of amino acids can occur in the presence of α-dicarbonyl compounds formed during the Maillard reaction or lipid peroxidation [19]. To this regard, literature data confirmed that asparagine, phenylalanine, and histidine changed in the corresponding amines 3-aminopropionamide, PHE, and HIS either in cocoa or in model systems [47].

As far as samples 4^{nr}-^{r3} are concerned, the impact of temperature on BAs concentrations during roasting showed a different behavior. Once again, all the amines exhibited higher quantities at the end of the thermal treatment mainly HIS (increasing factor 3.3) and PUT (increasing factor 2.8), followed by CAD (increasing factor 1.6) and SPM (increasing factor 1.3). To this regard, Hidalgo et al. (2013) [47] reported that the thermal degradation of histidine was more easily produced in comparison with that of phenylalanine. This effect could explain the higher increasing factors of HIS set against with those of PHE, for both samples series 6^{nr}-^{r2} and 4^{nr}-^{r3}.

As can be seen in Table 4, before roasting, sample 4^{nr} did not contain TYR and PHE, both appearing respectively only after a thermal treatment at 110 and 125 °C, supporting the idea that PHE is generated mainly by thermal decarboxylation of phenylalanine and not by biochemical reactions [44]. Additionally, in the case of TYR, traces of this compound, absent in green coffee (Rio quality), were detected in roasted samples after 16 min at 220 °C [48], thus demonstrating its "thermogenic" formation.

The different situations underlined by data in Table 4 probably depend on the complexity of the heat-induced formation of BAs. In fact, amines and amino acid-derived Strecker aldehydes, are simultaneously produced in food products during roasting, due to parallel pathways through the same key intermediates. Reactive carbonyl compounds started these degradations and the ratio between both aldehydes and amines generated is related to the carbonyl compound involved in the reaction and the experimental conditions, including amount of oxygen, pH, temperature, time, as well as the presence of other compounds such as antioxidants or amino acids [19]. In particular, additional amino acids were shown to play an important role in the preferential formation of either Strecker aldehydes or amino acid-derived amines by amino acid degradation in the presence of reactive carbonyl compounds. In this sense, the formation of PHE and phenylacetaldehyde in mixtures of phenylalanine, a lipid oxidation product, and a second amino acid was studied to determine the role of the second amino acid in the degradation of phenylalanine produced by lipid-derived reactive carbonyls. The presence of the second amino acid usually increased the formation of the amine and reduced the formation of the Strecker aldehyde to a differ extent depending on the considered amino acid [19]. The reasons for this behavior are not fully understood, although the obtained results suggested that they seem to be related to the other functional groups (mainly amino or similar groups) present in the side chains of the amino acid. To this regard, the limited aldehydes concentrations, especially at 125 °C (Table 3), could support this hypothesis.

Finally, the effect of antioxidants on BAs formation during roasting should be also considered. To this regard, the effect of the presence of phenolic compounds [49] on the degradation of phenylalanine, initiated by lipid-derived carbonyls was studied, to determine the structure-activity relationship of phenolics on the protection of amino compounds against modifications produced by carbonyl compounds. The obtained results showed that, among the different phenolic compounds assayed, the most efficient phenolic compounds were flavan-3-ols followed by single m-diphenols. The efficiency of these molecules was dependent on their ability to rapidly trap the carbonyl compounds. In this way the reaction of the carbonyl compound with the amino acid was avoided. This implies that the carbonyl-phenol reactions involving lipid-derived reactive carbonyls can be produced more rapidly than carbonyl-amine reactions, supporting the idea that antioxidants can provide a protection of amino compounds during thermal treatments of cocoa beans. In this sense, the loss of flavan-3-ols as the roasting temperature increased (Table 2) might be responsible of the limited BAs accumulation in the roasted cocoa beans.

4. Conclusions

Many classes of compounds present in cocoa nibs can be evaluated as indicators of quality and safety of raw materials and consequently of the final products.

In particular, along with a high [epicatechin]/[catechin] ratio, indicating a better bioavailability of flavanols, a high content on polyphenols could be considered as a favorable attribute of cocoa beans. This is related either to the health qualities of these compounds or to their capacity of preserving other compounds from chemical oxidation or enzymatic degradation, thus increasing stability and general characteristics of the product. According with the obtained results and taking into consideration that cocoa beans used for producing chocolate are usually roasted, the sample 6^{nr} (O'Payo 2016) appears to be the one with the best quality, showing a good content in polyphenols also after roasting at 110 °C (12.96 mg g^{-1} raw sample vs. 3.04 mg g^{-1} roasted sample). On the contrary, although showing the highest [epicatechin]:[catechin] ratio (27.9), the sample 2^{nr} seems to possess a lower quality among considered samples, in relation to its low polyphenols content (1.44 mg g^{-1}).

The monitoring of the volatile aromatic fraction, as reported for the not volatile one, suggested the same conclusions. Sample 2^{nr}, showed lower quality having high levels of acids that influence, in a negative way, the final aroma of chocolate. Besides, among the analyzed raw samples, low level of acetic acid and the highest levels of the aldehydes with chocolate and almond aroma confirmed the high quality of sample 6^{nr} (O'Payo 2016), as described from polyphenols analysis. The analysis of roasted beans confirmed changes in VOCs during roasting, as the decrease of acetic acid, especially in sample 6, and the increase of pyrazines associated with the nutty, cocoa, peanut-like aroma. The roasting temperature at 125 °C seemed to cause a loss of some minor compounds involved in the aroma of chocolate such as alcohols, aldehydes, and esters, resulting therefore excessive for the tested variety.

Considering BAs as cocoa quality markers as well, their total levels seem to indicate an opposite trend in comparison to that underlined by polyphenols and aroma compounds. In fact, among raw cocoa nibs, sample 6^{nr} showed the second higher BAs total concentration, indicating a medium quality among considered samples. However, it should be underlined that, after roasting at 110 °C, amine total amounts showed an increasing factor of 2.22 (6^{nr} vs. 6^{r2}) and of 2.37 (4^{nr} vs. 4^{r2}) implying, among the analyzed samples, a lower attitude of sample 6^{nr} to form amines during heat treatment. Anyway, from the food safety point of view, not alarming BAs amounts were found in all samples, both raw and roasted. All BAs concentrations increased after roasting, although to a different extent depending on the sample and on the considered amine. The latter aspect supports the idea that heat induced amines formation/accumulation probably during the Strecker degradation where aldehydes and amines compete to be formed, and at the same time BAs accumulation was lowered by the polyphenols intervention.

Author Contributions: Conceptualization, A.R. and D.R.; Methodology, U.G.S., F.I., M.C., D.R. and A.R.; Software, U.G.S., F.I. and M.C.; Validation, U.G.S., F.I. and M.C.; Formal Analysis, U.G.S., F.I., M.C. and D.P.; Investigation, U.G.S., F.I., M.C. and D.P.; Resources, U.G.S., F.I., M.C., D.R. and A.R.; Data Curation, U.G.S., F.I., M.C. and D.P.; Writing—Original Draft Preparation, U.G.S., F.I., M.C., D.R. and A.R.; Writing—Review and Editing, U.G.S., F.I., M.C., D.R. and A.R.; Visualization, U.G.S., F.I. and M.C.; Supervision, A.R., D.R.; Project Administration, A.R.; Funding Acquisition, A.R.

Funding: This research received no external funding

Acknowledgments: We thank Giorgio Sergio of Meraviglie S.r.l., Sommacampagna (VR), Italy for supplying us with cocoa beans and technical support and we thank Sixtus (BANDO A—POR CREO FESR 2014–2020. Linea 1.1.2) and project BIOSINOL—PSR 2014–2200 for financial support.

Conflicts of Interest: The authors declare no conflict of interest.

References

1. Schwan, R.F.; Wheals, A.E. The microbiology of cocoa fermentation and its role in chocolate quality. *Crit. Rev. Food Sci. Nutr.* **2004**, *44*, 205–221. [CrossRef] [PubMed]
2. Ding, E.L.; Hutfless, S.M.; Ding, X.; Girotra, S. Chocolate prevention of cardiovascular disease: A systematic review. *Nutr. Metab.* **2006**, *3*, 1–12. [CrossRef] [PubMed]
3. Pereira-Caro, G.; Borges, G.; Nagai, C.; Jackson, M.C.; Yokota, T.; Crozier, A.; Ashihara, H. Profiles of Phenolic Compounds and Purine Alkaloids during the Development of Seeds of *Theobroma cacao* cv. Trinitario. *J. Agric. Food Chem.* **2013**, *61*, 427–434. [CrossRef] [PubMed]
4. Camu, N.; De Winter, T.; Addo, S.K.; Takrama, J.S.; Bernaert, H.; De Vuyst, L. Fermentation of cocoa beans: Influence of microbial activities and polyphenol concentrations on the flavour of chocolate. *J. Sci. Food Agric.* **2008**, *88*, 2288–2297. [CrossRef]
5. do Carmo Brito, B.D.N.; Campos Chisté, R.; da Silva Pena, R.; Abreu Gloria, M.B.; Santos Lopes, A. Bioactive amines and phenolic compounds in cocoa beans are affected by fermentation. *Food Chem.* **2017**, *228*, 484–490. [CrossRef] [PubMed]
6. Hurst, W.J.; Krake, S.H.; Bergmeier, S.C.; Payne, M.J.; Miller, K.B.; Stuart, D.A. Impact of fermentation, drying, roasting and Dutch processing on flavan-3-ol stereochemistry in cacao beans and cocoa ingredients. *Chem. Cent. J.* **2011**, *5*, 53–62. [CrossRef]

7. Kothe, L.; Zimmermann, B.F.; Galensa, R. Temperature influences epimerization and composition of flavanol monomers, dimers and trimers during cocoa bean roasting. *Food Chem.* **2013**, *141*, 3656–3663. [CrossRef]
8. Arlorio, M.; Locatelli, M.; Travaglia, F.; Coïsson, J.D.; Del Grosso, E.; Minassi, A.; Appendino, G.; Martelli, A. Roasting impact on the contents of clovamide (N-caffeoyl-L-DOPA) and the antioxidant activity of cocoa beans (*Theobroma cacao* L.). *Food Chem.* **2008**, *106*, 967–975. [CrossRef]
9. Bailey, S.; Mitchell, D.; Bazinet, M.; Weurman, C. Studies of the volatile components of different varieties of cocoa beans. *J. Food Sci.* **1962**, *27*, 165–170. [CrossRef]
10. Clapperton, J.; Yow, S.; Chan, J.; Lim, D.; Lockwood, R.; Romanczyk, L.; Hammerstone, J. The contribution of genotype to cocoa (*Theobroma cacao* L.) flavour. *Trop. Agric.* **1994**, *71*, 303–308.
11. Van der Wals, B.; Kettenes, D.; Stoffelsma, J.; Sipma, G.; Semper, A. New volatile components of roasted cocoa. *J. Agric. Food Chem.* **1971**, *19*, 276–280.
12. Counet, C.; Callemien, D.; Ouwerx, C.; Collin, S. Use of gas chromatography-olfactometry to identify key odorant compounds in dark chocolate: Comparison of samples before and after conching. *J. Agric. Food Chem.* **2002**, *50*, 2385–2391. [CrossRef] [PubMed]
13. Restuccia, D.; Spizzirri, U.G.; Puoci, F.; Picci, N. Determination of biogenic amine profiles in conventional and organic cocoa-based products. *Food Addit. Contam. Part A Chem. Anal. Control Expo. Risk Assess.* **2015**, *32*, 1156–1163. [CrossRef] [PubMed]
14. Jairath, G.; Singh, P.K.; Dabur, R.S.; Rani, M.; Chaudhari, M. Biogenic amines in meat and meat products and its public health significance: A review. *J. Food Sci. Technol.* **2015**, *52*, 6835–6846. [CrossRef]
15. Araujo, Q.R.D.; Gattward, J.N.; Almoosawi, S.; Parada Costa Silva, M.D.G.C.; Dantas, P.A.D.S.; Araujo Júnior, Q.R.D. Cocoa and human health: From head to foot—A review. *Crit. Rev. Food Sci. Nutr.* **2016**, *56*, 1–12. [CrossRef] [PubMed]
16. Restuccia, D.; Spizzirri, U.G.; De Luca, M.; Parisi, O.I.; Picci, N. Biogenic amines as quality marker in organic and fair-trade cocoa-based products. *Sustainability* **2016**, *8*, 856. [CrossRef]
17. Bandanaa, J.; Egyir, I.S.; Asante, I. Cocoa farming households in Ghana consider organic practices as climate smart and livelihoods enhancer. *Agric. Food Secur.* **2016**, *5*, 29. [CrossRef]
18. Ormanci, H.B.; Arik Colakoglu, F. Changes in biogenic amines levels of lakerda (*Salted Atlantic Bonito*) during ripening at different temperatures. *J. Food Process. Preserv.* **2017**, *41*, e12736. [CrossRef]
19. Hidalgo, F.J.; León, M.; Zamora, R. Amino acid decarboxylations produced by lipid-derived reactive carbonyls in amino acid mixtures. *Food Chem.* **2016**, *209*, 256–261. [CrossRef]
20. Guillén-Casla, V.; Rosales-Conrado, N.; León-González, M.E.; Pérez-Arribas, L.V.; Polo-Díez, L.M. Determination of serotonin and its precursors in chocolate samples by capillary liquid chromatography with mass spectrometry detection. *J. Chromatogr. A* **2012**, *1232*, 158–165. [CrossRef]
21. Romani, A.; Ieri, F.; Turchetti, B.; Mulinacci, N.; Vincieri, F.F.; Buzzini, P. Analysis of condensed and hydrolysable tannins from commercial plant extracts. *J. Pharm. Biomed. Anal.* **2006**, *41*, 415–420. [CrossRef]
22. Sànchez-Rabaneda, F.; Jàuregui, O.; Casals, I.; Andrès-Lacueva, C.; Izquierdo-Pulido, M.; Lamuela-Raventòs, R.M. Liquid chromatographic/electrospray ionization tandem mass spectrometric study of the phenolic composition of cocoa (*Theobroma cacao*). *J. Mass Spectrom.* **2003**, *38*, 35–42. [CrossRef]
23. Hammerstone, J.F.; Lazarus, S.A.; Schmitz, H.H. Procyanidin Content and Variation in Some Commonly Consumed Foods. *J. Nutr.* **2000**, *130*, 2086S–2092S. [CrossRef] [PubMed]
24. Shumov, L.; Bodor, A. An industry consensus study on an HPLC fluorescence method for the determination of (±)-catechin and (±)-epicatechin in cocoa and chocolate products. *Chem. Cent. J.* **2011**, *5*, 39–45. [CrossRef] [PubMed]
25. Spizzirri, U.G.; Parisi, O.I.; Picci, N.; Restuccia, D. Application of LC with evaporative light scattering detector for biogenic amines determination in fair trade cocoa-based products. *Food Anal. Methods* **2016**, *9*, 2200–2209. [CrossRef]
26. Hümmer, W.; Schreier, P. Analysis of proanthocyanidins. *Mol. Nutr. Food Res.* **2008**, *52*, 1381–1398. [CrossRef] [PubMed]
27. Payne, M.J.; Hurst, W.J.; Miller, K.B.; Rank, C.; Stuart, D.A. Impact of fermentation, drying, roasting, and Dutch processing on epicatechin and catechin content of cacao beans and cocoa ingredients. *J. Agric. Food Chem.* **2010**, *58*, 10518–10527. [CrossRef]

28. Ioannone, F.; Di Mattia, C.D.; De Gregorio, M.; Sergi, M.; Serafini, M.; Sacchetti, G. Flavanols, proanthocyanidins and antioxidant activity changes during cocoa (*Theobroma cacao* L.) roasting as affected by temperature and time of processing. *Food Chem.* **2015**, *174*, 256–262. [CrossRef]
29. Counet, C.; Ouwerx, C.; Rosoux, D.; Collin, S. Relationship between procyanidin and flavor contents of Cocoa liquors from different origins. *J. Agric. Food Chem.* **2004**, *52*, 6243–6249. [CrossRef]
30. Di Mattia, C.D.; Sacchetti, G.; Mastrocola, D.; Serafini, M. From Cocoa to Chocolate: The impact of Processing on In Vitro Antioxidant Activity and the effects of Chocolate on Antioxidant Markers In Vivo. *Front. Immunol.* **2017**, *8*, 1207. [CrossRef]
31. Oracz, J.; Zyzelewicz, D.; Nebesny, E. The content of polyphenolic compounds in cocoa beans (*Theobroma cacao* L.), depending on variety, growing region and processing operations: A review. *Crit. Rev. Food Sci. Nutr.* **2015**, *55*, 1176–1192. [PubMed]
32. Tomas-Barberaän, F.A.; Cienfuegos-Jovellanos, E.; Marìn, A.; Muguerza, B.; Gil-Izquierdo, A.; Cerdà, B.; Zafrilla, P.; Morillas, J.; Mulero, J.; Ibarra, A.; et al. A New Process to Develop a Cocoa Powder with Higher Flavonoid Monomer Content and Enhanced Bioavailability in Healthy Humans. *J. Agric. Food Chem.* **2007**, *55*, 3926–3935. [CrossRef]
33. Afoakwa, E.O.; Quao, J.; Takrama, J.; Simpson Budu, A.; Saalia, F.K. Chemical composition and physical quality characteristics of Ghanaian cocoa beans as affected by pulp pre-conditioning and fermentation. *J. Food Sci. Technol.* **2013**, *50*, 1097–1105. [CrossRef]
34. Ducki, S.; Miralles-Garcia, J.; Zumbé, A.; Tornero, A.; Storey, D.M. Evaluation of solid-phase micro-extraction coupled to gas chromatography–mass spectrometry for the headspace analysis of volatile compounds in cocoa products. *Talanta* **2008**, *74*, 1166–1174. [CrossRef] [PubMed]
35. Heinzler, M.; Eichner, K. The role of amodori compounds during cocoa processing—Formation of aroma compounds under roasting conditions. *Z. Lebensm.-Unters.-Forsch.* **1992**, *21*, 445–450.
36. Kongor, J.E.; Hinneha, M.; Van deWalle, D.; Ohene Afoakwa, E.; Boeckx, P.; Dewettinck, K. Factors influencing quality variation in cocoa (*Theobroma cacao*) bean flavour profile—A review. *Food Res. Int.* **2016**, *82*, 44–52. [CrossRef]
37. Cambrai, A.; Marcic, C.; Morville, S.; Sae Houer, P.; Bindler, F.; Marchioni, E. Differentiation of chocolates according to the Cocoa's geographical origin using chemometrics. *J. Agric. Food Chem.* **2010**, *58*, 1478–1483. [CrossRef] [PubMed]
38. Ramli, N.; Hassan, O.; Said, M.; Samsudin, W.; Idris, N.A. Influence of roasting conditions on volatile flavor of roasted malaysian cocoa beans. *J. Food Process. Preserv.* **2006**, *30*, 280–298. [CrossRef]
39. Rohsius, C.; Matissek, R.; Lieberei, R. Free amino acid amounts in raw cocoas from different origins. *Eur. Food Res. Technol.* **2006**, *222*, 432–438. [CrossRef]
40. Adeyeye, E.I.; Akinyeye, R.O.; Ogunlade, I.; Olaofe, O.; Boluwade, J.O. Effect of farm and industrial processing on the amino acid profile of cocoa beans. *Food Chem.* **2010**, *118*, 357–363. [CrossRef]
41. Granvogl, M.; Bugan, S.; Schieberle, P. Formation of amines and aldehydes from parent amino acids during thermal processing of cocoa and model systems: New insights into pathways of the Strecker reaction. *J. Agric. Food Chem.* **2006**, *54*, 1730–1739. [CrossRef] [PubMed]
42. Lima, L.J.R.; Almeida, M.H.; Nout, M.J.R.; Zwietering, M.H. Theobroma cacao L., "the food of the gods": Quality determinants of commercial cocoa beans, with particular reference to the impact of the fermentation. *Crit. Rev. Food Sci. Nutr.* **2011**, *52*, 731–761.
43. Schwan, R.F.; Pereira, G.V.M.; Fleet, G.H. Microbial activities during cocoa fermentation. In *Cocoa and Coffee Fermentations*; Schwan, R.F., Fleet, G.H., Eds.; Taylor & Francis: London, UK, 2014; pp. 125–135.
44. Oracz, J.; Nebesny, E. Influence of roasting conditions on the biogenic amine content in cocoa beans of different *Theobroma cacao* cultivars. *Food Res. Int.* **2014**, *55*, 1–10. [CrossRef]
45. Caligiani, A.; Cirlini, M.; Palla, G.; Ravaglia, R.; Arlorio, M. GC/MS detection of chiral markers in cocoa beans of different quality and geographic origin. *Chirality* **2007**, *19*, 329–334. [CrossRef] [PubMed]
46. Shukla, S.; Park, H.K.; Kim, J.K.; Kim, M. Determination of biogenic amines in Korean traditional fermented soybean paste (Doenjang). *Food Chem. Toxicol.* **2010**, *48*, 1191–1195. [CrossRef] [PubMed]
47. Hidalgo, F.J.; Navarro, J.L.; Delgado, R.M.; Zamora, R. Histamine formation by lipid oxidation products. *Food Res. Int.* **2013**, *52*, 206–213. [CrossRef]

48. Oliveira, S.D.; Franca, A.S.; Gloria, M.B.A.; Borges, M.L.A. The effect of roasting on the presence of bioactive amines in coffees of different qualities. *Food Chem.* **2005**, *90*, 287–291. [CrossRef]
49. Hidalgo, F.J.; Delgado, R.M.; Zamora, R. Protective effect of phenolic compounds on carbonyl-amine reactions produced by lipid-derived reactive carbonyls. *Food Chem.* **2017**, *229*, 388–395. [CrossRef]

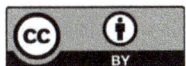

© 2019 by the authors. Licensee MDPI, Basel, Switzerland. This article is an open access article distributed under the terms and conditions of the Creative Commons Attribution (CC BY) license (http://creativecommons.org/licenses/by/4.0/).

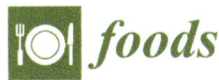

Article

Effect of Fermentation, Drying and Roasting on Biogenic Amines and Other Biocompounds in Colombian Criollo Cocoa Beans and Shells

Johannes Delgado-Ospina [1,2,*], Carla Daniela Di Mattia [1], Antonello Paparella [1], Dino Mastrocola [1], Maria Martuscelli [1,*] and Clemencia Chaves-Lopez [1]

[1] Faculty of Bioscience and Technology for Food, Agriculture and Environment, University of Teramo, Via R. Balzarini 1, 64100 Teramo, Italy; cdimattia@unite.it (C.D.D.M.); apaparella@unite.it (A.P.); dmastrocola@unite.it (D.M.); cchaveslopez@unite.it (C.C.-L.)
[2] Grupo de Investigación Biotecnología, Facultad de Ingeniería, Universidad de San Buenaventura Cali, Carrera 122 # 6-65, Cali 76001, Colombia
[*] Correspondence: jdelgado1@usbcali.edu.co (J.D.-O.); mmartuscelli@unite.it (M.M.)

Received: 21 March 2020; Accepted: 14 April 2020; Published: 21 April 2020

Abstract: The composition of microbiota and the content and pattern of bioactive compounds (biogenic amines, polyphenols, anthocyanins and flavanols), as well as pH, color, antioxidant and reducing properties were investigated in fermented Criollo cocoa beans and shells. The analyses were conducted after fermentation and drying (T1) and after two thermal roasting processes (T2, 120 °C for 22 min; T3, 135 °C for 15 min). The fermentation and drying practices affected the microbiota of beans and shells, explaining the great variability of biogenic amines (BAs) content. Enterobacteriaceae were counted in a few samples with average values of 10^3 colony forming units per gram (CFU g^{-1}), mainly in the shell, while *Lactobacillus* spp. was observed in almost all the samples, with the highest count in the shell with average values of 10^4 CFU g^{-1}. After T1, the total BAs content was found to be in a range of 4.9÷127.1 mg kg^{-1}_{DFW}; what was remarkable was the presence of cadaverine and histamine, which have not been reported previously in fermented cocoa beans. The total BAs content increased 60% after thermal treatment *T2*, and of 21% after processing at *T3*, with a strong correlation ($p < 0.05$) for histamine (ß = 0.75) and weakly correlated for spermidine (ß = 0.58), spermine (ß = 0.50), cadaverine (ß = 0.47) and serotonine (ß = 0.40). The roasting treatment of *T3* caused serotonin degradation (average decrease of 93%) with respect to unroasted samples. However, BAs were detected in a non-alarming concentration (e.g., histamine: n.d ÷ 59.8 mg kg^{-1}_{DFW}; tyramine: n.d. ÷ 26.5 mg kg^{-1}_{DFW}). Change in BAs level was evaluated by principal component analysis. PC1 and PC2 explained 84.9% and 4.5% of data variance, respectively. Antioxidant and reducing properties, polyphenol content and BAs negatively influenced PC1 with both polyphenols and BA increasing during roasting, whereas PC1 was positively influenced by anthocyanins, catechin and epicatechin.

Keywords: biogenic amines; polyphenols; histamine; microbiota; roasting

1. Introduction

In the last years, an increase in global cocoa production has been observed with a market demand of high-quality cocoa products [1]. Colombian cocoa was declared by the International Cocoa Organization as "fine" and "flavour" due to the agro-ecological characteristics of the areas in which it is cultivated and the adequate fermentation and drying processes that are carried out. In particular, Criollo is a variety of Colombia and other Latin American countries, known for its high quality.

Cocoa is produced from cocoa beans that undergo several processes such as fermentation, drying, roasting, dutching, conching, and tempering. In the first stages, cocoa pods (fruits) are picked from the trees (*Theobroma cacao*), collected in piles and immediately opened or left to stand for a few days (pod storage) to obtain positive effects on the quality of the final products. After harvesting, beans together with mucilage are removed from the pod, fermented, dried, and roasted [2].

Fermentation is essential for the degradation of mucilage thanks to the production of ethanol, which kills cocoa bean cotyledons, and to the production of different organic acids and important volatile compounds that diffuse into the interior of the beans and react with substances responsible for the flavour of final products during the subsequent roasting process. In addition, fermentation influences some functional properties such as antiradical activity and reduces the power of cocoa beans [3,4]. However, biogenic amines (BAs) can be formed during this step, with detrimental effects on cocoa quality and human health. The occurrence of BAs in food originates from decarboxylation of free amino acids, amination and transamination of ketones and aldehydes or during thermal processes. In fermented products, the concentration of BAs is the result of a balance between formation and degradation reactions in which several microorganisms are involved. In fact, cocoa microbiota may present strains with decarboxylase activity [5–8] and amino-oxidase activity [9].

A decrease of bioactive compounds, such as BAs and polyphenolic compounds, occurs in different steps of the cocoa beans processing, affecting their final content and functional properties in cocoa derivatives [10–12]. During roasting, physical and chemical changes occur in the beans, such as differences in colour, removal of undesirable volatile compounds, formation of desirable aroma and flavour, reduction of water content (up to 2%), and formation of a brittle structure, as well as changes in flavanols, proanthocyanidins and antioxidant activity [13,14]. In addition, peculiar cocoa volatile compounds are generated by Maillard reactions and their release is favoured by modifications of the matrix structure [15]. In spite of this, during roasting critical changes may also take place such as the formation of water-insoluble melanoidins, the degradation of catechin-containing compounds [16], the reduction of polyphenol content and antioxidant activity [17], and an increase of the biogenic amines content [12]. If some Maillard Reaction products, such as melanoidins, are required for the development of the peculiar cocoa sensory characteristics and brown colour, some furanic compounds are supposed to have negative effects on human health, as they can show cytotoxicity at high concentration and are "possibly carcinogenic to humans" [18]. Furthermore, since the presence of cocoa shell in cocoa beans derivatives adversely affects the final product quality [19], beans should be peeled before or after roasting [20,21].

The present research was aimed to study the effect of fermentation, drying and roasting on the microbiological, physical and chemical characteristics of Colombian Criollo cocoa (bean and shell), with a particular focus on the content of bioactive compounds such as BAs and polyphenols.

2. Materials and Methods

2.1. Origin of the Samples

Criollo cocoa bean samples were collected in spring 2018 directly from 18 farms (identified with a numerical code) located in three Departments of Colombia, with different environmental conditions and different fermentation and drying systems (Table 1). Thirteen samples were from Valle del Cauca, located in the western part of the country, between 3°05′ and 5°01′ N latitude, 75°42′ and 77°33′ W longitude; four samples from Cauca, located in the southwest of the country on the Andean and Pacific regions, between 0°58′54″ N and 3°19′04″ N latitude, 75°47′36″ W and 77°57′05″ W longitude; one sample from Nariño, located in the west of the country (1°16′0.01″ N latitude and 77°22′0.12″ W longitude) and, despite low altitude, affected by cold winds from the south of the continent.

Table 1. Geographical characteristics of the area of origin and fermentation and drying condition of the cocoa samples.

	Farm Location	Altitude (masl *)	Fermentation				Drying				
			T_{day} (°C)	T_{night} (°C)	Time (d)	Box	T_{day} (°C)	T_{night} (°C)	Time (d)	Drying Surface
1	Valle del Cauca	1000	27–31	18–20	4	plastic	28–30	17–18	4	wooden trays
2	Valle del Cauca	1000	27–31	18–20	3	plastic	28–30	17–18	5	wooden trays
3	Valle del Cauca	1000	25–27	17–18	6	wooden	25–27	18–19	3	wooden trays
4	Valle del Cauca	1000	27–31	18–20	6	plastic	28–30	17–18	3	wooden trays
5	Cauca	990	29–30	19–20	4	wooden	29–30	18–19	5	wooden trays
6	Valle del Cauca	1000	27–31	18–20	6	wooden	28–30	17–18	6	floors
7	Valle del Cauca	1000	25–27	17–18	6	plastic	25–27	18–19	4	wooden trays
8	Valle del Cauca	1000	25–27	17–18	6	plastic	25–27	18–19	4	metal trays
9	Cauca	990	29–30	19–20	4	wooden	29–30	18–19	6	floors
10	Cauca	990	28–33	19–20	4	wooden	28–33	17–20	7	floors
11	Valle del Cauca	1000	27–31	18–20	6	plastic	28–30	17–18	4	floors
12	Valle del Cauca	1000	27–31	18–20	6	plastic	28–30	17–18	3	floors
13	Valle del Cauca	1000	25–27	17–18	6	plastic	25–27	18–19	3	wooden trays
14	Cauca	990	29–30	19–20	4	wooden	29–30	18–19	5	wooden trays
15	Valle del Cauca	1000	27–31	18–20	6	plastic	28–30	17–18	5	wooden trays
16	Nariño	30	21–25	12–22	4	wooden	20–25	11–15	4	floors
17	Valle del Cauca	1000	27–31	18–20	6	plastic	28–30	17–18	4	floors
18	Valle del Cauca	1000	25–27	17–18	6	plastic	25–27	18–19	3	wooden trays

* meters above sea level.

2.2. Samples Preparation and Defatting

The samples were collected at the final stage of fermentation and drying (step T1). Moreover, dried cocoa beans were divided into two batches and treated in a convection oven (Memmert UN110, Büchenbach, Germany) in two different commercial roasting conditions: T2, 120 °C for 22 min; T3, 135 °C for 15 min.

After cooling, the shell was removed manually from the cocoa beans. After the removal of the external skin and grinding (IKA M20, Staufen, Germany), cocoa samples were defatted by three cycles of hexane washing (8 g of cocoa sample in 50 mL of hexane), following the method described by Di Mattia et al. [4]. Four grams of sample were weighed and 25 mL of hexane added, then the mixture was vortexed for 1 min and centrifuged ($2325\times g$ for 10 min), each time discharging the supernatant. To completely remove the hexane from the sample, the lipid-free solids were air-dried at room temperature. The fat-free samples were then used for the extraction of the phenolic fraction and other chemical determinations.

2.3. Moisture and pH Determination

The pH of defatted cocoa nibs was measured by diluting in distilled water (1:1) by using an electrode probe connected to a pHmeter (FE20, Mettler Toledo, Columbus, OH, USA).

Moisture content was determined according to the official procedure adopted by the Association of Official Analytical Chemists (AOAC) [22]. In particular, 1 g of sample was dried in a forced-air drying oven at 105 °C up to a constant weight.

2.4. Microbiological Analyses

Microbiological analyses were performed according to Chaves et al. [23]. From samples of dried cocoa beans, the beans (from here they are beans without shell) and the shells were obtained by manual separation. Twenty grams of cocoa nibs and separate shells were homogenized in a Stomacher Lab-blender (Thomas Scientific, Swedesboro, NJ, USA) in 90 mL phosphate buffer solution (PBS, Biolife, Milan, Italy) sterile solution, pH 7.4. Decimal dilutions of the suspension were prepared in PBS, plated and incubated as follows: Enterobacteriaceae were counted and isolated in Violet Red Bile Glucose Agar (Oxoid, Basingstoke, UK) at 37 °C in anaerobiosis for 48 h; mesophilic aerobic bacteria in Plate Count Agar (PCA) at 30 °C for 48 h; thermophilic aerobic bacteria in PCA and incubated at 45 °C for 48 h; lactobacilli in De Man Rogose and Sharp (MRS) Broth (Oxoid, Basingstoke, UK) at 37 °C in anaerobiosis for 72 h; lactic streptococci in M17 agar (Oxoid, Basingstoke, UK) at 37 °C in anaerobiosis for 72 h; yeasts in Yeast Extract-Peptone-Dextrose (YPD) agar medium and Walerstein Laboratory (WL) medium agar (Biolife, Milan, Italy) at 25 °C for 48 h; moulds in DG18 Agar (Oxoid, Basingstoke, UK) and Czapec-Agar (Biolife, Milan, Italy) added with 150 ppm chloramphenicol (Sigma-Aldrich Italy, Milan, IT) for 5 days.

2.5. Biogenic Amines Determination

Defatted samples were subjected to BAs extraction, detection, identification and quantification by high-performance liquid chromatography (HPLC) using an Agilent 1200 Series (Agilent Technologies, Milano, Italy), optimizing the method described by Chaves-Lopez et al. [23]. Shortly after, 1.0 g of sample was added of 5.0 mL of 0.1 N HCl and stirred in vortex (1 min) and ultrasound (20 min). It was centrifuged (Hettich Zentrifugen, Tuttlingen, Germany) at relative centrifugal force of $2325\times g$ for 10 min and the supernatant recovered. Then, 150 µL of saturated $NaHCO_3$ was added to 0.5 mL of the supernatant, adjusting the pH to 11.5 with 0.1 N NaOH. For derivatization, 2.0 mL of dansyl chloride/acetone (10 mg mL^{-1}) was added and incubated at 40 °C for 1 h under agitation (195 stokes) (Dubnoff Bath-BSD/D, International PBI, Milano, Italy). To remove excess of dansyl chloride, 200 µL of 30% ammonia was added, allowed to stand for 30 min at room temperature, and diluted with 1950 µL of acetonitrile.

In a Spherisorb S30ODS Waters C18-2 column (3 µm, 150 mm × 4.6 mm ID), 10 µl of sample were injected with gradient elution, acetonitrile (solvent A) and water (solvent B) as follows: 0–1 min 35% B isocratic; 1–5 min, 35%–20% B linear; 5–6 min, 20%–10% linear B; 6–15 min, 10% B isocratic; 15–18 min, 35% linear B; 18–20 min, 35% B isocratic. Identification and quantification of cadaverine (CAD), dopamine (DOP), ethylamine (ETH), histamine (HIS), 2-phenylethylamine (PHE), putrescine (PUT), serotonin (SER), spermidine (SPD), spermine (SPM), and tyramine (TYR) was performed by comparing retention times and calibration curves of pure standards. The results were reported as mg of BA kg^{-1} of defatted dry weight (of DFW).

2.6. Colour Analysis

Colour analysis of the cocoa samples was carried out by a Minolta Bench-top Colorimeter CR-5 (Konica Minolta, Tokyo, Japan) CM-500 spectrophotometer. Before analysis, two calibrations were carried out, one with black standard and the other one with white standard. For each measurement, a single layer of grounded cocoa beans was spread on a Petri dish. The analysis was repeated three times on each sample.

The instrument gave the results in terms of CIE L* a* b* parameters (CIELAB is a colour space specified by the International Commission on Illumination, French Commission Internationale de l'éclairage, CIE), where L* indicates the lightness within the range from 0 (black) to 100 (white); a* ranges from −60 (green) to +60 (red); b* ranges from −60 (blue) to +60 (yellow). a* and b* indicate colour direction and from these values we obtained the Hue angle (h°), calculated as h° = arctan(b*/a*)

2.7. Anthocyanin Determination

The total anthocyanins content was determined by the method described by do Carmo Brito et al. [11]. In brief, 1.0 mL of 95% ethanol and 1.5 N hydrochloric acid solution (85:15 v/v) were added to 0.1 g of defatted cocoa sample, then stirred in vortex for two min and allowed to stand overnight. The sample was centrifuged at 10,000× g, and the supernatant was suitably diluted to measure its absorbance at 535 nm by a spectrometer (Eppendorf Biospectrometer kinetic, Hamburg, Germany. The results were reported as mg of anthocyanins g^{-1} of sample.

2.8. Extraction of the Phenolic Fraction

The defatted samples were further ground with mortar and pestle to reduce the powder size and to allow better contact of the extracting solvent with the sample. The sample extraction was carried out according to Di Mattia et al. [4] with some modifications. One gram of defatted sample was added to 5 mL of 70:29.5:0.5 acetone/water/acetic acid; the mixture was vortexed for 1 min, then sonicated in an ultrasonic bath (Labsonic LBS 1, Falc, Treviglio, Bergamo, Italy) at 20 °C for 10 min and finally centrifuged (2325× g for 10 min). The surnatant liquid was recovered and filtrated through cellulose filters. The extracted polyphenols were then stored in the freezer at −32 °C until analyses. This extract was used for the evaluation of total polyphenol content, radical scavenging activity and ferric reducing properties. For flavanols analysis, samples were extracted, kept at −80 °C and analysed on the same day or at the latest a few days after extraction.

2.8.1. Total Polyphenols Content (TPC)

The total polyphenol content (TPC) was determined according to a procedure modified from Di Mattia et al. [10]. To a volume of 0.1 mL of diluted defatted sample extract, water was added up to a volume of 5 mL, and 500 µL of Folin–Ciocalteu reagent was added. After 3 min, 1.5 mL of a 25% (w/v) Na_2CO_3 solution was added and then deionized water up to 10 mL of the final volume. Solutions were maintained at room temperature under dark conditions for 60 min and the total polyphenols content was determined at 765 nm using a spectrophotometer (Lambda Bio 20 Perkin Elmer, Waltham, MA, USA) Gallic acid standard (Fluka, Buchs, Switzerland) solutions were used for calibration. Results were expressed as milligrams of gallic acid equivalents (GAE) per gram of defatted and dry weight.

2.8.2. Flavanols Identification and Quantification

HPLC (high-performance liquid chromatography) was used for separation, quantitative determination and identification of flavonoids. The chromatographic analyses were performed on a 1200 Agilent Series HPLC (Agilent Technologies, Milano, Italy) equipped with a quaternary pump, a degasser, a column thermostat, an autosampler injection system and a diode array detector (DAD). The system was controlled by Agilent ChemStation for Windows (Agilent Technologies). Flavanols determination was carried out according to Ioannone et al. [13]. The sample (20 µL) was injected into a C18 reversed-phase column. Separation of phenolic compounds was carried out at a flow rate of 1 mL/min with a non-linear gradient from A (1% acetic acid solution) to B (ACN). Gradient elution was as follows: from 6% to 18% B from 0 to 40 min, from 18% to 100% B from 40 to 45 min, from 100% to 6% B from 45 to 50 min, isocratic from 50 to 53 min. The DAD acquisition range was set from 200 to 400 nm. The calibration curves were made with epicatechin and catechin, and the results were expressed as mg per gram of defatted and dry weight.

2.8.3. ABTS (2,2′-azino-bis(3-ethylbenzthiazoline-6-sulfuric acid)) Assay

The radical scavenging activity was measured by ABTS (2,2′-azino-bis(3-ethylbenzthiazoline-6-sulfuric acid)) radical cation decoloration assay, as described by Re et al. [24]. The ABTS radical stock solution was prepared by dissolving ABTS in water to a 7 mM concentration and by making this solution react with 2.45 mM of potassium persulfate. The mixture was then left in the dark at room temperature for 12–16 h before use. The ABTS+• stock solution was diluted in water to an Abs of 0.70 ± 0.02 for the analysis, and the reaction was started by the addition of 30 µL of cocoa extract to 2.97 mL of ABTS+• radical solution. The bleaching rate of ABTS+• in the presence of the sample was monitored at 25 °C at 734 nm using a spectrophotometer (Lambda Bio 20, Perkin Elmer, Boston, MA, USA) and decoloration after 5 min was used as the measure of antioxidant activity. Radical scavenging activity was expressed as Trolox Equivalents Antioxidant Capacity (TEAC-µmol of Trolox equivalents per g of defatted and dry weight), calculated by the ratio between the correlation coefficient of the dose–response curve of the sample and the correlation coefficient of the dose–response curve of Trolox, the standard compound.

2.8.4. Ferric Reducing Antioxidant Power (FRAP)

The reducing activity of the samples was determined according to the method described by Benzie and Strain [25] with some modifications. One hundred microliters of suitably diluted sample extract were added to 2900 µL of the FRAP reagent obtained by mixing acetate buffer (300 mM, pH 3.6), TPTZ (2,4,6-tripyridyl-s-triazine), 10 mM solubilized in HCl 40 mM and FeCl$_3$ 20 mM in the ratio 10:1:1. The absorbance change was followed at 593 nm for 6 min. A calibration plot based on FeSO$_4$·7H$_2$O was used, and results were expressed as mmols of Fe^{2+} per gram of defatted and dry weight.

2.9. Statistical Analyses

All determinations were done in triplicate, except where differently indicated. Means and relative standard deviations were calculated. Analysis of variance (ANOVA) was performed to test the significance of the effects of the factor variables (processing steps); differences among means were separated by the least significant differences (LSD) test. Statistical analysis of data was performed using XLSTAT software version 2019.1 for Microsoft Excel (Addinsoft, New York, NY, USA). All results were considered statistically significant at $p < 0.05$.

The multivariate descriptive analysis was used to understand the presence of the main descriptors related to the BAs content of cocoa. The principal components analysis (PCA) started with the analysis of a matrix (18 × 55) that consisted of 18 samples of Criollo cocoa. The analyses were performed in triplicate. The 55 conformations of the values of the evaluated variables were gathered by the following tests: roasting temperature (raw, 120 °C for 22 min and 135 °C for 15 min), pH, content of total polyphenols (TPC), anthocyanins, antioxidant activity (FRAP and TEAC), flavonols (catechin and epicatechin), levels of the main microorganisms groups in cocoa beans and shell, ethylamine (ETH), dopamine (DOP), 2-phenylethylamine (PHE), putrescine (PUT), cadaverine (CAD), serotonin (SER), histamine (HIS), tyramine (TYR), spermidine (SPD), and spermine (SPM).

3. Results

3.1. Characterization of Fermented and Dried Cocoa Beans

Several indicators are used to measure the quality of cocoa beans. These include, in addition to microbiota, composition, colour and acidity of the beans [26].

3.1.1. Microbiota

Some researchers found that variations in the content of BAs in cocoa are mainly affected by fermentation, which is directly correlated to the type and quantity of microbial populations [11]. Figure 1a,b shows the distribution of microorganism groups enumerated both in cocoa beans and cocoa shells of investigated samples. A large variability was observed, confirming that postharvest practices carried out in the different Colombian farms affected microbiota, which in turn can explain the great diversity of decarboxylation products, such as BAs content at the T1 step. The microbial load of the shell was determined because many of the metabolites produced in the shell during fermentation and drying can migrate to the beans, causing a pH decrease due to the accumulation of organic acids. The microbiological analyses showed the presence of enterobacteria, total aerobic mesophiles, total aerobic thermophiles, acetic bacteria, spore-forming bacteria, lactobacilli, lactococci, fungi, and yeasts that are mainly involved in fermentation and drying. Variations in microbial counts and species were observed in the different samples, likely due to different fermentation and drying practices (pod ripeness, postharvest pod storage, variations in pulp/bean ratio, fermentation method, batch size, frequency of bean mixing or turning, and fermentation time), as well as due to some characteristics of the environment where the cultivation takes place (farm, weather conditions, pod diseases) [27,28].

A great difference was also observed between the microbial community found in the shell and inside the beans. As expected, the shell contained a greater number of microorganisms because sugars and other rapidly degradable nutrients are concentrated here, while a smaller number of microbial populations could adapt to the conditions of the beans. According to Lima et al. [29], average levels of total aerobic microorganisms and aerobic total spores are reduced in the beans, while Enterobacteriaceae and fungi were not detected.

Generally, the production of BAs is attributed to certain species of Enterobacteriaceae, mainly *Clostridium* spp., *Lactobacillus* spp., *Streptococcus* spp., *Micrococcus* spp., and *Pseudomonas* spp. [30]. Two of these groups were found in cocoa samples; Enterobacteriaceae were counted in a few samples with average values of 10^3 CFU g^{-1}, mainly in the shell and probably due to contamination during outdoor drying, while *Lactobacillus* spp. was observed in almost all the samples, with the highest count in the shell with average values of 10^4 CFU g^{-1}.

3.1.2. pH, Moisture and Colour

The characteristics of Colombian Criollo cocoa samples at the end of fermentation and drying (T1) are shown in Table 2. The great variability found in the samples depends on several factors, namely fermentation and drying, as well as some intrinsic characteristics of the farming system. The organic acids produced by lactic and acetic bacteria during fermentation diffuse within the beans and cause a pH decrease; low pH values are considered an index of appropriate fermentation while pH values above 5.5 may indicate an inadequate or incomplete fermentation [31]. The pH of the samples ranged between 4.43 and 6.17 (C.V. 10%). With the exception of sample 18, it can be stated that the samples coming from Valle de Cauca were generally characterized by lower pH values compared to Cauca samples.

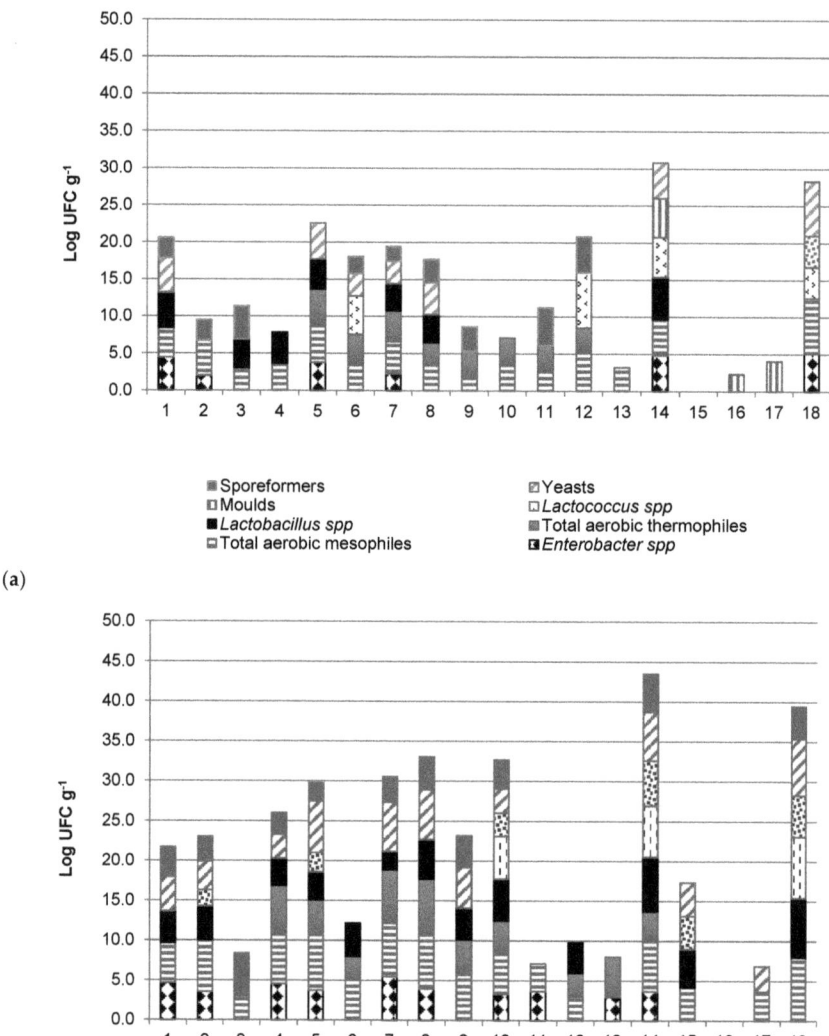

Figure 1. Levels of the main microorganisms groups in beans (**a**) and shells (**b**) of Colombian Criollo cocoa samples (after fermentation and drying, step T1).

Table 2. Chemico-physical and colour parameters (L*, a*, b* and h°) for fermented and dried samples (T1). The data are expressed as mean ± standard deviation.

Samples	Origin	pH	Moisture (%)	Colour			
				L*	a*	b*	h°
1	Valle de Cauca	5.01 ± 0.02	3.4 ± 0.3	40.83 ± 0.80	7.06 ± 0.08	11.17 ± 0.35	57.67 ± 0.01
2	Valle de Cauca	4.79 ± 0.11	3.9 ± 0.2	48.92 ± 0.27	3.64 ± 0.08	9.38 ± 0.10	68.77 ± 0.02
3	Valle de Cauca	4.43 ± 0.08	4.2 ± 0.4	41.78 ± 0.43	9.87 ± 0.12	12.35 ± 0.22	51.35 ± 0.06
4	Valle de Cauca	4.49 ± 0.03	3.8 ± 0.3	38.40 ± 0.16	9.49 ± 0.12	9.57 ± 0.13	45.24 ± 0.02
5	Cauca	5.85 ± 0.06	5.0 ± 0.2	41.42 ± 0.30	9.21 ± 0.05	10.25 ± 0.16	48.07 ± 0.01
6	Valle de Cauca	4.54 ± 0.10	1.2 ± 0.1	38.76 ± 0.67	9.05 ± 0.32	6.70 ± 0.54	36.49 ± 0.02
7	Valle de Cauca	4.99 ± 0.07	3.5 ± 0.2	41.71 ± 0.65	8.29 ± 0.15	10.85 ± 0.16	52.62 ± 0.01
8	Valle de Cauca	5.05 ± 0.05	4.8 ± 0.4	43.26 ± 0.37	8.25 ± 0.27	13.43 ± 0.20	58.45 ± 0.01
9	Cauca	5.11 ± 0.18	2.5 ± 0.1	36.84 ± 0.30	7.30 ± 0.16	11.79 ± 0.41	58.22 ± 0.01
10	Cauca	5.52 ± 0.15	1.7 ± 0.1	38.89 ± 0.68	4.37 ± 0.02	8.30 ± 0.09	62.22 ± 0.01
11	Valle de Cauca	4.41 ± 0.08	2.5 ± 0.2	39.85 ± 0.34	9.60 ± 0.24	10.27 ± 0.38	46.90 ± 0.01
12	Valle de Cauca	4.62 ± 0.03	2.2 ± 0.0	44.50 ± 0.38	7.31 ± 0.16	11.34 ± 0.18	57.19 ± 0.00
13	Valle de Cauca	4.67 ± 0.33	4.9 ± 0.4	37.54 ± 0.18	10.04 ± 0.05	15.77 ± 0.03	57.53 ± 0.00
14	Cauca	5.45 ± 0.09	6.2 ± 0.3	38.44 ± 1.02	8.18 ± 0.09	12.07 ± 0.26	55.87 ± 0.01
15	Valle de Cauca	5.07 ± 0.12	2.5 ± 0.2	38.23 ± 0.91	8.33 ± 0.14	9.30 ± 0.08	48.15 ± 0.00
16	Nariño	4.68 ± 0.13	3.9 ± 0.1	43.78 ± 0.07	5.34 ± 0.09	12.25 ± 0.25	66.43 ± 0.01
17	Valle de Cauca	4.44 ± 0.10	2.8 ± 0.2	48.89 ± 0.73	5.34 ± 0.09	12.25 ± 0.25	66.43 ± 0.01
18	Valle de Cauca	6.17 ± 0.27	4.7 ± 0.7	32.96 ± 0.89	9.39 ± 0.32	12.93 ± 0.46	54.00 ± 0.00

The moisture in bean samples ranged between 1.2% (sample 6) and 6.2% (sample 14), with differences depending on process conditions (solar or artificial dryers) and processing time. However, for all the samples, moisture content was below 12% which is considered the threshold value for optimal beans storage, corresponding to inhibition of both enzymatic reactions and fungal growth that can produce undesired metabolites during storage, such as mycotoxins.

The lightness (L*) of the 18 samples had a mean value of 40.8 (±4.03), ranging from 48.92, observed in sample 2, to 32.96 in sample 18. For redness values (a*), a mean of 7.78 (±1.94) was detected with 10.04 as the maximum value (in sample 13) and 3.64 as the minimum (in sample 2). For yellowness (b*), we observed the highest value in sample 13 (11.11 ± 2.07) and the lowest value in sample 6 (6.70 ± 0.54). Finally, for hue angle (h°), a mean value of 55.12 ± 8.26 was determined with a range from 68.77 (sample 2) to 36.49 (sample 6). Other authors reported L* values quite different from those obtained in the present study, while results for parameters of a* and b* were similar [32]. The values obtained for h° were similar to those reported by Sacchetti et al. [14].

3.2. Biogenic Amines Profile

The BAs profile of the Criollo cocoa beans under investigation is described in Table 3. In unroasted samples (T1), the total BAs amount was found to be 57.5 (±37.5) mg kg^{-1}$_{DFW}$, with a minimum value of 4.9 mg kg^{-1}$_{DFW}$ (in sample 16, from Nariño region) and a maximum of 127.1 mg kg^{-1}$_{DFW}$ (in sample 4, from Valle de Cauca). As far as the BAs pattern is concerned, the most represented BAs in unroasted beans (T1) were CAD, SER, HIS, SPD, and SPM (Table 3); DOP was also detected in unroasted sample 15 (from Cauca).

The Pearson correlation coefficient between total BAs content and each single BA was calculated. A strong correlation was only found with HIS (ß = 0.75); tot BAs correlated weakly with SPD (ß = 0.58), SPM (ß = 0.50), CAD (ß = 0.47), and SER (ß = 0.40), while no significant correlation was found with other amines.

Table 3. Biogenic amines (mg kg^{-1}$_{DFW}$) in Criollo cocoa bean samples after fermentation and drying (T1) and after roasting (T2, 120 °C for 22 min; T3, 135 °C for 15 min).

Sample		Biogenic Amines Content (mg kg^{-1}$_{DFW}$)									
		ETH *	DOP	PHE	PUT	CAD	SER	HIS	TYR	SPD	SPM
1	T1	nd	nd	nd	nd	49.75 ± 1.4	3.06 ± 0.0	5.96 ± 1.2	nd	30.85 ± 3.6	nd
	T2	14.72 ± 2.3	nd	12.2 ± 0.1	1.32 ± 0.2	nd	17.18 ± 4.2	0.21 ± 3.1	17.02 ± 0.2	nd	14.30 ± 2.2
	T3	15.56 ± 5.2	nd	26.23 ± 0.3	59.02 ± 3.5	5.38 ± 0.6	nd	13.25 ± 1.1	11.11 ± 0.0	nd	36.84 ± 5.2
2	T1	nd	nd	nd	nd	48.62 ± 0.2	0.60 ± 0.0	nd	nd	4.67 ± 0.3	nd
	T2	24.77 ± 0.7	33.27 ± 0.2	11.18 ± 0.1	nd	nd	17.70 ± 0.0	nd	26.51 ± 4.2	nd	46.42 ± 8.4
	T3	19.22 ± 0.4	1.99 ± 0.0	25.98 ± 1.2	62.58 ± 6.2	nd	2.95 ± 0.2	17.13 ± 0.9	11.27 ± 0.8	2.50 ± 0.0	52.82 ± 3.9
3	T1	nd	nd	nd	nd	nd	nd	3.56 ± 1.1	nd	13.91 ± 0.2	0.37 ± 0.0
	T2	0.89 ± 0.3	nd	12.55 ± 0.5	nd	nd	9.11 ± 0.6	0.44 ± 0.5	25.22 ± 1.7	nd	nd
	T3	1.08 ± 0.4	nd	9.69 ± 136	nd	nd	nd	0.80 ± 1.2	8.29 ± 0.3	nd	nd
4	T1	nd	nd	nd	nd	22.60 ± 0.6	11.65 ± 1.1	41.9 ± 2.2	nd	42.06 ± 2.8	8.86 ± 3.2
	T2	2.74 ± 0.1	nd	11.77 ± 0.1	nd	2.22 ± 0.1	3.07 ± 0.0	0.82 ± 0.5	14.96 ± 1.1	nd	2.03 ± 1.8
	T3	1.68 ± 0.2	nd	17.22 ± 0.0	nd	nd	1.01 ± 0.0	1.01 ± 1.2	15.98 ± 0.4	nd	nd
5	T1	nd	nd	nd	nd	66.57 ± 0.7	0.36 ± 0.0	39.8 ± 7.1	nd	5.99 ± 0.0	nd
	T2	29.17 ± 0.3	65.12 ± 0.1	10.36 ± 0.5	6.46 ± 0.3	3.28 ± 0.0	25.63 ± 2.3	0.46 ± 0.7	20.80 ± 0.5	nd	60.04 ± 8.4
	T3	17.06 ± 1.2	95.03 ± 0.1	10.67 ± 0.1	2.51 ± 0.1	3.87 ± 0.0	nd	0.38 ± 0.2	9.87 ± 0.0	1.15 ± 0.0	nd
6	T1	nd	nd	nd	nd	1.50 ± 0.0	6.98 ± 0.1	38.90 ± 5.3	nd	48.66 ± 2.1	13.61 ± 2.2
	T2	2.95 ± 1.2	nd	11.36 ± 0.1	nd	3.14 ± 0.0	nd	17.13 ± 2.2	17.03 ± 0.7	nd	5.38 ± 0.4
	T3	2.17 ± 0.7	nd	14.75 ± 0.1	nd	nd	nd	nd	13.50 ± 0.4	nd	nd
7	T1	nd	nd	nd	nd	1.80 ± 0.0	0.11 ± 0.0	5.96 ± 1.2	nd	18.53 ± 6.2	1.12 ± 0.0
	T2	0.98 ± 0.1	nd	13.85 ± 0.0	nd	3.14 ± 0.0	nd	13.55 ± 3.0	20.51 ± 0.2	nd	nd
	T3	1.24 ± 0.1	nd	15.72 ± 0.2	nd	nd	nd	nd	13.12 ± 0.8	nd	nd
8	T1	nd	nd	nd	nd	15.86 ± 0.1	nd	nd	nd	12.81 ± 2.5	0.12 ± 0.1
	T2	3.61 ± 0.4	nd	12.70 ± 0.1	nd	nd	nd	48.18 ± 1.9	14.88 ± 0.1	nd	1.05 ±
	T3	3.36 ± 0.3	nd	12.81 ± 0.1	nd	nd	nd	nd	10.82 ± 0.0	nd	nd
9	T1	nd	nd	nd	nd	51.77 ± 0.5	0.85 ± 0.1	nd	nd	11.93 ± 1.1	0.37 ± 0.3
	T2	13.67 ± 0.5	nd	14.14 ± 0.1	nd	nd	nd	37.73 ± 2.8	18.16 ± 7.7	0.51 ± 0.0	nd
	T3	11.3 ± 0.1	nd	14.98 ± 0.1	1.50 ±	2.31 ± 0.0	nd	nd	15.85 ± 1.6	0.03 ± 0.0	nd

Table 3. Cont.

Sample		ETH *	DOP	PHE	PUT	CAD	SER	HIS	TYR	SPD	SPM
10	T1	nd	nd	nd	nd	nd	nd	7.76 ± 4.1	nd	12.37 ± 0.0	2.37 ± 0.2
	T2	21.65 ± 0.1	76.92 ± 0.1	12.04 ± 0.1	3.99 ± 0.4	2.22 ± 0.0	3.71 ± 0.1	0.27 ± 0.7	14.97 ± 1.1	1.87 ± 0.0	nd
	T3	12.55 ± 0.2	56.68 ± 0.1	8.42 ± 0.5	nd	nd	nd	1.25 ± 0.2	11.5 ± 2.7	nd	nd
11	T1	nd	nd	nd	nd	5.54 ± 0.1	0.24 ± 0.0	5.04 ± 0.1	nd	23.15 ± 1.2	4.37 ± 0.6
	T2	2.63 ± 0.1	nd	13.35 ± 0.0	nd	nd	nd	21.53 ± 3.1	14.20 ± 0.7	nd	nd
	T3	2.89 ± 0.1	nd	14.83 ± 0.6	nd	nd	nd	0.27 ± 0.5	14.49 ± 5.7	nd	0.37 ± 0.2
12	T1	nd	nd	nd	nd	7.56 ± 0.1	4.28 ± 0.1	16.74 ± 3.1	nd	44.48 ± 4.2	9.61 ± 1.1
	T2	4.55 ± 0.4	nd	13.94 ± 3.2	nd	nd	nd	59.78 ± 6.4	19.68 ± 0.3	nd	nd
	T3	3.19 ± 0.2	nd	16.16 ± 4.1	nd	nd	nd	1.24 ± 0.2	8.54 ± 0.6	nd	nd
13	T1	nd	nd	nd	nd	0.61 ± 0.0	4.41 ± 1.1	4.76 ± 2.6	nd	40.75 ± 2.7	4.86 ± 0.2
	T2	8.38 ± 0.1	nd	11.81 ± 2.9	nd	nd	nd	0.60 ± 0.3	16.24 ± 0.5	nd	nd
	T3	7.46 ± 0.1	nd	13.43 ± 1.6	nd	nd	nd	0.17 ± 0.4	14.42 ± 0.8	nd	nd
14	T1	nd	nd	nd	nd	nd	15.33 ± 1.2	2.96 ± 0.3	nd	18.31 ± 3.1	0.62 ± 0.1
	T2	6.47 ± 0.2	nd	14.65 ± 2.8	nd	nd	5.62 ± 0.1	0.79 ± 0.7	18.51 ± 1.0	nd	nd
	T3	6.33 ± 0.3	nd	12.50 ± 3.1	nd	2.87 ± 0.0	nd	2.70 ± 0.5	12.41 ± 3.4	nd	nd
15	T1	nd	57.35 ± 01	nd	nd	0.83 ± 0.0	3.55 ± 0.0	nd	0.19 ± 0.0	24.47 ± 2.2	8.86 ± 0.8
	T2	11.92 ± 0.0	nd	16.27 ± 2.1	nd	nd	4.90 ± 0.0	nd	13.65 ± 0.3	nd	nd
	T3	6.102 ± 0.2	nd	10.81 ± 1.0	nd	nd	nd	nd	12.14 ± 0.6	nd	nd
16	T1	nd	nd	nd	nd	2.85 ± 0.0	1.34 ± 0.0	nd	nd	0.28 ± 0.0	0.42 ± 0.0
	T2	27.00 ± 0.2	92.17 ± 0.1	18.78 ± 1.2	nd	nd	nd	29.87 ± 5.6	9.64 ± 0.0	2.62 ± 0.2	3.35 ± 0.7
	T3	9.41 ± 0.8	55.76 ± 0.1	6.02 ± 0.0	nd	nd	nd	1.18 ± 9.4	0.79 ± 0.0	nd	nd
17	T1	nd	nd	nd	nd	5.77 ± 0.3	9.68 ± 0.4	5.36 ± 0.7	nd	14.79 ± 2.1	1.19 ± 0.5
	T2	23.52 ± 0.4	77.52 ± 0.1	11.81 ± 0.8	nd	5.45 ± 0.2	nd	27.27 ± 4.9	11.37 ± 0.4	2.30 ± 0.0	nd
	T3	22.27 ± 0.0	16.27 ± 0.1	11.73 ± 0.3	4.44 ± 1.1	5.45 ± 0.7	nd	8.12 ± 0.9	12.51 ± 0.0	2.60 ± 0.0	2.85 ± 0.0
18	T1	nd	nd	nd	nd	nd	nd	nd	nd	15.45 ± 0.0	0.87 ± 0.0
	T2	25.66 ± 0.1	nd	17.24 ± 2.1	nd	nd	nd	nd	15.14 ± 3.2	nd	nd
	T3	11.77 ± 0.1	nd	20.60 ± 1.6	nd	nd	nd	nd	16.94 ± 1.9	nd	nd

* Legend: ethylamine (ETH), dopamine (DOP), 2-phenylethylamine (PHE), putrescine (PUT), cadaverine (CAD), histamine (HIS), serotonin (SER), tyramine (TYR), spermidine (SPD), and spermine (SPM); nd, not detectable.

To the best of our knowledge, there are no studies reporting the occurrence of CAD and HIS in raw cocoa beans, although there are few studies where BAs are identified in cocoa. Some authors [12] found tyramine, 2-phenylethylamine, tryptamine, serotonin, and dopamine in different varieties of raw cocoa beans; other authors [11] also found spermidine and spermine in Brazilian samples during fermentation.

Most of the analysed samples presented similar profiles of BAs that might be explained by the fact that they belong to the same variety. However, variations in their concentration were found and can be explained by the difference between cultivars, different growth, fermentation and drying conditions, as well as the microbiota of beans and shell (see Figure 1a,b).

Polyamines can also occur naturally due to the large proliferation of cells that occur in the early stages of growth or germination caused by physiological changes in tissues [33,34]. In fact, being that the cocoa bean is a seed and germination does not start if the optimal fermentation conditions are not present, a consequence of this could be that secondary metabolites such as the aliphatic amines (PUT, CAD, SPM and SPD) could be accumulated in cells. To our best knowledge, very few studies have been published on the relation between the physiological conditions and the BAs content in cocoa seeds, thus these aspects should be thoroughly investigated.

Although the development of microorganisms with amino acid decarboxylases activity occurs in environments with optimal pH between 4.0 and 5.5, no correlation was observed between BAs content and low pH.

No direct relationship was found between the content of polyphenols and the content of BAs in cocoa beans (see below). However, it is possible to hypothesize that the presence of metabolites as polyamines may influence antioxidant activity in cocoa samples or exhibit pro-oxidant properties [35].

3.3. Effect of Roasting on the BAs Content

A significant effect of both the roasting processes on total BAs content was found in all the samples; in particular, the beans treated at T2 (120 °C for 22 min) showed an increase of 60% with respect to the raw beans samples (T1), whilst the roasting process T3 (135 °C, 15 min) caused an increase of 21% compared to T1 samples.

In our experiments, we observed a large variability in the behaviour of each BA in the samples (Table 3); after the high temperature treatment, we determined the presence of TYR, 2-PHE, ETH, and PUT that were not detected in unroasted beans (T1). On the other hand, the roasting treatment increased the concentration of DOP and SPM with the increase of the temperature, while CAD and SPD levels decreased dramatically.

Several factors could affect the final accumulation of BAs. In particular, some authors have reported that Strecker degradation is responsible for the formation of BAs during the thermal decarboxylation of amino acids in the presence of α-dicarbonyl compounds formed during the Maillard reaction [12,36] or lipid peroxidation [37].

After treatment at 120 °C (T2), total BAs concentration correlated significantly with SPM (ß = 0.77), SPD (ß = 0.67) and PUT (ß = 0.60), while at 135 °C (T3) there was a strong correlation between tot BAS and SPD (ß = 0.85), HIS (ß = 0.81), and PUT, CAD and SPM (ß > 0.70).

Some authors suggested that serotonin could be formed as a result of the transformation of its precursors (tryptophan and 5-hydroxytryptophan) at very high temperatures [38]. In this study, we detected an increase in the concentration of serotonin only in three samples after T2 treatment, while this monoamine neurotransmitter in most of the samples decreased considerably after roasting at 135 °C (T3) with respect to unroasted samples (T1); a similar behaviour was observed for histamine in 50% of investigated samples. These results are in contrast with other authors who demonstrated the histamine thermostability during cooking processes [39,40].

It was also observed that the histamine level increased in foods after frying and grilling [41]. However, other authors elucidated the mechanism by which certain cooking ingredients and common organic acids destroy histamine [42], so it could be very interesting to deepen this aspect by considering

3.4. Anthocyanins, Total Polyphenols and Flavanols Content

The results on the content of anthocyanins, total polyphenols and flavanols of the eighteen cocoa samples at different process steps (T1, T2 and T3) are reported in Table 4.

After fermentation and drying treatment (T1), the anthocyanin concentration was between 0.17 and 3.36 mg g^{-1}_{DFW}, with an average value of 1.02 mg g^{-1}_{DFW}; these pigments disappeared during fermentation [11], reaching low values on the sixth day of fermentation, and they are a good parameter to determine the progress or status of the fermentation. The contents found are similar to other cocoa varieties from Colombia [43], but inferior to those found in other studies conducted on Ghana cocoa varieties [44]. In unroasted samples (T1), the average content of total polyphenols was 45.50 mg GAE g^{-1}_{DFW}, values that are similar to other cocoa varieties planted in Colombia [43,45], with the only exception being sample 4 which presented higher contents (over 80 mg GAE g^{-1}_{DFW}). These are more similar to the values found in other studies carried out on varieties planted in Ghana, as well as in other varieties planted in Colombia [44,46]. It is important to point out that these results may have been affected by the fact that each single phenol shows a different response to the Folin-Ciocalteau reagent [14].

According to Carrillo et al. [45], the cocoa-producing region can have a significant effect on the total polyphenol content, as a proportional relationship was found between polyphenols content and altitude of plant crops. Their results suggest that plants grown at lower altitude accumulate more polyphenols compared to plants grown at higher altitude. In the present study, the TPC determined for sample 16 (from geographical area at 30 m.a.s.l) was lower than other cocoa samples so it seems that the theory proposed by Carillo et al. is not confirmed by our data, although this aspect would be worth investigating with a large number of samples.

Roasting did not cause a statistically significant decrease in anthocyanin content in samples from all the three regions, with the following exception: a decrease of 50%–60% was observed in roasted cocoa beans in the sample of the Narino region (sample 16) due to its highest values at the end of fermentation. The decrease in anthocyanin content is in accordance with data observed by other authors [12,43] for different roasting temperatures. Regarding the TPC, a not statistically significant increase was found from 45.50 mg GAE g^{-1}_{DFW} for T1 to 55.26 mg GAE g^{-1}_{DFW} (+21%) for T2 and 62.01 mg GAE g^{-1}_{DFW} (+14%) for T3. However, an increase in TPC values after the roasting process is consistent with the data reported by Ioannone et al. [13]; these authors suggested that an increase in TPC is dependent on temperature and exposure time, as a series of condensation and polymerization reactions occur with the formation of complex molecules such as pro-anthocyanidins from lower molecular weight compounds such as phenols and anthocyanins. Additionally, through Maillard reactions, melanoidins can be formed from reducing sugars and free amino acids; as a consequence, melanoidins can have reducing properties that affect the response to the Folin-Ciocalteu reagent, thus causing an overestimation of the TPC values [14].

The occurrence of flavanols before and after roasting was also investigated in Criollo cocoa samples and the results are reported in Table 3. Moreover, Table S1 shows the epicatechin to catechin ratio (epi/cat) for both unroasted and roasted samples. Catechin was found in all unroasted samples (ranging from n.d. to 4.43 ± 0.13) with the exception of the samples 1, 5 and 9. Epicatechin was detected in all the samples with a maximum value of 5.7 ± 0.17 mg g^{-1} (in sample 12) and a minimum of 0.45 ± 0.01 mg g^{-1} (in sample 11). Similar catechin contents were found by Loureiro et al. in dried cocoa beans from Latin America [47].

Table 4. Anthocyanins, total polyphenols (TPC) and flavanols content of the Criollo cocoa samples after fermentation and drying (T1) and after roasting (T2, 120 °C for 22 min; T3, 135 °C for 15 min). The data are expressed as mean of triplicate analysis.

Sample	Anthocyanins (mg g^{-1}$_{DFW}$)			Sign.	TPC (mg GAE g^{-1}$_{DFW}$)			Sign.	Catechin (mg g^{-1}$_{DFW}$)			Sign.	Epicatechin (mg g^{-1}$_{DFW}$)			Sign.
	T1	T2	T3		T1	T2	T3		T1	T2	T3		T1	T2	T3	
1	2.28 ^{a}	1.36 ^{c}	2.08 ^{b}	*	43.00 ^{c}	68.79 ^{b}	83.85 ^{a}	*	nd	8.41 ^{b}	11.49 ^{a}	**	0.5 ^{b}	0.87 ^{a}	0.51 ^{b}	*
2	3.36 ^{a}	1.77 ^{b}	2.00 ^{b}	*	22.97 ^{b}	100.73 ^{a}	110.17 ^{a}	***	0.18 ^{b}	4.36 ^{a}	nd	***	0.76	0.9	0.54	**
3	0.24 ^{c}	0.31 ^{b}	0.37 ^{a}	*	47.38 ^{b}	33.54 ^{a}	45.56 ^{b}	*	1.47 ^{b}	1.64 ^{b}	2.17 ^{a}	*	1.72 ^{a}	nd	0.7 ^{b}	**
4	0.76 ^{a}	0.59 ^{b}	0.51 ^{b}	*	85.75 ^{a}	48.56 ^{c}	56.42 ^{b}	*	1.82 ^{b}	2.23 ^{b}	3.72 ^{a}	*	1.41	nd	nd	*
5	2.33 ^{a}	1.79 ^{b}	1.80 ^{b}	*	40.66 ^{b}	79.91 ^{a}	83.76 ^{a}	*	n.d	3.36 ^{b}	4.66 ^{a}	*	1.16 ^{a}	nd	1.1 ^{a}	*
6	0.36 ^{b}	0.50 ^{a}	0.56 ^{c}	*	65.12 ^{a}	68.36 ^{a}	60.39 ^{b}	*	2.16 ^{b}	5.93 ^{a}	6.12 ^{a}	**	1.07 ^{a}	0.47 ^{b}	nd	*
7	0.35 ^{b}	0.33 ^{b}	0.45 ^{a}	*	70.61 ^{a}	33.29 ^{b}	44.41 ^{b}	*	0.16 ^{b}	1.69 ^{a}	0.16 ^{b}	**	1.29	nd	nd	*
8	0.29 ^{c}	0.33 ^{b}	0.45 ^{a}	*	34.04 ^{b}	29.33 ^{b}	43.24 ^{a}	*	0.49 ^{a}	0.17 ^{b}	0.18 ^{b}	*	1.22	nd	nd	*
9	1.42 ^{a}	0.97 ^{c}	0.86 ^{b}	*	47.34 ^{b}	83.17 ^{a}	57.77 ^{b}	*	nd	0.65	nd	*	1.26	nd	nd	*
10	1.94 ^{c}	1.86 ^{b}	2.29 ^{a}	*	54.73 ^{c}	75.15 ^{b}	89.98 ^{a}	***	0.03 ^{b}	13.02 ^{a}	0.19 ^{b}	*	0.45 ^{b}	nd	0.83 ^{a}	*
11	0.57 ^{a}	0.49 ^{b}	0.52 ^{ab}	*	53.02 ^{a}	40.38 ^{c}	46.23 ^{b}	*	4.35 ^{a}	3.06 ^{b}	0.13 ^{c}	*	5.7 ^{a}	nd	3.58 ^{b}	**
12	0.46	0.48	0.44	n.s.	49.59 ^{b}	55.46 ^{a}	58.36 ^{a}	**	3.42 ^{b}	4.39 ^{a}	0.42 ^{c}	*	1.61 ^{b}	nd	5.26 ^{a}	***
13	0.17 ^{c}	0.23 ^{b}	0.31 ^{a}	*	22.62 ^{b}	18.99 ^{b}	38.49 ^{a}	*	4.43 ^{a}	0.74 ^{b}	0.05 ^{c}	*	0.59 ^{b}	nd	2.07 ^{a}	**
14	0.92 ^{b}	0.48 ^{c}	1.15 ^{a}	*	42.02 ^{b}	28.78 ^{c}	48.02 ^{a}	**	0.66	0.13	0.33	n.s.	0.79 ^{b}	nd	2.62 ^{a}	**
15	0.52 ^{b}	0.64 ^{a}	0.66 ^{a}	*	32.90 ^{c}	46.56 ^{b}	57.72 ^{a}	**	4.43 ^{b}	6.61 ^{a}	nd	**	2.34 ^{a}	1.62 ^{b}	nd	**
16	1.39 ^{a}	0.63 ^{c}	0.84 ^{b}	*	23.89 ^{b}	60.64 ^{a}	62.91 ^{a}	**	4.00 ^{b}	0.50 ^{b}	nd	**	0.97 ^{b}	5.87 ^{a}	0.78 ^{b}	***
17	0.72 ^{a}	0.71 ^{a}	0.35 ^{b}	*	33.83 ^{b}	87.43 ^{a}	88.57 ^{a}	***	0.65 ^{b}	0.27 ^{b}	nd	*	0.7 ^{c}	2.27 ^{a}	1.14 ^{b}	*
18	0.35 ^{b}	0.52 ^{a}	0.60 ^{a}	*	49.53 ^{a}	35.56 ^{c}	40.32 ^{b}	*	0.09 ^{b}	0.11 ^{b}	1.65 ^{a}	*	1.58 ^{a}	0.95 ^{b}	0.53 ^{c}	*

Legend: nd, not detectable; data followed by different superscript letters, in the same line, are significantly different (LSD test, $p < 0.05$); asterisks indicate significance at * $p < 0.05$; ** $p < 0.01$; *** $p < 0.001$; n.s. not significant.

The epi/cat ratio is a widely used index as it may be associated with the degree of cocoa processing [48,49] (Table S1). Generally, with the increase of temperature the epi/cat ratio tends to decrease due to isomerization reactions and the faster degradation of epicatechin with respect to catechin [50]. The major flavanol present in unroasted samples was (−)-epicatechin. According to Hurst et al. [51], the high temperatures may induce the epimerization of this flavanol to (−)-catechin, and (+)-catechin to (+)-epicatechin. This behaviour was noticed in many samples, even though in other cases the opposite was observed. Moreover, in many cases the ratio could not be calculated since either catechin or epicatechin was not detected. Finally, it can be said that both roasting conditions had a similar effect on flavanols.

3.5. Trolox Equivalent Antioxidant Capacity (TEAC) and the Ferric Reducing Antioxidant Power (FRAP) Assays

Table 5 shows the effect of the different roasting treatments on the radical scavenging activity (TEAC) and the reducing activity (FRAP) assays with respect to unroasted cocoa bean samples. The Pearson correlation coefficient was calculated: a strong correlation was found between TPC content and TEAC (ß = 0.88, $p < 0.05$) and between TPC content and FRAP (ß = 0.92, $p < 0.05$).

Table 5. Results of Trolox Equivalent Antioxidant Capacity (TEAC) and the Ferric Reducing Antioxidant Power (FRAP) assays on the Criollo cocoa samples after fermentation and drying (T1) and after roasting (T2, 120 °C for 22 min; T3, 135 °C for 15 min). The data are expressed as mean of triplicate analysis.

Sample	TEAC (μmol TE g^{-1})			Sign.	FRAP (μmol Fe^{2+} g^{-1})			Sign.
	T1	T2	T3		T1	T2	T3	
1	293.6 [b]	270.6 [c]	374.0 [a]	*	374.9 [c]	594.7 [a]	439.4 [b]	*
2	125.0 [c]	529.8 [b]	578.6 [a]	***	144.6 [c]	714.8 [b]	790.6 [a]	**
3	380.1 [a]	100.9 [c]	193.5 [b]	*	382.4 [a]	217.5 [c]	261.9 [b]	*
4	304.7 [a]	181.7 [b]	158.2 [c]	*	486.6 [a]	301.5 [c]	405.6 [b]	*
5	200.4 [c]	313.5 [b]	384.6 [a]	*	249.2 [b]	521.5 [a]	488.0 [a]	*
6	268.4 [a]	220.7 [b]	260.9 [a]	*	510.1	481.2	488.3	n.s.
7	411.0 [a]	94.5 [c]	170.6 [b]	***	562.3 [a]	242.3 [b]	243.0 [b]	*
8	101.5 [b]	91.4 [b]	187.9 [a]	*	259.2 [a]	187.0 [b]	269.9 [a]	*
9	161.4 [c]	396.9 [a]	188.9 [b]	*	282.6 [c]	321.0 [b]	431.2 [a]	*
10	217.1 [c]	389.0 [b]	459.3 [a]	*	432.2 [c]	562.7 [b]	703.5 [a]	**
11	238.4 [a]	135.2 [c]	168.3 [b]	*	401.9 [a]	282.0 [b]	279.5 [b]	*
12	246.3 [b]	284.8 [a]	279.2 [a]	*	313.8 [c]	352.0 [b]	440.1 [a]	*
13	98.2 [b]	69.6 [c]	141.3 [a]	**	174.5 [b]	135.7 [c]	222.1 [a]	***
14	195.5 [a]	136.1 [c]	161.1 [b]	*	264.3 [b]	252.8 [b]	334.3 [a]	*
15	161.3 [b]	202.5 [a]	111.3 [c]	*	205.6 [c]	349.9 [b]	466.3 [a]	**
16	184.1 [c]	224.8 [b]	351.0 [a]	*	151.1 [c]	388.4 [b]	498.8 [a]	***
17	191.0 [c]	391.9 [b]	441.5 [a]	***	214.6 [c]	636.9 [b]	789.1 [a]	***
18	231.0 [a]	167.2 [b]	122.3 [c]	*	275.3	229.1	273.8	n.s.

Legend: data followed by different superscript letters, in the same line, are significantly different (LSD test, $p < 0.05$); asterisks indicate significance at * $p < 0.05$; ** $p < 0.01$; *** $p < 0.001$; n.s. not significant.

Regarding the reducing capacity as evaluated by FRAP assay (Table 5), a mean value of 395 μmol Fe^{2+}/g was determined in unroasted samples, which is in agreement with other authors [4,52].

The trend of values of FRAP was similar to those obtained in the ABTS assay. Moreover, in roasted samples results of TEAC and FRAP were comparable with values found by Ioannone et al. [13]. Generally, the antioxidant activity was higher in roasted samples compared with unroasted ones, with the exception of some cases (samples 3, 4, 7, 11, 14 and 18).

The improvement in the antioxidant and reducing properties after the roasting process may be related to the formation of reducing molecules, not quantified in the present work, as well as to the occurrence of condensation reactions among polyphenols, as evidenced by the results reported in Table 4.

3.6. Principal Component Analysis

A principal component analysis (PCA) was performed to highlight how factors or variables can influence the changes in the BA level in raw cocoa beans after roasting. Figure 2 shows the distribution of the variables analysed in the two first principal components which represent 90.1% of data variance. Usually, the two first principal components are sufficient to explain the maximum variation in all data [31]. PC1 and PC2 explained 84.9% and 5.2% of date variance related to the BA content of cacao. In order to better describe the data set, the following results and information were included: microbial counts, polyphenols (TPC), anthocyanins, antioxidant activity (FRAP and TEAC), flavonols (catechin and epicatechin), BA content at different processing conditions (T1, T2, and T3) and origin of the samples.

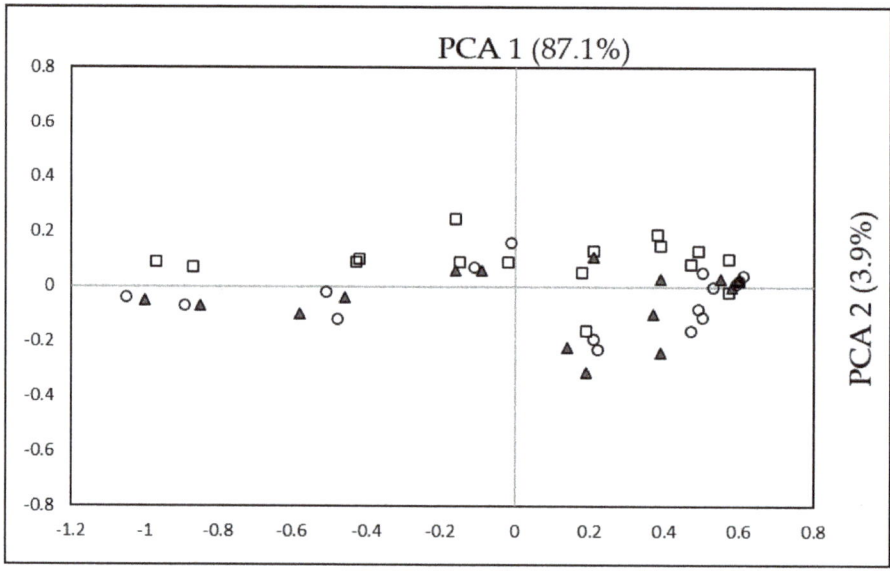

Figure 2. Principal component analysis related to the content of biogenic amines in Colombian criollo cocoa samples. Legend: empty square, T1 (raw cocoa beans); gray triangle, T2 (120 °C for 22 min); empty circle, T3 (135 °C for 15 min).

Concerning PC1, antioxidant activity (FRAP and TEAC) (−1.23 to −1.01), polyphenol content (TPC), and BA (−0.72 to −0.56) showed a negative influence on this component, while FRAP, TEAC, and TPC showed a significant increase in concentration in the same way as BA during roasting conditions. On the other side, anthocyanins, catechin, and epicatechin (0.43 to 0.55) showed a positive influence on this component. The anthocyanin content is a good parameter to determine if fermentation is carried out properly since they decrease as the fermentation progresses; therefore, the correlation found between a high anthocyanin content in raw cocoa (T1) and a high BA content may be related to a non-ideal fermentation process in which, for different reasons, the enzymatic activity of the grains remained active, generating metabolic intermediates such as BAs.

As for the individual BAs, a positive influence was found for DOP (0.51) under initial conditions (T1) after treatment at 120 °C (T2) for PUT, CAD, and SPD (0.49 to 0.54), and at 135 °C (T3) for CAD, SPD, SER, HIS, and SPM (0.44 to 0.56), while the other BAs showed no influence on this component.

The variables pH (0.1), region (0.41), shell microbiota (−0.26), and bean microbiota (−0.12) showed a weak correlation with each other. The pH is important to select the type of microorganisms that can grow and therefore quantity, and on the type of BAs they can generate [53]; in the present study, the values found for pH were not low enough to inhibit Enterobacteriaceae, which is one of the main groups that can produce BAs [31]. Moreover, pH values were in the optimal range that can favour BAs accumulation. The synthesis of polyamines, such as spermine and spermidine, occurs in response to high pH environments; these BAs act as inhibitors of carbonic anhydrase enzymes that catalyse the interconversion of carbon dioxide and water into bicarbonate and protons and vice versa [54].

According to Lima et al. [29], average levels of microorganisms are lower in the beans compared to those found in the shell due to the lower availability of nutrients, which can cause the activation of metabolic pathways in some groups of microorganisms that can lead to the accumulation of decarboxylation products such as BAs; however, no influence was observed in this component. Regarding the origin, the difference between cultivars, different growth, and postharvest conditions may be related to the presence of these BAs, but no influence in this component was established between the different sites where the samples were taken.

Concerning PC2, this component was mainly influenced by roasting. On the positive axis, the characteristics of the beans without heat treatment (T1) were located predominantly, differing from the samples T2 and T3 that were located on the negative axis of the component. Although a statistically significant difference was found in the content of BAs at T1, T2 and T3 in most of the samples, in the PC2 component only a small correlation was evident among them.

4. Conclusions

The present study aimed to evaluate the accumulation of bioactive compounds in eighteen Criollo cocoa beans samples from Colombia, with a special focus on biogenic amines and polyphenols, after fermentation and drying and after two different roasting processes commonly used in cocoa factories.

The samples showed a similar BAs profile, with a variability in their concentration as a consequence of both cocoa beans and shell microbiota, as well as differences among cultivars, growth conditions and fermentation and drying treatments. High temperature seems to correlate with the occurrence of TYR, PHE, ETH and PUT; moreover, the roasting process significantly increased the concentration of DOP and SPM, whilst CAD and SPD levels generally decreased. The total phenolic content was positively affected by the roasting processes; even without a statistically significant difference a remarkable improvement in the antioxidant and reducing properties were observed, showing an enhancement of their functionality.

No direct relationship was found between the content of polyphenols and the content of BAs in cocoa beans, even if it can be speculated that polyamines could have a role by influencing the antioxidant activity or exhibiting pro-oxidant properties in cocoa beans. Therefore, the correlation found between a high anthocyanin content and a high BAs content in unroasted cocoa samples (T1) could be attributable to a non-ideal fermentation process. One important result that it is worth pointing out is that the quantities of BAs found in the unroasted cocoa beans were not alarming, especially with regard to HIS and TYR, the amines of toxicological interest.

Moreover, low BAs amounts were also found in roasted samples, which is of crucial importance considering that such values that were calculated for defatted samples will be further processed and used as ingredients in complex formulations.

Supplementary Materials: The following are available online at http://www.mdpi.com/2304-8158/9/4/520/s1, Table S1: The ratio of epicatechin to catechin (epi/cat) in cocoa bean samples, fermentation and drying (T1) and after roasting (T2 and T3).

Author Contributions: Conceptualization, C.C.-L., M.M., C.D.D.M. and J.D.O.; methodology, M.M., C.D.D.M. and C.C.-L.; software, M.M. and J.D.-O.; formal analysis, J.D.-O., C.D.D.M., M.M.; investigation, J.D.-O., C.D.D.M., and M.M.; resources, J.D.-O., C.D.D.M. and M.M.; data curation, M.M.; writing—original draft preparation, J.D.-O., M.M.; writing—review and editing, M.M. and C.D.D.M.; visualization, M.M. and C.C.-L.; supervision, D.M., A.P.; project administration, C.C.-L.; funding acquisition, J.D.-O. All authors have read and agreed to the published version of the manuscript.

Funding: This research was funded by "Colciencias, Patrimonio Autónomo Fondo Nacional de Financiamiento para la Ciencia, la Tecnología y la Innovación Francisco José de Caldas" (C. 808-2018. Agreement 240-2019. Number 123280864259).

Conflicts of Interest: The authors declare no conflict of interest.

References

1. International Cocoa Organization. *Quarterly Bulletin of Cocoa Statistics*; International Cocoa Organization: London, UK, 2019; Volume 45, p. 101. Available online: http:www.icco.org (accessed on 12 December 2019).
2. Beg, M.S.; Ahmad, S.; Jan, K.; Bashir, K. Status, supply chain and processing of cocoa—A review. *Trends Food Sci. Technol.* **2017**, *66*, 108–116. [CrossRef]
3. Afoakwa, E.O. The chemistry of flavour development during Cocoa processing and chocolate manufacture. In *Chocolate Science and Technology*, 1st ed.; Afoakwa, E.O., Ed.; Wiley online library: Hoboken, NJ, USA, 2016; p. 296.
4. Di Mattia, C.; Martuscelli, M.; Sacchetti, G.; Scheirlinck, I.; Beheydt, B.; Mastrocola, D.; Pittia, P. Effect of fermentation and drying on procyanidins, antiradical activity and reducing properties of cocoa beans. *Food Bioprocess. Technol.* **2013**, *6*, 3420. [CrossRef]
5. Coton, E.; Coton, M. Evidence of horizontal transfer as origin of strain to strain variation of the tyramine production trait in *Lactobacillus brevis*. *Food Microbiol.* **2009**, *26*, 52–57. [CrossRef] [PubMed]
6. Lucas, P.M.; Blancato, V.S.; Claisse, O.; Magni, C.; Lolkema, J.S.; Lonvaud-Funel, A. Agmatine deiminase pathway genes in *Lactobacillus brevis* are linked to the tyrosine decarboxylation operon in a putative acid resistance locus. *Microbiology* **2007**, *153*, 2221–2230. [CrossRef] [PubMed]
7. Lucas, P.M.; Wolken, W.A.M.; Claisse, O.; Lolkema, J.S.; Lonvaud-Funel, A. Histamine-producing pathway encoded on an unstable plasmid in *Lactobacillus hilgardii* 0006. *Appl. Environ. Microbiol.* **2005**, *71*, 1417–1424. [CrossRef] [PubMed]
8. Marcobal, Á.; De Las Rivas, B.; Moreno-Arribas, M.V.; Muñoz, R. Evidence for horizontal gene transfer as origin of putrescine production in *Oenococcus oeni* RM83. *Appl. Environ. Microbiol.* **2006**, *72*, 7954–7958. [CrossRef] [PubMed]
9. Martuscelli, M.; Crudele, M.A.; Gardini, F.; Suzzi, G. Biogenic amine formation and oxidation by *Staphylococcus xylosus* strains from artisanal fermented sausages. *Lett. Appl. Microbiol.* **2000**, *31*, 228–232. [CrossRef] [PubMed]
10. Di Mattia, C.; Martuscelli, M.; Sacchetti, G.; Beheydt, B.; Mastrocola, D.; Pittia, P. Effect of different conching processes on procyanidin content and antioxidant properties of chocolate. *Food Res. Int.* **2014**, *63*, 367–372. [CrossRef]
11. Do Carmo Brito, B.D.N.; Campos Chisté, R.; da Silva Pena, R.; Abreu Gloria, M.B.; Santos Lopes, A. Bioactive amines and phenolic compounds in cocoa beans are affected by fermentation. *Food Chem.* **2017**, *228*, 484–490. [CrossRef]
12. Oracz, J.; Nebesny, E. Influence of roasting conditions on the biogenic amine content in cocoa beans of different *Theobroma cacao* cultivars. *Food Res. Int.* **2014**, *55*, 1–10. [CrossRef]
13. Ioannone, F.; Di Mattia, C.D.; De Gregorio, M.; Sergi, M.; Serafini, M.; Sacchetti, G. Flavanols, proanthocyanidins and antioxidant activity changes during cocoa (*Theobroma cacao* L.) roasting as affected by temperature and time of processing. *Food Chem.* **2015**, *174*, 263–269. [CrossRef] [PubMed]
14. Sacchetti, G.; Ioannone, F.; De Gregorio, M.; Di Mattia, C.; Serafini, M.; Mastrocola, D. Non enzymatic browning during cocoa roasting as affected by processing time and temperature. *J. Food Eng.* **2016**, *169*, 44–52. [CrossRef]
15. Hinneh, M.; Abotsi, E.E.; Van De Walle, D.; Tzompa-Sosa, D.A.; De Winne, A.; Simonis, J.; Messens, K.; Van Durme, J.; Afoakwa, E.O.; De Cooman, L.; et al. Pod storage with roasting: A tool to diversifying the flavor profiles of dark chocolates produced from 'bulk' cocoa beans? (part I: Aroma profiling of chocolates). *Food Res. Int.* **2019**, *119*, 84–98. [CrossRef] [PubMed]
16. Oliviero, T.; Capuano, E.; Cämmerer, B.; Fogliano, V. Influence of roasting on the antioxidant activity and HMF formation of a cocoa bean model systems. *J. Agric. Food Chem.* **2009**, *57*, 147–152. [CrossRef]

17. Djikeng, F.T.; Teyomnou, W.T.; Tenyang, N.; Tiencheu, B.; Morfor, A.T.; Touko, B.A.H.; Houketchang, S.N.; Boungo, G.T.; Karuna, M.S.L.; Ngoufack, F.Z.; et al. Effect of traditional and oven roasting on the physicochemical properties of fermented cocoa beans. *Heliyon* **2018**, *4*, e00533. [CrossRef]
18. International agency for research on cancer (IARC). Monographs on the evaluation of carcinogenic risks to humans. In *Dry Cleaning, Some Chlorinated Solvents and Other Industrial Chemicals*; IARC Publications: Lyon, France, 1995; Volume 63, pp. 3194–3407.
19. Codex Alimentarius Commission. Standard for Cocoa (Cacao) Mass (Cocoa/Chocolate Liquor) and Cocoa Cake Codex Stan 141-1983; 2014. Available online: http://www.fao.org/input/download/standards/69/CXS_141e.pdf (accessed on 1 March 2020).
20. Okiyama, D.C.G.; Navarro, S.L.B.; Rodrigues, C.E.C. Cocoa shell and its compounds: Applications in the food industry. *Trends Food Sci. Technol.* **2017**, *63*, 103–112. [CrossRef]
21. Quelal-Vásconez, M.A.; Lerma-García, M.J.; Pérez-Esteve, É.; Arnau-Bonachera, A.; Barat, J.M.; Talens, P. Fast detection of cocoa shell in cocoa powders by near infrared spectroscopy and multivariate analysis. *Food Control* **2019**, *99*, 68–72. [CrossRef]
22. Association of Official Analytical Chemists. *Official Methods of Analysis*, 17th ed.; AOAC: Gaithersburg, MD, USA, 2002.
23. Chaves-López, C.; Serio, A.; Montalvo, C.; Ramirez, C.; Peréz-Álvarez, J.A.; Paparella, A.; Mastrocola, D.; Martuscelli, M. Effect of nisin on biogenic amines and shelf life of vacuum packaged rainbow trout (*Oncorhynchus mykiss*) fillets. *J. Food Sci. Technol.* **2017**, *54*, 3268–3277. [CrossRef] [PubMed]
24. Re, R.; Pellegrini, N.; Proteggente, A.; Pannala, A.; Yang, M.; Rice-Evans, C. Antioxidant activity applying an improved ABTS radical cation decolorization assay. *Free Radic. Biol. Med.* **1999**, *26*, 1231–1237. [CrossRef]
25. Benzie, I.F.F.; Strain, J.J. Ferric reducing/antioxidant power assay: Direct measure of total antioxidant activity of biological fluids and modified version for simultaneous measurement of total antioxidant power and ascorbic acid concentration. *Methods Enzymol.* **1999**, *299*, 15–27.
26. Kongor, J.E.; Hinneh, M.; Van de Walle, D.; Afoakwa, E.O.; Boeckx, P.; Dewettinck, K. Factors influencing quality variation in cocoa *Theobroma cacao* bean flavour profile: A review. *Food Res. Int.* **2016**, *82*, 44–52. [CrossRef]
27. Schwan, R.F.; Pereira, G.D.M.; Fleet, G.H. Microbial activities during cocoa fermentation. In *Cocoa and Coffee Fermentations*, 1st ed.; Shwan, R.F., Fleet, G.H., Eds.; Taylor & Francis: Boca Raton, FL, USA, 2014; pp. 129–192.
28. Schwan, R.F.; Wheals, A.E. The microbiology of cocoa fermentation and its role in chocolate quality. *Crit. Rev. Food Sci. Nutr.* **2004**, *44*, 205–221. [CrossRef] [PubMed]
29. Lima, L.J.R.; van der Velpen, V.; Wolkers-Rooijackers, J.; Kamphuis, H.J.; Zwietering, M.H.; Rob Nout, M.J. Microbiota dynamics and diversity at different stages of industrial processing of cocoa beans into cocoa powder. *Appl. Environ. Microbiol.* **2012**, *78*, 2904–2913. [CrossRef] [PubMed]
30. Baraggio, N.G.; Velázquez, N.S.; Simonetta, A.C. Aminas biógenas generadas por cepas bacterianas provenientes de alimentos lácteos y cárnicos. *Rev. Cienc. Tecnol.* **2010**, *13*. Available online: http://www.scielo.org.ar/scielo.php?script=sci_arttext&pid=S1851-75872010000100012 (accessed on 20 March 2020).
31. Rodriguez-Campos, J.; Escalona-Buendía, H.B.; Orozco-Avila, I.; Lugo-Cervantes, E.; Jaramillo-Flores, M.E. Dynamics of volatile and non-volatile compounds in cocoa (*Theobroma cacao* L.) during fermentation and drying processes using principal components analysis. *Food Res. Int.* **2011**, *44*, 250–258. [CrossRef]
32. García-Alamilla, P.; Lagunes-Gálvez, L.M.; Barajas-Fernández, J.; García-Alamilla, R. Physicochemical changes of cocoa beans during roasting process. *J. Food Qual.* **2017**, *12*, 1–11. [CrossRef]
33. Gloria, M.B.A.; Tavares-Neto, J.; Labanca, R.A.; Carvalho, M.S. Influence of cultivar and germination on bioactive amines in soybeans (*Glycine max* L. Merril). *J. Agric. Food Chem.* **2005**, *53*, 7480–7485. [CrossRef]
34. Bandeira, C.M.; Evangelista, W.P.; Gloria, M.B.A. Bioactive amines in fresh, canned and dried sweet corn, embryo and endosperm and germinated corn. *Food Chem.* **2012**, *131*, 1355–1359. [CrossRef]
35. Albertini, B.; Schoubben, A.; Guarnaccia, D.; Pinelli, F.; Della Vecchia, M.; Ricci, M.; Di Renzo, G.C.; Blasi, P. Effect of fermentation and drying on cocoa polyphenols. *J. Agric. Food Chem.* **2015**, *63*, 9948–9953. [CrossRef]
36. Granvogl, M.; Bugan, S.; Schieberle, P. Formation of amines and aldehydes from parent amino acids during thermal processing of cocoa and model systems: New insights into pathways of the Strecker reaction. *J. Agric. Food Chem.* **2006**, *54*, 1730–1739. [CrossRef]
37. Zamora, R.; Delgado, R.M.; Hidalgo, F.J. Formation of β-phenylethylamine as a consequence of lipid oxidation. *Food Res. Int.* **2012**, *46*, 321–325. [CrossRef]

38. Martins, A.C.C.L.; Gloria, M.B.A. Changes on the levels of serotonin precursors - tryptophan and 5-hydroxytryptophan-during roasting of Arabica and Robusta coffee. *Food Chem.* **2010**, *118*, 529–533. [CrossRef]
39. Luten, J.B.; Bouquet, W.; Seuren, L.A.J.; Burggraaf, M.M.; Riekwel-Booy, G.; Durand, P.; Etienne, M.; Gouyou, J.P.; Landrein, A.; Ritchie, A.; et al. Biogenic amines in fishery products: Standardization methods within E.C. In *Quality Assurance in the Fish Industry*; Elsevier Science Publishers, B.V.: Amsterdam, The Netherlands, 1992; pp. 427–439.
40. Wendakoon, C.N.; Sakaguchi, M. Combined effect of sodium chloride and clove on growth and biogenic amine formation of *Enterobacter aerogenes* in Mackerel muscle extract. *J. Food Prot.* **1993**, *56*, 410–413. [CrossRef] [PubMed]
41. Chung, B.Y.; Park, S.Y.; Byun, Y.S.; Son, J.H.; Choi, Y.W.; Cho, H.S.; Kim, H.O.; Park, C.W. Effect of different cooking methods on Histamine levels in selected foods. *Ann. Dermatol.* **2017**, *296*, 706–714. [CrossRef]
42. Thadhani, V.M.; Jansz, E.R.; Peiris, H. Destruction of histamine by cooking ingredients-an artifact of analysis. *J. Natl. Sci. Found. Sri Lanka* **2001**, *29*, 129–135. [CrossRef]
43. Zapata-Bustamante, S.; Tamayo-Tenorio, A.; Rojano, B.A. Effect of roasting on the secondary metabolites and antioxidant activity of Colombian cocoa clones. *Rev. Fac. Nac. Agron. Medellín* **2015**, *68*, 7497–7507. [CrossRef]
44. Afoakwa, E.O.; Ofosu-Ansah, E.; Budu, A.S.; Mensah-Brown, H.; Takrama, J.F. Roasting effects on phenolic content and free-radical scavenging activities of pulp preconditioned and fermented cocoa (*Theobroma cacao*) beans. *Afr. J. Food Agric. Nutr. Dev.* **2015**, *15*, 9635–9650.
45. Carrillo, L.C.; Londoño-Londoño, J.; Gil, A. Comparison of polyphenol, methylxanthines and antioxidant activity in *Theobroma cacao* beans from different cocoa-growing areas in Colombia. *Food Res. Int.* **2014**, *60*, 273–280. [CrossRef]
46. Porras Barrientos, L.D.; Torres Oquendo, J.D.; Gil Garzón, M.A.; Martínez Álvarez, O.L. Effect of the solar drying process on the sensory and chemical quality of cocoa (*Theobroma cacao* L.) cultivated in Antioquia, Colombia. *Food Res. Int.* **2019**, *115*, 259–267. [CrossRef]
47. Loureiro, G.A.H.A. Qualidade de solo e Qualidade de Cacau. Master's Thesis, Universidade Estadual de Santa Cruz, Ilhéus, Bahia, Brazil, 2014.
48. Janszky, I.; Mukamai, K.J.; Ljung, R.; Ahnve, S.; Ahlbom, A.; Hallqvist, J. Chocolate consumption and mortality following a first acute myocardial infarction: The Stockholm Heart Epidemiology Study. *J. Intern. Med.* **2009**, *266*, 248–257. [CrossRef]
49. Payne, M.J.; Hurst, W.J.; Miller, K.B.; Rank, C.; Stuart, D.A. Impact of fermentation, drying, roasting, and dutch processing on epicatechin and catechin content of cacao beans and cocoa ingredients. *J. Agric. Food Chem.* **2010**, *58*, 10518–10527. [CrossRef] [PubMed]
50. Caligiani, A.; Cirlini, M.; Palla, G.; Ravaglia, R.; Arlorio, M. GC-MS detection of chiral markers of cocoa beans of different quality and geographic origin. *Chirality* **2007**, *19*, 329–334. [CrossRef]
51. Hurst, W.J.; Krake, S.H.; Bergmeier, S.C.; Payne, M.J.; Miller, K.B.; Stuart, D.A. Impact of fermentation, drying, roasting and Dutch processing on flavan-3-ol stereochemistry in cacao beans and cocoa ingredients. *Chem. Cent. J.* **2011**, *5*, 53. [CrossRef] [PubMed]
52. Bauer, D.; de Abreu, J.P.; Oliveira, H.S.S.; Goes-Neto, A.; Koblitz, M.G.B.; Teodoro, A.J. Antioxidant activity and cytotoxicity effect of cocoa beans subjected to different processing conditions in human lung carcinoma cells. *Oxid. Med. Cell. Longev.* **2016**, *2016*, 7428515. [CrossRef] [PubMed]
53. Tabanelli, G.; Montanari, C.; Gardini, F. Biogenic amines in food: A review of factors affecting their formation. In *Encyclopedia of Food Chemistry*; Melton, L., Shahidi, F., Varelis, P., Eds.; Academic Press: New York, NY, USA, 2019; pp. 337–343.
54. Carta, F.; Temperini, C.; Innocenti, A.; Scozzafava, A.; Kaila, K.; Supuran, C.T. Polyamines inhibit carbonic anhydrases by anchoring to the zinc-coordinated water molecule. *J. Med. Chem.* **2010**, *53*, 511–522. [CrossRef] [PubMed]

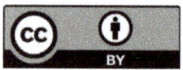

© 2020 by the authors. Licensee MDPI, Basel, Switzerland. This article is an open access article distributed under the terms and conditions of the Creative Commons Attribution (CC BY) license (http://creativecommons.org/licenses/by/4.0/).

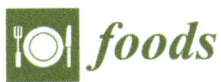

Article

Effects of Soaking and Fermentation Time on Biogenic Amines Content of *Maesil* (*Prunus Mume*) Extract

So Hee Yoon [1], Eunmi Koh [2], Bogyoung Choi [2] and BoKyung Moon [1,*]

[1] Department of Food and Nutrition, Chung-Ang University, Gyeonggi-do 17546, Korea; kisingserpe@naver.com
[2] Major of Food & Nutrition, Division of Applied Food System, Seoul Women's University, Seoul 01797, Korea; kohem7@swu.ac.kr (E.K.); 5326460@hanmail.net (B.C.)
* Correspondence: bkmoon@cau.ac.kr; Tel.: +82-31-670-3273

Received: 30 October 2019; Accepted: 15 November 2019; Published: 19 November 2019

Abstract: *Maesil* extract, a fruit-juice concentrate derived from *Prunus mume* prepared by fermenting with sugar, is widely used with increasing popularity in Korea. Biogenic amines in *maesil* extract were extracted with 0.4 M perchloric acid, derivatized with dansyl chloride, and detected using high-performance liquid chromatography. Among 18 home-made *maesil* extracts collected from different regions, total biogenic amine content varied from 2.53 to 241.73 mg/L. To elucidate the effects of soaking and fermentation time on biogenic amine content in *maesil* extract, *maesil* was soaked in brown sugar for 90 days and the liquid obtained was further fermented for 180 days at 15 and 25 °C, respectively. The main biogenic amines extracted were putrescine and spermidine and the total biogenic amine content was higher at 25 °C than at 15 °C. Soaking at 15 and 25 °C increased the total biogenic amines content from 14.14 to 34.98 mg/L and 37.33 to 69.05 mg/L, respectively, whereas a 180 day fermentation decreased the content from 31.66 to 13.59 mg/L and 116.82 to 57.05 mg/L, respectively. Biogenic amine content was correlated with total amino acid content (particularly, arginine content). Based on these results, we have considered that biogenic amine synthesis can be reduced during *maesil* extract production by controlling temperature and fermentation time.

Keywords: biogenic amine; *maesil*; amino acids; soaking; fermentation; temperature

1. Introduction

Maesil (*Prunus mume*) known as Japanese *Ume* has been used not only as a food but also as a medicine on account of its various functionalities [1–3]. As the seed of *maesil* has a toxic substance called amygdalin [4], *maesil* has been processed into various products such as alcoholic beverage, juice, pickle or extract rather than eaten raw [5]. *Maesil* extract is a fruit-juice concentrate produced by the fermentation of *maesil* and sugar. Recently, it has been increasingly used as a seasoning to impart sweetness and a unique flavor to foods [5–8]. Traditionally, *maesil* extract is soaked for a long period (90 days) at room temperature and fermented naturally under different conditions in individual households. Therefore, uncontrolled fermentation can lead to the formation of biogenic amines, which are produced by molds and bacteria.

As biogenic amines are mainly produced by the microbial decarboxylation of free amino acids, they are easily found in fermented foods [9,10]. These biogenic amines have been reported to be abundant and they have been found in a wide range of food products, including fish products, soy sauce, *Chunjang* (traditional fermented soybean paste in Korea and China), and agricultural products [11–15]. As a high intake of biogenic amines can cause various detrimental effects such as migraine and gastrointestinal problems, their ingestion needs to be restricted [16,17]. Indeed, their content is currently regulated in certain food products. For example, the histamine content in fish products is regulated by the US Food and Drug Administration (FDA, 50 mg/kg) and the European

Union (100 mg/kg) in fish products [18]. The formation of biogenic amines is influenced by microbial flora and their growth as well as the fermentation conditions used in the production of fermented foods [19,20]. To date, however, studies on the changes in biogenic amines during fruit fermentation have mainly focused on wine [9]. Moreover, little research has been conducted on the fermentation of biogenic amines during the fermentation of other fruits.

Therefore, in this study, we tried to monitor the biogenic amine content of *maesil* extracts and determine the effect of fermentation conditions on the changes in biogenic amines in *maesil* extracts during fermentation. For this purpose, we (i) determined the content of biogenic amines content in 18 home-made *maesil* extracts collected from different households in Korea and (ii) monitored the content of biogenic amines during the fermentation of *maesil* extracts at two different temperatures, 15 and 25 °C, over a period of 9 months.

2. Materials and Methods

2.1. Chemicals

Biogenic amine standards (histamine dihydrochloride (HIS), tryptamine hydrochloride (TRP), 2-phenylethylamine (2-PHE), putrescine dihydrochloride (PUT), cadaverine dihydrochloride (CAD), tyramine hydrochloride (TYR), spermidine trihydrochloride (SPD), and spermine tetrahydrochloride (SPM)) and dansyl chloride were obtained from Sigma-Aldrich Chemical Co. (St. Louis, MO, USA). Perchloric acid, 25% ammonium hydroxide solution, sodium hydroxide sodium hydrogen carbonate, and diethyl ether were acquired from Daejung Chemical Co. (Siheung, Korea). Acetone and acetonitrile (High-performance liquid chromatography (HPLC) grade) were purchased from Tedia Co. (Fairfield, OH, USA). Compound mixtures of amino acids, borate buffer, *o*-phthalaldehyde (OPA) and 9-fluorenylmethoxycarbonyl chloride (FMOC-Cl) were obtained from Agilent Technologies (Andover, MA, USA).

2.2. Preparation of Food Samples

During the period from 2010 to 2014, we collected samples 18 *maesil* extracts from different households in Korea for analysis of biogenic amines content. We also prepared our own *maesil* extract, following the method of Choi and Koh (2016) [5], and the process of preparation is shown in Figure 1. *Maesil* fruits obtained from a local market were washed with pure water, and drained at room temperature (23 ± 1 °C). To the 400 g of *maesil*, we added 400 g of brown sugar and the mixture was then placed in 1 L clear plastic jars, which were maintained in incubators set at 15 °C and 25 °C, respectively. After the *maesil* fruits were taken out from the jar after 90 days of soaking, the obtained liquid (490 mL at 15 °C and 476 mL at 25 °C) was further fermented for the next 180 days in the same jar. Biogenic amines were analyzed at 30, 45, 75, and 90 days of soaking period and 30, 60, 120, 150, and 180 days of fermentation.

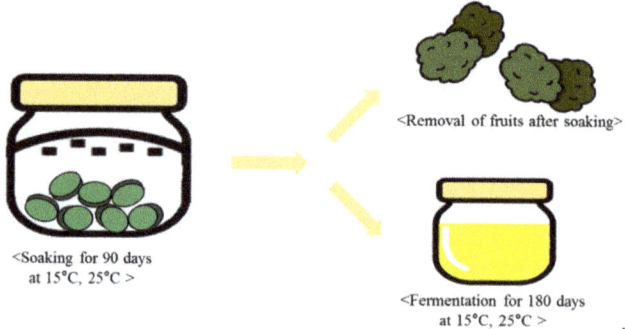

Figure 1. The fermentation process used for producing *maesil* extract.888.

2.3. pH Measurement

To measure the pH, *maesil* extract (10 g) was mixed with 10 mL deionized water for 3 min and then filtered through Whatman paper No.2 filter paper (Advantec, Tokyo, Japan). The pH was measured using a pH meter (Beckman Coulter, FL, USA) following the method of Shukla et al. [21].

2.4. Amino Acids Analysis

Amino acids in the *maesil* extract were analyzed using an HPLC system (Dionex Ultimate 3000, Thermo Fisher Scientific, Waltham, MA, USA), equipped with a 1260 Infinity fluorescence detector (Agilent Technologies, Waldbronn, Germany), following the method described by Jajic et al. (2013) [22] with slight modifications. The samples were derivatized with OPA and FMOC via a programmed autosampler. After derivatization, samples (0.5 µL) were injected into an Inno-C_{18} column (4.6 × 50 mm, 5 µm, Youngin Biochrom, Korea) at 40 °C. The fluorescence was detected at excitation and emission wavelengths of 340 and 450 mm, respectively for OPA, and at 266 and 305 nm, respectively, for FMOC. Primary and secondary amino acids were analyzed based on the OPA and FMOC derivatives, respectively. The mobile phase solvent A was 40 mM sodium phosphate (pH 7), and solvent B was a 10:45:45 (*v/v*) mixture of distilled water, acetonitrile, and methanol. The gradient program was run at a flow rate of 1.0 mL/min as follows: 5% B for 3 min; followed by elution with 5% to 55% B in 24 min; 55% to 90% B in 25 min; maintained 90% of B for next 6 min; and 90% to 5% B for 3.5 min, maintained for 0.5 min.

2.5. Biogenic Amine Analysis

2.5.1. Extraction of Biogenic Amines

Biogenic amines were extracted from the *maesil* extract using the method of Shukla et al. (2014) [21] with slight modifications. Briefly, 10 mL of 0.4 M perchloric acid solution was mixed with 5 g *maesil* extract, homogenized for 3 min, and then centrifuged at 3000× *g* for 10 min at 4 °C. The residue was re-extracted with 0.4 M perchloric acid solution (10 mL). After the supernatants were combined and 0.4 M perchloric acid solution was added to adjust the final volume to 50 mL. After filtering through Whatman filter paper No.1 (11 µm, Adventec, Tokyo, Japan), 1 mL of the extract was used for derivatization with dansyl chloride.

2.5.2. Derivatization of Biogenic Amines

Biogenic amines were derivatized following the methods described by Shukla et al. (2010) [23] and Frias et al. (2007) [24]. An extract sample (1 mL) or standard solution mixture (1 mL) was mixed with 200 µL 2 M sodium hydroxide; next, 300 µL of sodium hydrogen carbonate solution was added to saturate the solution. To the mixture, 1 mL of a dansyl chloride solution (10 mg/mL in acetone) was added and kept for 45 min at 40 °C. To stop the reaction, 100 µL of 25% ammonium hydroxide was added to the mixture and reacted for 30 min at 25 °C. Then, the derivatized biogenic amines were extracted twice with 1 mL of diethyl ether. Subsequent to drying in a nitrogen stream, the extract was redissolved in acetonitrile (1 mL) and filtered through a 0.22 µm polyvinylidene fluoride (PVDF) filter (Millipore Co., Bedford, MA, USA) for injection into the HPLC system.

2.5.3. HPLC Analysis of Biogenic Amines

Biogenic amines were analyzed using an HPLC system consisting of an Alliance 2695 separations module (Waters, Milford, MA, USA) and Ultra violet (UV)/Visible detector 2487 (Waters, Milford, MA, USA) with a Capcell Pak C18 column (4.6 × 250 mm i.d., 5 µm; Shiseido, Kyoto, Japan), thermostated at 30 °C, and detected at 210 nm [24–26]. The injection volume was 20 µL and the mobile phase consisted of solvent A (water) and B (acetonitrile) run at a flow rate of 0.8 mL/min with the following gradient elution program for 35 min: 65:35 (A:B, *v*/*v*), followed by 45% B for 5 min, elution with 45% to 65% B in 10.05 min, 65% to 80% B in 17.05 min, 80% to 90% B up to 26.25 min, and 90% to 35% B in 35 min.

2.6. Method Validation

The HPLC method for biogenic amines analysis was validated for linearity, limits of detection (LOD) and limits of quantification (LOQ), accuracy, and precision [22]. The linearity was evaluated using five concentrations (0.5, 1, 2, 5, and 10 mg/L) of each the biogenic amine standards (PUT, CAD, HIS, TRP, 2-PHE, TYR, SPD, and SPM) by constructing a calibration curve. The LOD and LOQ values were calculated using the following equations: LOD = 3.3 × (standard deviation (SD)/slope of calibration curve) and LOQ = 10 × (SD/slope of calibration curve). The accuracy of the method was verified by triplicate analysis of spiked samples at two different levels (5 and 10 mg/L) and expressed as % recovery. The recoveries were calculated by contrasting the peak area of measured concentration with the peak area of the spiked concentrations. To evaluate the precision, repeatability, inter-day, and intra-day were performed and expressed as the percentage relative standard deviation (RSD) of the peak area measurements. Repeatability was estimated by analysis of six consecutively injected samples. The inter-day precision was determined at two different levels, 5 and 10 mg/L, and the analyses were performed over a period of three consecutive days. The intra-day precision was determined by spiking five blank samples at concentrations levels of 5 and 10 mg/mL and the evaluation was based on the results obtained using the method operating over a single day under the same conditions.

2.7. Statistical Analysis

Quantitative data are expressed as the means ± SD of at least three measurements. Statistical analysis was performed using a one-way analysis of variance (ANOVA) and Duncan's multiple range test by SAS software, version 8.0 for Windows (SAS Institute, Cary, NC, USA). The probability value of $p < 0.05$ was considered statistically significant.

3. Results and Discussion

3.1. Method Validation

The results obtained from the different method validations are presented in Table 1. Standard curves for biogenic amines were constructed from triplicate analyses of five concentrations in the range 0.5–10 mg/L. With the exception of spermine (correlation coefficient (R^2) > 0.998), the linearity of the calibration curves for each biogenic amine was >0.999. The precision, expressed as %RSD, of inter-day variation was between 0.17% and 5.20%, and the RSD values for intra-day variation were between 0.07% and 6.46%. The LOD and LOQ of the biogenic amines ranged from 0.01 to 0.20 mg/L and 0.02 to 0.61 mg/L, respectively. The accuracy of the method with regard to recovery was between 89.4% and 110.8%.

Table 1. Summary results relating to validation of the high-performance liquid chromatography (HPLC) method used for biogenic amines.

Compound	R^2	LOD (mg/L)	LOQ (mg/L)	Precision (%RSD)				Accuracy	
				Inter-Day		Intra-Day		Recovery (%)	
				Low	High	Low	High	Low	High
HIS	1.0000	0.02	0.04	3.82	5.20	0.49	6.46	97.9	89.4
TRP	1.0000	0.01	0.02	0.66	0.19	0.10	0.09	101.8	105.3
2-PHE	1.0000	0.16	0.22	0.22	0.74	0.07	0.64	101.3	97.9
PUT	1.0000	0.01	0.02	0.45	0.34	0.25	0.76	99.8	104.0
CAD	1.0000	0.01	0.02	0.14	0.19	0.25	0.49	100.1	100.0
TYR	1.0000	0.07	0.10	0.27	0.17	0.09	0.22	99.7	99.3
SPM	0.9981	0.20	0.61	2.27	1.86	1.07	2.21	95.1	110.8
SPD	1.0000	0.04	0.08	0.14	0.40	0.16	0.11	107.1	99.6

LOD: Limits of detection; LOQ: Limits of quantification; RSD: Relative standard deviation HIS: Histamine; TRP: Tryptamine; PUT: Putrescine; 2-PHE: 2-phenylethylamine; CAD: Cadaverine; TYR: Tyramine; SPM: Spermine; SPD: Spermidine.

3.2. Content of Biogenic Amines in Home-Made Maesil Extract

Among the 18 home-made maesil extracts analyzed, the total content of biogenic amines ranged from 2.5 to 241.7 mg/L, the major individual biogenic amines were putrescine (not detectable (ND)-80.82 mg/L) and spermidine (ND-219.20 mg/L), followed by tryptamine (Table 2). Putrescine, histamine, tyramine, cadaverine, 2-phenylethylamine, spermidine, spermine, agmatine, and tryptamine are the main biogenic amines in wine [27]. Among these amines, putrescine has been reported to be generated from the raw material or by microbial decarboxylation [28]. In the case of wine, putrescine content has been found to be influenced by geographical region and grape variety [29]. Histamine and spermine detected in wine [27,29,30] are known to have toxicity or play a role in enhancing toxicity [11,31]. However, we were unable to detect either of these two amines in the 18 maesil extracts examined in the present study. These results imply that the amount and composition of biogenic amines may differ widely among different fruit-derived products and that these differences could be attributed to differences in manufacturing practice and fruit material.

Table 2. Biogenic amines content (mg/L) in 18 home-made *maesil* extracts prepared in individual households.

Sample	HIS	TRP	2-PHE	PUT	CAD	TYR	SPM	SPD	Total
A	ND	ND	ND	19.7 ± 0.53	2.9 ± 1.01	ND	ND	219.2 ± 6.30	241.8 ± 4.89
B	ND	3.0 ± 0.53	ND	12.4 ± 0.67	ND	ND	ND	44.5 ± 1.96	60.0 ± 1.64
C	ND	ND	ND	15.3 ± 0.74	ND	ND	ND	14.9 ± 0.91	30.2 ± 1.64
D	ND	1.9 ± 0.36	ND	8.8 ± 0.42	ND	ND	ND	25.6 ± 0.74	36.2 ± 0.18
E	ND	3.2 ± 0.47	ND	15.9 ± 1.69	ND	ND	ND	44.3 ± 2.31	63.4 ± 4.07
F	ND	ND	ND	13.1 ± 0.99	ND	ND	ND	83.5 ± 6.28	96.5 ± 6.21
G	ND	2.9 ± 0.65	ND	25.8 ± 2.33	17.3 ± 3.79	ND	ND	44.6 ± 3.11	90.6 ± 4.93
H	ND	5.7 ± 1.32	ND	ND	12.7 ± 0.42	ND	ND	35.9 ± 1.22	54.3 ± 2.09
I	ND	2.5 ± 0.48	ND	ND	ND	ND	ND	ND	2.5 ± 0.48
J	ND	3.5 ± 0.35	5.26 ± 1.47	ND	ND	ND	ND	ND	8.8 ± 1.19
K	ND	5.3 ± 0.45	ND	21.8 ± 0.70	ND	0.8 ± 0.02	ND	77.9 ± 1.81	105.8 ± 1.38
L	ND	ND	ND	ND	ND	1.0 ± 0.12	ND	ND	1.0 ± 0.12
M	ND	5.4 ± 0.38	ND	ND	ND	ND	ND	ND	5.4 ± 0.38
N	ND	ND	ND	17.5 ± 0.15	ND	ND	ND	71.8 ± 4.60	89.3 ± 4.45
O	ND	3.2 ± 035	ND	6.8 ± 0.26	ND	ND	ND	ND	9.9 ± 0.46
P	ND	ND	ND	80.8 ± 4.72	ND	ND	ND	17.1 ± 1.76	97.9 ± 4.29
Q	ND	4.1 ± 0.83	ND	5.9 ± 0.70	ND	0.7 ± 0.07	ND	10.1 ± 1.44	20.8 ± 3.10
R	ND	3.4 ± 0.45	ND	8.4 ± 0.97	ND	ND	ND	41.3 ± 1.41	53.1 ± 2.01

HIS: Histamine; TRP: Tryptamine; PUT: Putrescine; 2-PHE: 2-phenylethylamine; CAD: Cadaverine; TYR: Tyramine; SPM: Spermine; SPD: Spermidine; ND: Not detected.

The content of biogenic amines is known to be affected by fermentation conditions, including temperature, microorganisms, and the synthetic pathways of the biogenic amine formation [32–35]. In wine, cadaverine, histamine, putrescine, and tyramine are mainly detected, the content of which can vary depending on fermentation factors, storage, microbial decarboxylase activity, and vinification [27,30,36]. Marcobal et al. (2006) have reported that the content of biogenic amines in wine ranged from ND to 54.02 mg/L [31]. Garai et al. (2006) found that the main biogenic amine in commercial apple ciders was putrescine and that the total biogenic amine content ranged from ND to 23.26 mg/L [12]. In comparison, the results of this study indicate that the biogenic amine content in home-made *maesil* extracts is considerably higher than that reported in wine or apple ciders [12,27,30], thereby emphasizing the necessity to control biogenic amines productions during the fermentation of *maesil* extract.

3.3. Content of Biogenic Amines During Soaking and Fermentation

During the 90 day soaking of *maesil* examined in the present study, we found that the total biogenic amines content increased from 14.1 to 35.0 mg/L and 37.3 to 69.1 mg/L at 15 and 25 °C, respectively, indicating that the content was higher at the latter temperature throughout the soaking period (Figure 1a). Previous studies have reported that biogenic amines are generated via the catalytic activity of decarboxylase enzymes produced during the growth of microorganisms such as lactic acid bacteria [37], and thus, the increase in biogenic amines during the soaking period might be caused by microbial decarboxylase activity. At both incubation temperatures we assessed, the predominant biogenic amines detected in *maesil* extract were putrescine and spermidine (Figure 2b,c), and the latter comprised approximately 80% of the total biogenic amines.

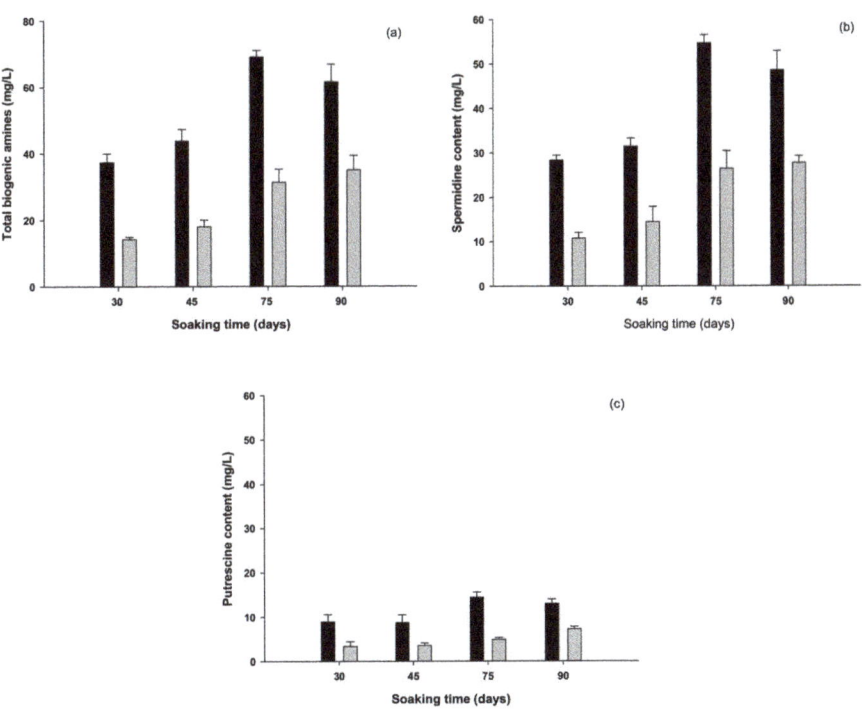

Figure 2. The content (mg/L) of total biogenic amines (**a**), spermidine (**b**), and putrescine (**c**) during soaking at 25 °C (■) and 15 °C (■).

After removing the *maesil* fruit from the sample jars at the end of the soaking period, the residual liquid was subsequently fermented for 180 days, during which, the content of biogenic amines decreased from 31.7 to 13.6 mg/L and 116.8 to 57.1 mg/L at 15 and 25 °C, respectively (Table 3). Generally, the extracts fermented at 25 °C exhibited biogenic amines content that was twice as high as that obtained at 15 °C. Moreover, at the end of the fermentation period, the total biogenic amines content at 15 °C was 23.8% of that at 25 °C. In addition to putrescine and spermidine, tryptamine was also detected at 0.33 mg/L when *maesil* was fermented at the higher temperature for 30 days. In this regard, Chong et al. (2011) have reported that temperature was the most important factor affecting biogenic amines formation [38], and Pinho et al. (2001) reported a higher increase in biogenic amines at a storage temperature of 21 °C than at 4 °C [35]. In addition, Kim et al. (2002) found that 25 °C was the optimum temperature for histamine production in fish muscles [39]. *Maesil* extract is typically produced by natural fermentation without controlling the temperature or starter culture. Moreover, it is sometimes consumed immediately after a 90 day soaking without subsequent fermentation. On the basis of the results obtained in this study, we recommend that, to yield a product with lower levels of biogenic amines, *maesil* extract should be fermented at a relatively low temperature and for a long period of time.

3.4. Effects of Processing Factors on Biogenic Amines Formation

The pathways implicated in the synthesis of biogenic amines can vary depending on the temperature, sugar content, precursors, and microorganisms involved in the fermentation of various food items [16,32,40]. Generally, putrescine is derived from the decarboxylation of arginine and ornithine or is already present in raw materials [28,32], whereas, spermidine is produced from arginine and ornithine or is converted from putrescine by spermidine synthase [16,31]. Poveda (2019) and Bardocz (1995) reported that most putrescine is either converted to spermidine or spermine, or is catabolized to succinate and other amino acids via succinate [28,31].

In the present study, to determine the effects of the factors influencing biogenic amines formation, we performed Pearson's correlation. Among these factors, we detected no significant correlation between biogenic amines content and pH, which had a narrow range (pH 2.9–3.3) during the fermentation.

Arena et al. (2008) reported a negative correlation between biogenic amines and sugar concentration and found that; the additions of glucose and fructose at 5 and 20 g/L reduced biogenic amines production by 82%–93% and 61%–99%, respectively [40]. Cid et al. (2008) reported that lower glucose concentration is associated with a high activity of ornithine-decarboxylase produced by *Lactobacillus* [41]. In our study, we found that, although there was a negative correlation between sugar content and biogenic amines content (Figure 3a), the relationship was not significant, which could be attributable to the narrow range of sugar content (61 to 81 °Brix) during fermentation.

Table 3. Biogenic amines content (mg/L) during fermentation at different temperatures.

Biogenic amine	Fermentation Days at 15 °C						Fermentation Days at 25 °C					
	30	60	120	150	180	30	60	120	150	180
TRP	ND	ND	ND	ND	ND	0.33 ± 0.09	ND	ND	ND	ND
PUT	8.1 ± 1.18 [a]	12.8 ± 1.15 [b]	13.8 ± 0.67 [b]	12.5 ± 1.95 [b]	7.4 ± 0.01 [a]	30.9 ± 0.77 [c]	23.9 ± 1.56 [b]	14.5 ± 0.76 [a]	20.0 ± 0.34 [b]	15.6 ± 4.03 [a]
CAD	ND	ND	ND	ND	ND	ND	ND	ND	ND	ND
SPD	23.6 ± 1.19 [b]	26.6 ± 2.32 [c]	22.2 ± 0.66 [b]	22.2 ± 0.65 [b]	6.2 ± 0.74 [a]	84.8 ± 0.68 [d]	74.9 ± 2.36 [c]	52.3 ± 3.25 [b]	46.5 ± 4.93 [a,b]	41.4 ± 2.58 [a]
Total	31.7 ± 2.15 [b]	39.4 ± 3.30 [d]	36.0 ± 1.33 [c,d]	34.7 ± 2.69 [b,c]	13.6 ± 0.75 [a]	116.8 ± 4.17 [d]	98.8 ± 0.93 [c]	66.8 ± 3.96 [b]	66.5 ± 4.59 [b]	57.0 ± 6.43 [a]

TRP: Tryptamine; PUT: Putrescine; CAD: Cadaverine; SPD: Spermidine; ND: Not detected. Each value expressed the mean of triplicates ± standard deviation (SD). Different superscript letters in the same row indicate significant difference ($p < 0.05$).

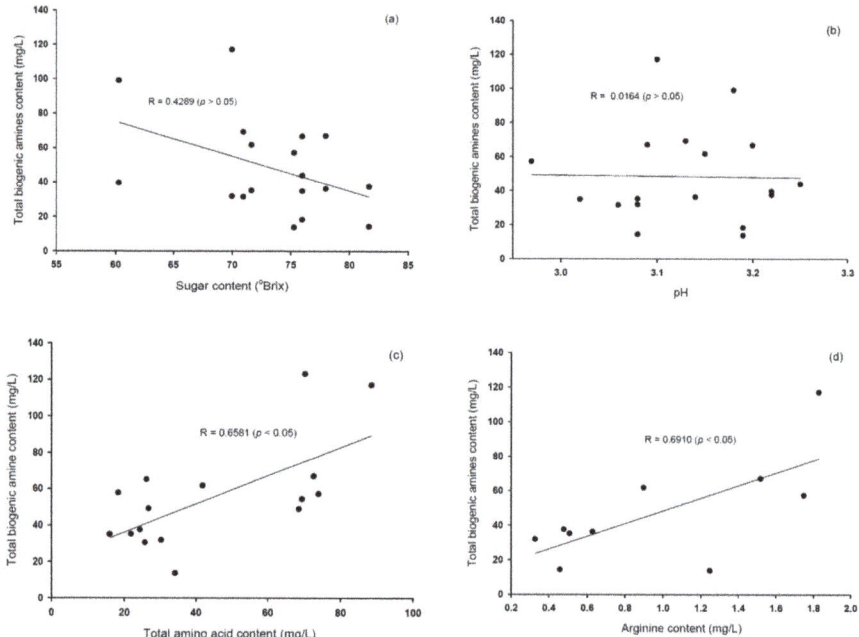

Figure 3. Correlations between sugar content and biogenic amine content (mg/L) (**a**); pH and biogenic amine content (mg/L) (**b**); the content (mg/L) of total amino acid and total biogenic amines (**c**); and the content (mg/L) of biogenic amines and arginine (**d**).

The total biogenic amines content showed a positive correlation with the total amounts of amino acids ($R = 0.6581$, $p < 0.05$), which could be explained by the fact that amino acids are precursors of biogenic amines [42]. We also detected a strong positive correlation between the amounts of putrescine and spermidine ($R = 0.9277$, $p < 0.01$; data not shown), consistent with the findings of Bardocz (1995) [31] and Nuriez et al. (2016) [16], which indicates that putrescine is a precursor of spermidine. However, apart from a positive correlation between arginine and total biogenic amines content ($R = 0.6910$, $p < 0.05$), we detected no correlation between individual biogenic amines and their respective precursor amino acid, which is consistent with the findings reported by Soufleros et al. (1998) [43]. Gezginc et al. (2013) reported that arginine serves as a precursor of putrescine, which can, in turn, be converted to spermidine [32]. Furthermore, it has been found that, in plants and some microorganisms, there are alternative pathways in which putrescine is generated from arginine via agmatine [33]. These results indicate that the fermentation of *maesil* extract at low temperature could reduce the production of biogenic amines. In addition, biogenic amine formation in *maesil* extract could be affected by the origin of *maesil*, the number of amino acids as well as the content of biogenic amine precursors.

4. Conclusions

The present study was conducted to evaluate the changes in biogenic amines formation and the relationship between biogenic amines and amino acids in *maesil* extract during the fermentation of this product. Although the consumption of *maesil* extract is currently increasing, there has, to date, been a lack of studies on the changes that biogenic amines undergo during *maesil* extract fermentation. The results of this study showed that the biogenic amines content in *maesil* extract is affected by both the inherent amino acids content and fermentation temperature and time. Moreover, the content of some biogenic amines may also be affected by the presence of other biogenic amines. We found that both amino acids and biogenic amines content was lower during fermentation at 15 °C than at 25 °C and decreased with increasing fermentation time. Accordingly, these observations indicate that employing protracted low-temperature fermentations could be an effective approach for reducing the production of biogenic amines in *maesil* extract. In further research, it will be necessary to study the types of microorganisms and formation on biogenic amines in *maesil* extract.

Author Contributions: Conceptualization, S.H.Y. and B.C.; methodology, S.H.Y. and B.C.; validation, S.H.Y., B.C., and E.K.; formal analysis, S.H.Y., B.C., and E.K.; investigation, S.H.Y. and B.C.; resources, B.M.; data curation, S.H.Y. and B.C.; writing—original draft preparation, S.H.Y. and B.C.; writing—review and editing, B.M.; supervision, B.M.; project administration, B.M.

Funding: This research received no external funding.

Acknowledgments: This research did not receive any specific grant from funding agencies in the public, commercial, or not-for-profit sectors.

Conflicts of Interest: The authors declare no conflict of interest.

References

1. Kang, M.Y.; Jeong, Y.H.; Eun, J.B. Physical and chemical characteristics of flesh and pomace of Japanese Apricots (*Prunus mume* Sieb. et Zucc). *Korean J. Food Sci. Technol.* **1999**, *31*, 1434–1439.
2. Ko, M.S.; Yang, J.B. Antimicrobial activities of extracts of *Prunus mume* by sugar. *Korean Soc. Food Preser.* **2009**, *16*, 759–764.
3. Miyazawa, M.; Yamada, T.; Utsunomiya, H. Suppressive effect of the SOS-inducing activity of chemical mutagen by citric acid esters from *Prunus mume* Sieb. et Zucc. using the *Salmonella typhimurium* Ta1535/Psk1002 Umu test. *Nat. Prod. Res.* **2003**, *17*, 319–323. [CrossRef] [PubMed]
4. Bolarinwa, I.F.; Orfila, C.; Morgan, M.R.A. Amygdalin content of seeds, kernels and food products commercially-available in the UK. *Food Chem.* **2014**, *152*, 133–139. [CrossRef]
5. Choi, B.G.; Koh, E. Changes of ethyl carbamate and its precursors in maesil (*Prunus mume*) extract curing one-year fermentation. *Food Chem.* **2016**, *209*, 318–322. [CrossRef]
6. Kim, H.W.; Han, S.H.; Lee, S.W.; Suh, H.J. Effect of isomaltulose used for osmotic extraction of Prunus mume fruit juice substituting sucrose. *Food Sci. Technol.* **2018**, *27*, 1599–1605. [CrossRef]
7. Ko, Y.J.; Jeong, D.Y.; Lee, J.O.; Park, M.H.; Kim, E.J.; Kim, J.W.; Kim, Y.S.; Ryu, C.H. The establishment of optimum fermentation conditions for *Prunus mume* vinegar and its quality evaluation. *Korean Soc. Food Sci. Nutr.* **2007**, *36*, 361–365. [CrossRef]
8. Yan, X.T.; Lee, S.H.; Li, W.; Sun, Y.N.; Yang, S.Y.; Jang, H.D.; Kim, Y.H. Evaluation of the antioxidant and anti-osteoporosis activities of chemical constituents of the fruits of *Prunus mume*. *Food Chem.* **2014**, *156*, 408–415. [CrossRef]
9. Henriquez-Aedo, K.; Galarce-Bustos, O.; Aqueveque, P.; Garcia, A.; Aranda, M. Dynamic of biogenic amines and precursor amino acids during cabernet sauvignon vinification. *LWT Food Sci. Technol.* **2018**, *97*, 238–244. [CrossRef]
10. Shalaby, A.R. Significance of biogenic amines to food safety and human health. *Food Res. Int.* **1996**, *29*, 675–690. [CrossRef]
11. Bai, X.; Byun, B.Y.; Mah, J.H. Formation and destruction of biogenic amines in Chunjang (a black soybean sauce) and Jajang (a blck soybean sauce). *Food Chem.* **2013**, *141*, 1026–1031. [CrossRef] [PubMed]
12. Garai, G.; Duenas, M.T.; Irastorza, A.; Martin-Alvarez, P.J.; Moreno-Arribas, M.V. Biogenic amines in natural ciders. *J. Food Prot.* **2006**, *69*, 3006–3012. [CrossRef] [PubMed]
13. Kim, J.H.; Park, H.J.; Kim, M.J.; Ahn, H.J.; Byun, M.W. Survey of biogenic amine contents in commercial soy sauce. *Korean J. Food Sci. Technol.* **2003**, *35*, 325–328.
14. Mohan, C.O.; Ravishankar, C.N.; Srinivasa Gopal, T.K.; Ashok Kumar, K.; Lalitha, K.V. Biogenic amines formation in seer fish (*Scomberomoruscommerson*) steaks packed with O_2 scavenger during chilled storage. *Food Res. Int.* **2009**, *42*, 411–416. [CrossRef]
15. Yoon, H.; Park, J.H.; Choi, A.; Hwang, H.J.; Mah, J.H. Validation of an HPLC analytical method for determination of biogenic amines in agricultural products and monitoring of biogenic amines in Korean fermented agricultural products. *Toxicol. Res.* **2015**, *31*, 299–305. [CrossRef] [PubMed]

16. Nuriez, M.; del Olmo, A.; Calzada, J. Biogenic amines. *Encycl. Food Health* **2016**, 416–423.
17. Zarei, M.; Najafzadeh, H.; Enayati, A.; Pashmforoush, M. Biogenic amines content of canned tuna fish marketed in Iran. *Am. Eurasian J. Toxicol. Sci.* **2011**, *3*, 190–193.
18. Nadeem, M.; Naveed, T.; Rehman, F.; Xu, Z. Determination of histamine in fish without derivatization by indirect reverse phase-HPLC method. *Microchem. J.* **2019**, *144*, 209–214. [CrossRef]
19. Carelli, D.; Centonze, D.; Palermo, C.; Quinto, M.; Rotunno, T. An interference free amperometric biosensor for the detection of biogenic amines in food products. *Biosens. Bioelectron.* **2007**, *23*, 64–647. [CrossRef]
20. Nout, M.J.R.; Ruikes, M.M.W.; Bouwmeester, H.M.; Belfaars, P.R. Effect of processing conditions on the formation of biogenic amines and ethyl carbamate in soybean Tempeh. *J. Food Saf.* **1993**, *13*, 293–303. [CrossRef]
21. Shukla, S.; Park, H.K.; Lee, J.S.; Kim, J.K.; Kim, M. Reduction of biogenic amines and aflatoxin in Doenjang samples fermented with various *Meju* as starter cultures. *Food Control.* **2014**, *42*, 181–187. [CrossRef]
22. Jajic, I.; Krstovic, S.; Glamocic, D.; Jaksic, S.; Abramovic, B. Validation of HPLC method for the determination of amino acids in feed. *J. Serb. Chem. Soc.* **2013**, *78*, 839–850. [CrossRef]
23. Shukla, S.; Park, H.K.; Kim, J.K.; Kim, M.H. Determination of biogenic amines in Korean traditional fermented soybean paste (Doenjang). *Food Chem. Toxicol.* **2010**, *48*, 1191–1195. [CrossRef] [PubMed]
24. Frias, J.; Martinez-Villaluenga, C.; Gulewicz, P.; Perez-Romero, A.; Pilarski, R.; Gulewicz, K.; Vidal-Valverde, C. Biogenic amines and HL 60 citotoxicity of alfalfa and fenugreek sprouts. *Food Chem.* **2007**, *105*, 959–967. [CrossRef]
25. Qiu, S.; Wang, Y.; Cheng, Y.; Liu, Y.; Yadav, M.P.; Yin, L. Reduction of biogenic amines in sufu by ethanol during ripening stage. *Food Chem.* **2018**, *239*, 1244–1252. [CrossRef]
26. Costa, M.P.; Balthazar, C.F.; Rodrigues, B.L.; Lazaro, C.A.; Silva, A.C.O.; Cruz, A.G.; Conte Junior, C.A. Determination of biogenic amines by high-performance liquid chromatography (HPLC-DAD) in probiotic cow's and goat's fermented milks and acceptance. *Food Sci. Nutr.* **2015**, *3*, 172–178. [CrossRef]
27. Jastrzebska, A.; Piasta, A.; Kowalska, S.; Krzeminski, M.; Szlyk, E. A new derivatization reagent for determination of biogenic amines in wines. *J. Food Compos. Anal.* **2016**, *48*, 111–119. [CrossRef]
28. Poveda, J.M. Biogenic amines and free amino acids in craft beers from the Spanish market: A statistical approach. *Food Control.* **2019**, *96*, 227–233. [CrossRef]
29. Landete, J.M.; Ferrer, S.; Polo, L.; Pardo, I. Biogenic amines in wines from three Spanish regions. *J. Agric. Food Chem.* **2005**, *53*, 1119–1124. [CrossRef]
30. Marcobal, A.; Martin-Alvarez, P.J.; Polo, M.C.; Moreno-Arribas, M.V. Formation of biogenic amines throughout the industrial manufacture of red wine. *J. Food Prot.* **2006**, *69*, 397–404. [CrossRef]
31. Bardocz, S. Polyamines in food and their consequences for food quality and human health. *Trends Food Sci. Technol.* **1995**, *6*, 341–346. [CrossRef]
32. Gezginc, Y.; Akyol, I.; Kuley, E.; Ozogul, F. Biogenic amines formation in *Streptococcus thermophiles* isolated from home-made natural yogurt. *Food Chem.* **2013**, *138*, 655–662. [CrossRef] [PubMed]
33. Karovicova, J.; Kohajdova, Z. Biogenic amines in food. *Chem. Pap.* **2005**, *59*, 70–79. [CrossRef]
34. Ozogul, F.; Hamed, I. The importance of lactic acid bacteria for the prevention of bacterial growth and their biogenic amines formation: A review. *Crit. Rev. Food Sci. Nutr.* **2018**, *58*, 1660–1670. [CrossRef]
35. Pinho, O.; Ferreira, I.M.P.L.V.O.; Mendes, E.; Oliveira, B.M.; Ferreira, M. Effect of temperature on evolution of free amino acid and biogenic amine contents during storage of Azeitao cheese. *Food Chem.* **2001**, *75*, 287–291. [CrossRef]
36. Santos, M.H.S. Biogenic amines: Their importance in foods. *Int. J. Food Microbiol.* **1996**, *29*, 213–231. [CrossRef]
37. Patel, M.A.; Ou, M.S.; Harbrucker, R.; Aldrich, H.C.; Buszko, M.L.; Ingram, L.O.; Shanmugam, K.T. Isolation and characterization of acid-tolerant, thermophilic bacteria for effective fermentation of biomass-derived sugars to lactic acid. *Appl. Environ. Micorobiol.* **2006**, *72*, 3228–3235. [CrossRef]
38. Chong, C.Y.; Abu Bakar, F.; Russly, A.R.; Jamilah, B.; Mahyudin, N.A. The effects of food processing on biogenic amines formation. *Int. Food Res. J.* **2011**, *18*, 867–876.
39. Kim, S.H.; Price, B.J.; Morrissey, M.T.; Field, K.G.; Wei, C.I.; An, H. Occurrence of histamine-forming bacteria in albacore and histamine accumulation in muscle at ambient temperature. *J. Food Sci.* **2002**, *67*, 1515–1521. [CrossRef]

40. Arena, M.E.; Landete, J.M.; Manca de Nadra, M.C.; Pardo, I.; Ferrer, S. Factors affecting the production of putrescine from agmatine by *Lactobacillus hilgardii* X1B isolated from wine. *J. Appl. Microbiol.* **2008**, *105*, 158–165. [CrossRef]
41. Cid, B.S.; Miguelez-Arrizado, M.J.; Becker, B.; Holzapfel, W.H.; Vidal-Carou, M.C. Amino acid decarboxylation by *Lactobacillus curvatus* CTC 273 affected by the pH and glucose availability. *Food Microbiol.* **2008**, *25*, 269–277. [PubMed]
42. Wang, Y.Q.; Ye, D.Q.; Zhu, B.Q.; Wu, G.F.; Duan, C.Q. Rapid HPLC analysis of amino acids and biogenic amines in wine during fermentation and evaluation of matrix effect. *Food Chem.* **2014**, *163*, 6–15. [CrossRef] [PubMed]
43. Soufleros, E.; Barrios, M.L.; Bertrand, A. Correlation between the content of biogenic amines and other wine compounds. *Am. J. Enol. Vitic.* **1998**, *49*, 266–278.

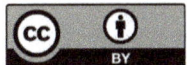

© 2019 by the authors. Licensee MDPI, Basel, Switzerland. This article is an open access article distributed under the terms and conditions of the Creative Commons Attribution (CC BY) license (http://creativecommons.org/licenses/by/4.0/).

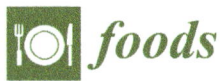

Article

Casing Contribution to Proteolytic Changes and Biogenic Amines Content in the Production of an Artisanal Naturally Fermented Dry Sausage

Annalisa Serio, Jessica Laika, Francesca Maggio, Giampiero Sacchetti, Flavio D'Alessandro, Chiara Rossi, Maria Martuscelli, Clemencia Chaves-López * and Antonello Paparella

Faculty of Bioscience and Technology for Food, Agriculture and Environment, University of Teramo, via Balzarini 1, 64100 Teramo, Italy; aserio@unite.it (A.S.); jessica.laika@hotmail.com (J.L.); fmaggio@unite.it (F.M.); gsacchetti@unite.it (G.S.); flavio_dale@live.it (F.D.); crossi@unite.it (C.R.); mmartuscelli@unite.it (M.M.); apaparella@unite.it (A.P.)
* Correspondence: cchaveslopez@unite.it

Received: 26 August 2020; Accepted: 8 September 2020; Published: 13 September 2020

Abstract: The effect of two kinds of casings on the production and characteristics of a dry fermented sausage was investigated. In detail, an Italian product, naturally fermented at low temperatures and normally wrapped in beef casing instead of the most diffused hog one, was selected. Two different productions (one traditionally in beef casing (MCB) and another in hog casing (MCH)) were investigated over time to determine the differences particularly regarding proteolytic changes during fermentation and ripening. First of all, the product in hog casing required a longer ripening time, up to 120 days, instead of 45–50 days, because of the lower drying rate, while the microbial dynamics were not significantly modified. Conversely, the proteolysis showed a different evolution, being more pronounced, together with the biogenic amines content up to 341 mg/Kg instead of 265 mg/Kg for the traditional products. The latter products were instead characterized by higher quantities of total free amino acids, 3-methyl butanoic acid, 3-Methyl-1-butanal, and 2-Methylpropanal, enriching the final taste and aroma. The traditional product MCB also showed lower hardness and chewiness than MCH. The results highlight how the choice of casing has a relevant impact on the development of the final characteristics of fermented sausages.

Keywords: proteolysis; dry fermented sausage; casing; biogenic amines; volatile compounds; texture; low temperature

1. Introduction

The characteristics of dry fermented sausages depend on many factors, including the ingredients, the recipe, the microbiota composition, and the different production steps. These factors, combined together, determine the variety of products widespread in different European countries [1]. Many fermented meats are produced in Italy; among them, a very particular one is produced during autumn and winter in the Abruzzo Region (Central Italy), and is called *"Mortadella di Campotosto"*. It is made of lean pork meat mixed with salt, pepper, and nitrite and it contains a bar of lard, previously cured with salt and spices for about two weeks. It shows a characteristic sub-ovoid shape and length about 15–20 cm, with a diameter of 8–10 cm. Among the typical characteristics, this product is handmade and wrapped (instead of being stuffed) into a natural beef casing; afterwards, it is fermented at low temperature without any starter addition. Traditionally, the product is exposed to dry cold northern winds that provide the ideal conditions for product ripening, which lasts about 40–50 days, with temperatures varying from −1 °C to about 10 °C.

As for this product, the traditional casing is made of beef middles, we decided to evaluate the effect of both the traditional casing and a more usual hog casing on the characteristics of the sausage.

In fact, although "*Mortadella di Campotosto*" sausage manufacturing does not have any particular specifications about the natural casing to use, most of the producers use beef casing, but some may use hog casing because of its larger availability.

As regards fermented sausages, besides containing the meat batter, the casing exerts mechanical protection and guarantees permeability, which is the basis of the exchange of water and oxygen necessary for adequate and homogeneous drying and ripening [2]. Many features affect the quality of natural casings, such as the portion of the intestinal tract used, the manipulation of the product [3] and the mechanical and physical characteristics such as casing elasticity, permeability to water and gases, diameter and its uniformity, adhesion, and resistance to temperature variations [2]. In addition, casing can be a relevant source of enzymes, while casing microbiota is important overall when starter cultures are not added for fermentation [4].

In light of these considerations, we hypothesized that different casings could affect ripening by modifying sausage microbiota, water diffusion, and proteolysis dynamics, with a potentially significant impact on the product quality. Therefore, in this research, we aimed to deepen the knowledge on the influence of the type of casing on the characteristics of "*Mortadella di Campotosto*"-like sausages and to highlight the effect of casing on specific quality traits of the product. For these reasons, the specific objectives were: to follow the evolution of the principal microbial groups during the production process; to evaluate the protein hydrolysis of the fermented meats soon after stuffing and during ripening; to evaluate the texture and flavor of the finished product; and to follow the production of biogenic amines during the process.

2. Materials and Methods

2.1. Samples Production

"*Mortadella di Campotosto*"-like sausages were manufactured in autumn–winter in Macelleria "L'Olmo", sited in Scanno (AQ), Italy. The sausages were produced according to the traditional formulation and procedure: pork lean meat (ham, shoulder, and loin) and bacon were first minced, then mixed with salt (20 g/Kg), black pepper (1.0 g/Kg), and a mixture of sucrose, glucose, ascorbic acid (E300), and potassium nitrite (E252) in a total quantity of 4.0 g/Kg. After 12 h at 4 °C, the meat mix was then minced again, and about 420 g was taken for each sausage. A stripe of back lard was previously cured at 4 °C with salt, spices (pepper, oregano, rosemary, pimento, juniper, and cilantro), and a mixture of sucrose, glucose, ascorbic acid, and potassium nitrite, for about 14 days, after which it was cut into portions of about $3 \times 3 \times 10$ cm that were inserted into the batter. Then, the product was shaped in its typical oval form. Successively, the meat balls were hand-wrapped with the natural casing, previously washed with water and vinegar, then air-dried for about 10 h. Then, the products were left in air for 3–4 h, to favor the sealing of the casing edges; afterward, they were linked with a cotton string of medium caliber and tied in pairs. Thirty-one samples for each batch were used. The size of the samples at T0 was 17 ± 2 cm in length $\times\ 9 \pm 2$ cm in width and the weight was 452 ± 18 g. At the end of ripening, the size was about 10 ± 1 cm in length $\times\ 6 \pm 1$ cm in width and about 20 ± 1.5 in diameter and a final weight of about 270 ± 10 g.

Two different batches were produced: batch A, named MCB, wrapped with beef casing (beef middles), and batch B, named MCH, wrapped with hog casing (hog bung). All samples were transferred to a fermentation room, in which the temperature varied from −2 and 5 °C for 5 days. The samples were then moved to a drying–ripening room, where they stayed up to 120 days. In the room, natural ventilation was favored, with variable relative humidity (depending on the external weather conditions) and temperatures below 12 °C.

2.2. Microbiological Analysis

Microbiological analyses were carried out on the batter section, excluding the lard, after casing removal. Ten grams of the sausages were homogenized with 90 mL of sterile 0.1% (*w/v*) peptone water for 2 min, using sterile plastic pouches in a Stomacher Lab-Blender 400 (PBI International Milan, Italy). Serial 10-fold dilutions were prepared in sterile peptone water solution and inoculated in duplicate in appropriate culture media. The following microbial groups were determined: aerobic mesophilic bacteria on Plate Count Agar (PCA) at 30 °C for 48 h; mesophilic lactobacilli (LAB) and cocci on MRS agar and M17, respectively, at 30 °C for 48–72 h under anaerobiosis; presumptive enterococci on Slanetz and Bartley agar (S&B) at 37 °C for 48 h; total enterobacteria on Violet Red Bile Glucose Agar (VRBGA) at 37 °C for 24 h; micrococci and staphylococci on Mannitol Salt Agar (MSA) at 30 °C for 72 h; yeasts on Yeast extract-Peptone-Dextrose agar (YPD), added with 150 ppm of chloramphenicol, at 30 °C for 72 h.

Mold development on the casing was evaluated by sampling 10 cm^2 of casing and determining mold growth on YPD added with 150 ppm of chloramphenicol. All the culture media were from Oxoid SpA (Rodano, Italy).

2.3. Physical Analyses

Measurement of water activity (a_w) was performed by the Aqualab instrument CX/2 (Series 3, Decagon Devices, Inc., Pullman, WA, USA). Samples (10 g) were randomly obtained from the sausage (batter section). Moisture (g water/100 g sample) was measured by drying a 3 g sample at 100 °C to constant weight [5], and the pH values were obtained using a MP 220 pH meter (Mettler-Toledo, Columbus, OH, USA).

The weight loss of *"Mortadella di Campotosto"*-like samples during drying was gravimetrically determined and calculated as shown in the following Equation (1):

$$\text{Weight loss (\%)} = [(m0 - mt)/m0] \times 100 \qquad (1)$$

where m0 is the weight of sausage obtained after filling and mt is the weight of the sausages after a specific processing time (0, 6, 11, 18, 30, 45, and 120 days).

The measurements of moisture were performed by air oven drying [6], while for the NaCl content, the method of Volhard (ISO 1841-2: 1996) was used [7].

2.4. Chemical Determinations

Total nitrogen content (TN, % w/w) was determined by the Kjeldahl method, while proteins were obtained by multiplying TN × 6.25 [8]. Non-protein nitrogen content (NPN, % w/w) was measured by the precipitation of proteins with trichloroacetic acid, followed by determination of the nitrogen in the extract by the Kjeldahl method. Proteolysis Index (PI, %) was calculated as the ratio between NPN and TN (PI % = 100 × NPN × TN^{-1}), as previously reported [9].

To evaluate the intensity of the primary proteolytic changes during the process, sarcoplasmic and myofibrillar proteins were extracted [10]. The protein concentrations were determined using Bradford reagent (Sigma-Aldrich, Milan, Italy) and bovine serum albumin (BSA, Sigma-Aldrich) as standard reference, according to Bradford (1976) [11]. Sodium dodecyl sulphate-polyacrylamide gel electrophoresis (SDS-PAGE) was used to analyze proteins [12] by Mini Protean III electrophoresis equipment (Bio-Rad, Segrate, Italy), as previously described [10]. The GS-800™ Calibrated Densitometer (Bio-Rad, Segrate, Italy) was used to quantify the relative abundance of each protein band.

Total amino acids were extracted and measured on 2 g of each sample, using the Cadmium-ninhydrin method [13]. For the extraction of the free amino acids, the method proposed by Berardo and colleagues [14] was followed and concentrations were determined by Reverse-phase high performance liquid chromatography (RP-HPLC), as previously reported [15], by using the Waters AccQ Tag method (Millipore Co-Operative, Milford, MA, USA). Amino acids were converted to stable fluorescent derivatives by reaction with AccQ·Fluor reagent (6-Aminoquinolyl-N-hydroxysuccinimidyl carbamate). RP-HPLC was performed using a Waters liquid chromatography system consisting of a Waters™ 626 pump, Waters™ 600 S controller, and Waters™ 717 S autosampler (Millipore Co-operative, Milford, MA, USA), by means of a Nova-Pak™ C18 column (4 μm, 3.9 × 4.6 mm), heated to 37 °C in a Shimadzu model

CTO-10AC column oven. Elution was performed in a gradient of solvent A (Waters AccQ·Tag eluent A), solvent B (acetonitrile: Aldrich Chemical Co., Milan, Italy), and solvent C (20% methanol in Milli-Q water), prepared as follows: initial eluent 100% A; 99% A and 1% B at 0.5 min; 95% A and 5% B at 18 min; 91% A and 9% B at 19 min; 83% A and 17% B at 29.5 min; 60% B and 40% C at 33 min and held under these conditions for 20 min before returning to 100% A. The concentration of A was maintained at 100% up to 65 min, after which the gradient was changed to 60% B and 40% C for 35 min, before returning to the starting conditions. The single amino acids were identified by comparing their retention times with calibration standards. Peak areas were processed using Millennium 32 software v.4.0 (Waters, Milford, MA, USA).

2.5. Determination of Volatile Compounds

Volatile compounds were determined by solid phase micro-extraction coupled with gas chromatography mass spectrometry (SPME/GC-MS) [16] on 5 g of MCB or MCH at the selected sampling times. Volatile peaks identification was carried out by computer matching of mass spectral data with those of the compounds contained in the Agilent Hewlett-Packard NIST 98 and Wiley v. 6 mass spectral database. The volatile compounds content was expressed as relative percentage area.

2.6. Determination of Biogenic Amines

The following eight biogenic amines were detected, identified, and quantified: tryptamine (TRP), β-phenylethylamine (β-PHE), putrescine (PUT), cadaverine (CAD), histamine (HIS), tyramine (TYR), spermidine (SPD), and spermine (SPM).

The procedure of amines extraction and derivatization was carried out as described by Martuscelli et al. [17]: an aliquot of 2 g was homogenized (in Stomacher Lab blender 400, International PBI, Milan, Italy) with 10 mL of 5% trichloroacetic acid (TCA) and centrifuged (Hettich Zentrifugen, Tuttlingen, Germany) at a relative centrifugal force of 2325× g for 10 min; the supernatant was recovered and the extraction was performed with 5% TCA acid. The two acid extracts were mixed and made up to 50 mL with 5% TCA acid; the final acid extract was filtered through Whatman 54 paper (Carlo Erba, Milan, Italy). For derivatization of the samples, an aliquot of each acid extract (0.5 mL) was mixed with 150 µL of a saturated $NaHCO_3$ solution and the pH was adjusted to 11.5 with about 150 µL NaOH 1.0 M. Dansyl chloride (Fluka, Milan, Italy) solution (2 mL of 10 mg/mL dansyl chloride/acetone) was added to the alkaline amine extract. Derivatized extracts were transferred to an incubator and kept for 60 min at 40 °C under agitation (195 stokes) (Dubnoff Bath-BSD/D, International PBI, Milano, Italy). The residual dansyl chloride was removed by adding 200 mL of 300 g/L ammonia solution (Carlo Erba). After 30 min at 20 ± 1 °C and protected from light, each sample was brought up to 5 mL with acetonitrile (Carlo Erba) and filtered through a 0.22 µm PTFE filter (Alltech, Sedriano, Italy).

Biogenic amines were determined, after extraction and derivatization, by high-performance liquid chromatography (HPLC) using an Agilent 1200 Series (Agilent Technologies, Milano, Italy). In a Spherisorb S30ODS Waters C18-2 column (3 µm, 150 mm × 4.6 mm ID), 10 µL of sample was injected with gradient elution, acetonitrile (solvent A), and water (solvent B) as follows: 0–1 min 35% B isocratic; 1–5 min, 35%–20% B linear; 5–6 min, 20%–10% linear B; 6–15 min, 10% B isocratic; 15–18 min, 35% linear B; 18–20 min, 35% B isocratic. Identification of the biogenic amines (BAs) was based on their retention times and BAs content was reported as mg/kg of product.

2.7. Texture Analysis

Textural properties were evaluated at room temperature (22 ± 2 °C) using an Instron Universal Testing Machine (mod. 5422, Instron LTD, Wycombe, UK) equipped with a 500 N load cell.

Slices (1 cm thick) were transversally cut from the central part of the sausage. Cubic samples (1 × 1 × 1 cm) were cut from the inner part of the slices placed between the lard and the casing. Samples were compressed by a plunger with a plane circular surface (35 mm diameter) using a crosshead speed of 0.5 mm/s. Two different tests were carried out for the textural characterization:

- Compression–relaxation test: samples were compressed by 30% of their initial height, then the run was stopped and the plunger was maintained at the maximum compression extension for 2 min, after which the load was removed. The maximum peak force in compression (N) was taken as a hardness index and the relaxation load was used to study the elastic behavior.
- Texture Profile Analysis (TPA) test: samples were submitted to a two-cycle compression test to 30% of their initial height in the first compression. After the first cycle, samples were left for 1 min to recover their deformation and then, the second cycle was started. Hardness (N), cohesiveness ($J\ J^{-1}$), springiness (mm), and chewiness (N mm) were determined as previously described [18].

Each test was carried out on 10 samples of each batch (MCB and MCH). Since, in both tests, the experimental conditions in the first compression stage were the same, 20 samples were used for hardness calculation.

2.8. Experimental Design and Statistical Analysis

Two batches of sausages characterized by different casings were analyzed over time. In detail, three sausages per batch were randomly taken and analyzed at each ripening time (0, 6, 11, 18, 30, and 45 days). Time zero was considered as the time in which the batter was just wrapped in the casings, thus samples of batter (which was the same for the two batches) were taken just before being wrapped. All the data were subjected to two-way analysis of variance (ANOVA) to test the significance of individual (casing, ripening time) and interactive (casing × ripening time) effect. The model used for the two-way ANOVA is presented in Equation (2):

$$Y_{ijk} = \mu + \alpha_i + \beta_j + \gamma_{ij} + \varepsilon_{ijk} \qquad (2)$$

where μ is the intercept; α the casing factor; β the time factor; γ the interaction; ε the error; i and j are the level of the first and second factor; k the number of within group replicates. The significance of the effects was tested by Fisher's F value and the associated p value.

Since the MCH batch was still not ripened after 45 days, an additional sampling was carried out only for this batch at 120 days. As the definitive experimental design was incomplete, data were further analyzed by the two-way nested ANOVA and the model used is presented in Equation (3):

$$Y_{ijk} = \mu + \alpha_i + \beta_{j(i)} + \varepsilon_{ijk} \qquad (3)$$

where β is the time factor nested with the casing factor. Post hoc mean comparison was carried out on the time nested with casing effect using the Tukey's HSD test.

The mold load and textural properties of the fully ripened sausages (MCB at 45 days and MCH at 120 days) were eventually compared among them using the Student's t-test for independent samples in order to test significant differences between the two groups of samples.

Statistical analyses were performed by using Statistica v. 6.1 (Statsoft Europe, Hamburg, Germany).

3. Results and Discussion

3.1. Effect of the Different Casings on Microbial Growth

Differently from other Mediterranean dry fermented sausages, in which the fermentation time is 1–2 days at 18–24 °C or 1 week at relatively low temperatures (10–12 °C), the fermentation of "*Mortadella di Campotosto*" sausages is carried out at very low temperatures, below 4 °C. These conditions, together with the absence of starters, cause a slow growth of lactic acid bacteria and therefore, an extension of the fermentation time.

Table 1 depicts the behavior of the different microbial groups during time. As evidenced, during the fermentation phase (up to 11 days) and the first week of ripening (day 18), no statistically significant differences were noticed in the growth dynamics of all microbial groups between MCB and MCH products. As expected, Enterobacteriaceae were not detected after 6 days of production, probably as a consequence of the progressive pH reduction. With the extension of the ripening time (from 30 days), statistically significant differences were observed in yeast and CNS counts that were lower in MCB. In detail, the yeast count increased in MCH samples at 30 days, probably because of a succession of different species. It has to be underlined that at 30 days, the a_w values of MCB and MCH samples were significantly different and the higher MCH a_w allowed a greater microbial growth with more abundant cells loads. After that, the number of cells progressively decreased during the ripening time.

In addition, in this study, we observed that the type of casing used can affect the colonization of molds, which reached values of 5.60 Log CFU/cm^2 in MCB and < 2.0 Log CFU/cm^2 in MCH at the end of the process.

3.2. Effect of the Different Casings on Physicochemical Parameters

In Table 1, the changes in pH values during fermentation and ripening of the samples in beef casing (MCB) and in hog casing (MCH) are reported. A significant ($p < 0.05$) pH decrease was detected in both cases up to day 11, which could thus be presumably considered as the end of fermentation. The pH decrease was concurrent with the increasing number of presumptive LAB that reached levels of 7.66 and 7.85 Log CFU/g for MCH and MCB, respectively. After that, pH slowly increased, due to the typical phenomena of ripening, starting with proteolysis in both batches, but with different rates throughout ripening. The end of ripening (45 days for MCB and 120 days for MCH, respectively) was first evaluated by professional manufacturers, who tested product hardness, as perceived by digital pressure, and flavor sniffing, and then, confirmed by textural analysis before final sampling. At the end of ripening, the pH reached levels of about 5.67 for MCB and of 5.90 for MCH, respectively.

The type of casing exerted a significant effect on the drying rate, as highlighted by moisture (Figure 1) and a_w (Table 1) data; no water losses were observed during fermentation but, during ripening, the moisture dramatically differed between the two batches. After 45 days of ripening (the end of the ripening for MCB products), MCB batches reached moisture (31.2%) and a_w (0.841) values significantly lower than MCH samples, in which the values of moisture and a_w were 53.7% and 0.923, respectively. These differences can be attributed to the physical characteristics of the two types of casing, such as the degree of casing permeability, which influences the level of exchange between the filling and the external environment. In fact, hog bung casings had greater thickness (about 3-fold) than MCB, leading to a lower water vapor transmission rate and higher a_w [4]. The degree of casing permeability to water, gas, and light affects water loss, fat hydrolysis, fat oxidation, as well as pH and a_w [2,4].

As regards NaCl content, given as g 100/g total solids, slightly significant differences were observed at the end of the ripening time in both types of sausages, which showed values of 4.77 ± 0.01% and 4.97 ± 0.16% for MCB and MCH, respectively.

Table 1. Physical-chemical and microbiological characteristics of "*Mortadella di Campotosto*"-like sausages produced with beef (MCB) and hog (MCH) casings over time.

Batch	Time (Days)	pH	a$_w$	MAB	Yeasts	LAB	LAC	ENTC	CNS	PSE	ENTB
						Complete design (CD)					
MCB	0	5.96 ± 0.04 [a]	0.957 ± 0.003 [a]	7.24 ± 0.08 [b]	7.14 ± 0.00 [a]	6.37 ± 0.11 [cd]	7.07 ± 0.06 [bc]	6.52 ± 0.38 [cd]	5.87 ± 0.36 [abc]	5.56 ± 0.38 [a]	3.09 ± 0.20 [a]
MCH	0	5.86 ± 0.12 [a]	0.959 ± 0.004 [a]	7.12 ± 0.18 [b]	7.02 ± 0.10 [a]	6.60 ± 0.08 [cd]	7.02 ± 0.10 [bc]	6.92 ± 0.10 [cd]	5.91 ± 0.48 [abc]	5.71 ± 0.46 [a]	3.42 ± 0.08 [a]
MCB	6	5.50 ± 0.09 [b]	0.956 ± 0.002 [a]	7.55 ± 0.21 [ab]	7.63 ± 0.13 [a]	7.53 ± 0.18 [abc]	7.80 ± 0.04 [ab]	7.29 ± 0.13 [cd]	6.98 ± 0.14 [d]	4.72 ± 0.39 [a]	0.95 ± 0.75 [b]
MCH	6	5.47 ± 0.17 [b]	0.956 ± 0.002 [a]	7.17 ± 0.07 [b]	7.63 ± 0.09 [a]	7.14 ± 0.13 [abcd]	8.13 ± 0.33 [ab]	7.84 ± 0.04 [b]	7.18 ± 0.13 [a]	4.41 ± 0.61 [a]	1.11 ± 0.31 [b]
MCB	11	5.48 ± 0.07 [b]	0.960 ± 0.006 [a]	7.91 ± 0.09 [ab]	7.80 ± 0.26 [a]	7.85 ± 0.04 [abc]	7.93 ± 0.09 [ab]	7.79 ± 0.04 [b]	6.29 ± 0.41 [a]	4.58 ± 0.49 [a]	<1.00 [b]
MCH	11	5.44 ± 0.08 [b]	0.944 ± 0.009 [a]	8.15 ± 0.33 [ab]	7.26 ± 0.08 [a]	7.66 ± 0.31 [abcd]	8.28 ± 0.22 [a]	8.09 ± 0.04 [b]	4.47 ± 0.31 [c]	4.45 ± 0.62 [a]	<1.00 [b]
MCB	18	5.62 ± 0.20 [ab]	0.960 ± 0.006 [a]	7.85 ± 0.21 [ab]	4.00 ± 0.04 [cd]	6.23 ± 0.27 [d]	7.83 ± 0.20 [bc]	7.64 ± 0.20 [bc]	5.11 ± 0.15 [bcd]	5.64 ± 0.01 [ab]	<1.00 [b]
MCH	18	5.55 ± 0.13 [ab]	0.952 ± 0.006 [a]	7.79 ± 0.12 [ab]	4.00 ± 0.16 [cd]	6.23 ± 0.27 [d]	7.83 ± 0.26 [abc]	7.64 ± 0.04 [bc]	5.18 ± 0.15 [bcd]	5.64 ± 0.27 [ab]	<1.00 [b]
MCB	30	5.65 ± 0.14 [ab]	0.890 ± 0.008 [b]	8.26 ± 0.15 [ab]	4.80 ± 0.39 [bc]	6.38 ± 0.06 [d]	8.14 ± 0.13 [ab]	8.03 ± 0.20 [b]	6.22 ± 0.29 [ab]	4.48 ± 0.95 [ab]	<1.00 [b]
MCH	30	5.56 ± 0.12 [ab]	0.940 ± 0.012 [a]	8.44 ± 0.20 [a]	5.36 ± 0.17 [b]	8.24 ± 0.20 [a]	8.48 ± 0.39 [a]	8.18 ± 0.08 [b]	6.78 ± 0.29 [ab]	3.95 ± 0.10 [bc]	<1.00 [b]
MCB	45	5.67 ± 0.11 [ab]	0.841 ± 0.006 [c]	8.08 ± 0.03 [ab]	2.47 ± 0.20 [e]	7.96 ± 0.22 [ab]	8.54 ± 0.29 [a]	6.31 ± 0.29 [d]	2.00 ± 0.20 [e]	5.11 ± 0.12 [ab]	<1.00 [b]
MCH	45	5.59 ± 0.09 [ab]	0.923 ± 0.008 [b]	7.97 ± 0.07 [ab]	3.54 ± 0.22 [e]	7.10 ± 0.14 [abcd]	7.72 ± 0.39 [abc]	7.76 ± 0.04 [bc]	3.98 ± 0.23 [d]	3.69 ± 0.10 [bc]	<1.00 [b]
F (C)		0.46	51.5 ***	0.20	93.5 ***	0.26	0.07	0.15	26.4 ***	2.90	0.06
F (t)		3.51 *	39.5 ***	9.10 ***	257 ***	1.7 **	7.93 ***	12.3 ***	4.38 **	5.38 **	65.9 ***
F (C × t)		0.04	15.4 ***	0.66	25.6 ***	7.59 ***	1.68	5.16 **	34.5 ***	0.96	0.06
						Incomplete Design (CD + MCH 120 d)					
MCH	120	5.90 ± 0.05 [a]	0.812 ± 0.006 [c]	7.55 ± 0.14 [ab]	3.50 ± 0.14 [d]	6.55 ± 0.36 [b]	6.60 ± 0.34 [a]	9.33 ± 0.11 [a]	3.32 ± 0.06 [de]	2.00 ± 0.20 [c]	<1.00
F (C)		0.01	135 ***	0.47		0.01	1.17	3.42	43.0 ***	12.3 **	0.26
F (t(C))		2.21 *	45.6 ***	4.60 ***		7.77 ***	6.51 ***	13.3 ***	19.8 ***	6.41 ***	33.3 ***

Means with different letters in the same column are significantly different ($p < 0.05$). Log CFU/g—Log Colony Forming Unit/gram of product a$_w$—water activity MAB—Mesophilic Aerobic Bacteria, LAB—Lactic acid bacteria; LAC—Lactococci; ENTC—Enterococci; PSE—Pseudomonas spp.; CNS—Coagulase negative Staphylococci; ENTB—Enterobacteriaceae. Fisher's F value of casing (F(C)), time (F(t)), combined casing and time (F(C × t)), and time nested with casing (F(t(C))) factors calculated for each analytical determination. ANOVA significant differences were indicated by F values. * $p < 0.05$, ** $p < 0.01$. *** $p < 0.005$.

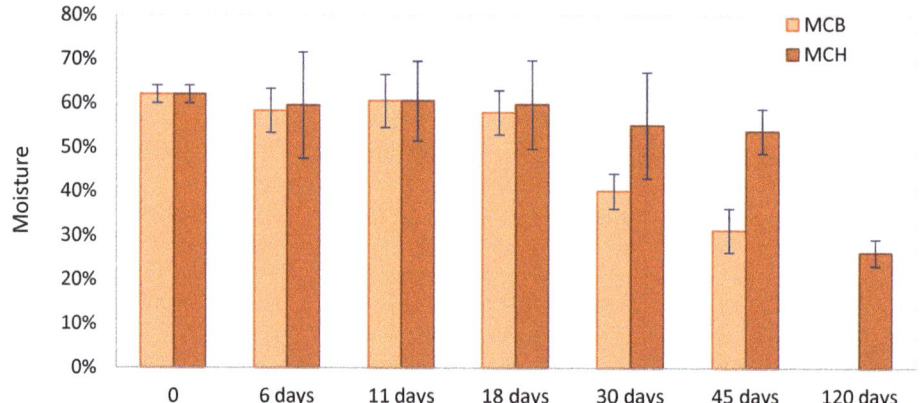

Figure 1. Evolution of the relative humidity of "*Mortadella di Campotosto*"-like sausages produced with beef (MCB) and hog (MCH) casings over time.

3.3. Effect on Proteolysis

Protein hydrolysis was evaluated by gel electrophoresis, as well as by measuring the content of total free amino acids, volatiles, and amines that greatly influence the texture, flavor, and safety of dry fermented sausages [19]. The hydrolysis of sarcoplasmic and myofibrillar proteins, determined via SDS-PAGE analysis, was influenced by the ripening time and the type of casing (Figure 2).

3.3.1. Sarcoplasmic Fraction

The electrophoretic separation of sarcoplasmic proteins of MCB and MCH at different processing stages is illustrated in Figure 2a. Proteolysis took place during fermentation, as revealed by the slight changes from the first fermentation phase; the bands most susceptible to degradation were those of about 61 and 56 kDa, followed by a huge band of about 48 kDa, and the most intensive degradation was observed in MCH samples. In addition, two fragments were generated at 36 and 35 KDa, which were assumed to be glyceraldehyde-3-phosphate dehydrogenase [20], and 18 KDa in both types of samples.

In addition, during ripening, starting from day 18, a more intense hydrolysis was observed in MCH samples, as indicated by the intensity decrease in the band at 45 kDa (data at 120 days not shown), which is assumed to be creatine kinase [21]. This band completely disappeared after 45 days, while the intensity of the bands of about 74, 37, 36, 18, and 12 KDa increased overall in the MCB samples. The appearance and increase in polypeptides in the range of 14–100 kDa have been observed also by other authors [10,22].

As a_w strongly affects the activities of all endogenous proteinases [23], the differences between MCB and MCH could be ascribable to the higher a_w values of MCH samples (Table 1). Thus, it could be possible that the highest a_w values in MCH batches could have favored the activity of cathepsins B, which are able to break down sarcoplasmic proteins [24]. However, the contribution of bacterial enzymes to protein degradation needs to be taken into account, since LAB counts at day 30 reached higher values in MCH samples (8.24 Log CFU/g) than in MCB samples (6.48 Log CFU/g). In this context, in addition to LAB microbial enzymes, also *Staphylococcus carnosus* and *Staphylococcus simulans* proteases are capable to hydrolyze sarcoplasmic proteins [25].

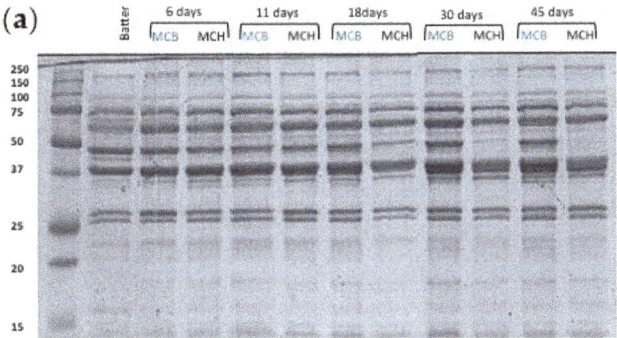

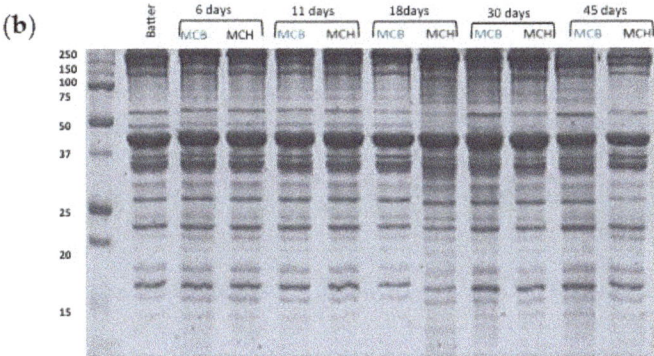

Figure 2. SDS-PAGE electrophoretic profiles of *"Mortadella di Campotosto"*-like sausages produced with beef (MCB) and hog (MCH) casings over time. Panel (**a**) sarcoplasmic fraction; panel (**b**) myofibrillar fraction. Batter: 0 days. Values on the ordinates refer to the marker and express the bands dimension in KDa.

3.3.2. Myofibrillar Fraction

Myofibrillar proteins play the most critical role during meat processing, as they are responsible for the cohesive structure and firm texture of meat products [26]. As evidenced, this protein fraction was less susceptible to degradation and the hydrolysis dynamics in MCB and MCH showed very similar profiles. Recently, Berardo et al. [14] reported that actin (45 kDa) is highly broken down during fermentation; nevertheless, we did not evidence any change of this protein during fermentation in both MCB and MCH samples, in agreement with other studies [27,28]. On the contrary, the generation of polypeptides and large peptides with molecular weight from 50 to 100 kDa was more evident at day 11.

During ripening, when the endogenous enzymes are affected by the a_w decrease, having particular impact on cathepsins and alanyl- and pyroglutamyl-amino-peptidases [29], an important degradation of the band of about 48 kDa was detected (day 18); afterwards, it disappeared in both batches. In the meantime, a band of about 33 KDa, probably corresponding to β-tropomyosin, appeared in MCH samples at day 18, while in MCB samples, it was detected at 30 days of ripening [30].

Differences between the two products were clear from the 30th day of the process, in which the a_w values were 0.890 ± 0.008 and 0.940 ± 0.012 for MCB and MCH, respectively.

As regards Myosin Heavy Chain (220 kDa), an important degradation for at least 45% in MCH samples was detected at day 45, in contrast with MCB samples, in which it remained almost unchanged during ripening. The hydrolysis of actin (45 kDa) was less severe than that of myosin (25 kDa), and it was clear from day 30 in MCB, in which the reduction was about 15%. These results are in accordance with other authors [31], who reported a lower degradation of actin in fermented sausages with higher pH, suggesting that this might be due to the low optimum pH of cathepsin D-like muscle enzymes, playing a major role in actin hydrolysis.

Additionally, changes in tropomyosin (35 kDa) were more intense in MCB samples that presented also hydrolysis of the bands at 48 and 54 kDa, probably corresponding to desmin. Moreover, the myosin II short-chain (about 18 kDa) showed an intensity increase of approximatively 10% in MCH samples; muscle proteinases predominate in proteolysis evolution along the dry fermented sausage ripening, while those from bacteria mainly act during fermentation [32]. Nevertheless, the major proteolysis of the myofibrillar fractions in MCH (presenting a_w values of 0.890 at day 30) could be attributed to particular bacteria or yeast species present in the meat or in the casing, well adapted to the particular environment of this sausage and probably dominating during fermentation and ripening. Moreover, on the MCB casing surface, the molds, reaching loads of 5.60 Log CFU/g, could have promoted the greater proteolysis [33]. In fact, during ripening, when a_w decreases, the molds, and especially strains of *Aspergillus* and *Penicillium* genera, tend to dominate due to their capability to overcome xerophilic and halophilic conditions. *Penicillium chrysogenum* and *P. nalgiovense* contribute to proteolytic activities [34] and *Penicillium chrysogenum* Pg222 proteolytic enzymes show activity on the principal myofibrillar proteins, including actin, myosin, tropomyosin, and troponin [35].

3.4. Total Amino Acids Content

The generation of free amino acids (FAA) is the final outcome of proteolysis, and it contributes to the specific taste and also to the generation of volatile compounds, which provide the flavor in fermented sausages. The FAA content, expressed as mM of leucine, of both kinds of samples, was analyzed during the experimental period. As expected, the low temperatures applied in the production of the samples resulted in a limited generation of FAA, and their content was significantly different ($p < 0.05$) depending on the type of casing.

The quantification of total free amino acids (TFAA) is reported in Table 2. As evidenced, the initial batter contained about 361.25 ± 13.32 mg amino acids/100 g of dry-matter, and during the process, this concentration changed over time to a final concentration of 84.35 ± 19.18 and 235.59 ± 6.59 mg/100 g of dry-matter for MCB and MCH, respectively, at 45 and 120 days, with the major contribution of arginine (Arg) and alanine (Ala), followed by leucine (Leu) and valine (Val). The observed fluctuations in the content of each individual amino acid could be ascribed to the balance between FAA produced by protein breakdown and microbial activity. Among the bacteria, coagulase-negative staphylococci (CNS), *Lactobacillus sakei*, *Lactobacillus curvatus*, and some yeasts such as *Saccharomyces cerevisiae* have been reported to be directly involved in meat proteolysis and in free amino acids generation [15]. At the same time, many of these microorganisms use free amino acids as substrate for further metabolic reactions (deamination, dehydrogenation, and transamination), which are related to the development of aroma and flavor that characterize the final fermented sausage [36,37]. Moreover, arginine reduction in MCH samples could also be correlated to decarboxylation reactions, with the consequent production of putrescine, starting from day 45.

Table 2. Free amino acids content (mg/100 g meat) in "*Mortadella di Campotosto*"-like sausages produced with beef (MCB) and hog (MCH) casings over time.

Batch	Time (Days)	Arg	Asp	Glu	His	Ser	Ala	Gly	Ile	Leu	Met	Phe	Val	TOTAL FAA
Complete Design														
MCB	0	254 ± 2 ^{a}	0.85 ± 0.04 ^{ab}	10.1 ± 0.24 ^{b}	n.d.	0.13 ± 0.08 ^{bcde}	21.0 ± 2.25 ^{d}	n.d.	2.36 ± 0.04 ^{de}	7.80 ± 0.57 ^{de}	59.4 ± 7.7 ^{ab}	2.36 ± 0.20 ^{f}	3.25 ± 0.20 ^{bc}	361.25 ± 13.32 ^{aa}
MCH	0	247 ± 2 ^{a}	0.70 ± 0.16 ^{ab}	11.8 ± 1.59 ^{b}	n.d.	0.13 ± 0.08 ^{bcde}	18.9 ± 0.53 ^{d}	n.d.	2.20 ± 0.17 ^{de}	6.70 ± 0.33 ^{de}	58.4 ± 6.9 ^{ab}	2.46 ± 0.13 ^{f}	2.90 ± 0.08 ^{bc}	351.19 ± 11.97 ^{a}
MCB	6	192 ± 7 ^{bcd}	0.69 ± 0.05 ^{ab}	n.d.	n.d.	0.23 ± 0.03 ^{bc}	4.50 ± 0.37 ^{e}	n.d.	2.1 ± 0.17 ^{de}	7.26 ± 0.30 ^{de}	55.7 ± 0.5 ^{b}	5.31 ± 3.10 ^{bcd}	2.27 ± 0.11 ^{c}	349.40 ± 10.10 ^{a}
MCH	6	158 ± 23 ^{d}	0.45 ± 0.07 ^{bc}	n.d.	37.9 ± 0.87 ^{b}	0.07 ± 0.01 ^{cde}	6.81 ± 1.47 ^{e}	37.9 ± 0.92 ^{e}	1.31 ± 0.27 ^{e}	5.46 ± 0.52 ^{ef}	55.3 ± 3.2 ^{b}	4.23 ± 0.39 ^{e}	2.24 ± 0.18 ^{c}	318.34 ± 15.66 ^{ab}
MCB	11	236 ± 7 ^{ab}	0.70 ± 0.05 ^{ab}	1.73 ± 0.23 ^{c}	n.d.	0.16 ± 0.01 ^{bcde}	32.7 ± 2.5 ^{c}	n.d.	2.46 ± 0.20 ^{cd}	7.00 ± 0.15 ^{de}	62.4 ± 1.8 ^{ab}	3.56 ± 0.26 ^{ef}	2.96 ± 0.37 ^{bc}	270.34 ± 19.75 ^{b}
MCH	11	220 ± 16 ^{abc}	0.63 ± 0.30 ^{ab}	2.80 ± 0.45 ^{c}	2.50 ± 0.08 ^{d}	0.09 ± 0.01 ^{bcde}	17.8 ± 1.5 ^{d}	3.95 ± 0.92 ^{d}	1.53 ± 0.27 ^{d}	6.26 ± 0.52 ^{de}	55.6 ± 1.8 ^{b}	3.73 ± 0.26 ^{ef}	2.70 ± 0.38 ^{bc}	310.07 ± 37.12 ^{b}
MCB	18	177 ± 4 ^{cd}	0.87 ± 0.08 ^{ab}	n.d.	15.5 ± 1.16 ^{c}	0.24 ± 0.02 ^{bc}	136 ± 2 ^{a}	15.5 ± 1.15 ^{bc}	2.40 ± 0.15 ^{cd}	8.44 ± 0.32 ^{cde}	73.6 ± 0.2 ^{a}	6.94 ± 0.17 ^{ab}	2.57 ± 0.21 ^{bc}	438.81 ± 6.61 ^{c}
MCH	18	13.8 ± 0.9 ^{e}	0.67 ± 0.07 ^{ab}	n.d.	35.6 ± 1.74 ^{b}	0.05 ± 0.01 ^{b}	123 ± 4 ^{b}	35.6 ± 2.57 ^{a}	3.22 ± 0.10 ^{c}	14.3 ± 0.30 ^{b}	7.20 ± 0.21 ^{c}	3.42 ± 0.20 ^{e}	3.11 ± 0.11 ^{b}	237.78 ± 1.72 ^{d}
MCB	30	186 ± 10 ^{bcd}	0.95 ± 0.12 ^{a}	n.d.	13.1 ± 1.02 ^{c}	0.26 ± 0.01 ^{b}	131 ± 1 ^{ab}	13.1 ± 0.41 ^{c}	3.35 ± 0.23 ^{bc}	9.23 ± 0.37 ^{c}	21.8 ± 0.6 ^{c}	8.42 ± 0.23 ^{a}	2.56 ± 0.17 ^{bc}	389.53 ± 20.13 ^{a}
MCH	30	4.15 ± 0.90 ^{f}	0.67 ± 0.06 ^{ab}	n.d.	38.4 ± 1.24 ^{ab}	1.07 ± 0.07 ^{a}	128 ± 2 ^{ab}	38.4 ± 2.02 ^{a}	3.49 ± 0.25 ^{ab}	13.4 ± 1.02 ^{b}	7.07 ± 1.02 ^{c}	4.31 ± 0.30 ^{cde}	3.47 ± 0.18 ^{b}	241.73 ± 9.05 ^{b}
MCB	45	63.5 ± 15 ^{e}	0.05 ± 0.11 ^{cd}	n.d.	2.03 ± 0.21 ^{d}	n.d.	1.61 ± 1.20 ^{e}	2.03 ± 1.20 ^{c}	3.61 ± 0.20 ^{ab}	2.74 ± 0.18 ^{f}	6.51 ± 0.88 ^{c}	2.13 ± 0.20 ^{f}	n.r.	84.35 ± 19.18 ^{e}
MCH	45	8.43 ± 0.20 ^{f}	0.97 ± 0.12 ^{a}	15.9 ± 1.65 ^{a}	45.9 ± 4.83 ^{a}	0.14 ± 0.02 ^{bcd}	135 ± 2 ^{a}	32.9 ± 3.06 ^{ab}	4.49 ± 0.19 ^{a}	21.0 ± 1.52 ^{a}	8.30 ± 0.41 ^{c}	5.82 ± 0.12 ^{bc}	5.16 ± 0.32 ^{a}	287.32 ± 30.97 ^{d}
F (C)		154 ***	0.12	48.8 ***	580 ***	34.5 ***	268 ***	109 ***	0.090	124 ***	65.3 ***	26.3 ***	76.9 ***	
F (t)		138 ***	3.58 *	96.2 ***	121 ***	143 ***	1808 ***	22.7 ***	45.5 ***	30.7 ***	119 ***	45.5 ***	4.87 **	
F (C × t)		27.8 ***	13.8 ***	41.9 ***	66.6 ***	98.6 ***	485 ***	10.7 ***	8.56 ***	63.0 ***	36.4 ***	43.3 ***	47.2 ***	
Incomplete design (CD + MCH 120d)														
MCH	120	1.61 ± 0.08 ^{f}	n.r.	14.0 ± 0.70 ^{ab}	33.0 ± 1.5 ^{b}	1.10 ± 0.08 ^{a}	123 ± 20 ^{ab}	33.0 ± 2.5 ^{a}	3.88 ± 0.20 ^{ab}	11.4 ± 0.7 ^{bc}	6.70 ± 0.67 ^{ef}	3.31 ± 0.26 ^{ef}	4.75 ± 0.29 ^{a}	235.59 ± 6.6 ^{d}
F (C)		263 ***	0.06	112 ***	690 ***	125 ***	596 ***	133 ***	3.60	131 ***	120 ***	34.3 ***	111 ***	
F (t(C))		90.7 ***	0.29 ***	75.8 ***	87.6 ***	113 ***	1130 ***	16.0 ***	27.1 ***	42.1 ***	81.7 ***	41.3 ***	25.6 ***	

Arg—arginine; Asp—aspartic acid; Glu—glutamine; His—histidine; Ser—serine; Ala—alanine; Gly—glycine; Ile—isoleucine; Leu—leucine; Met—methionine Phe—phenylalanine; Val—valine; FAA—free amino acids. Means with different letters in the same column are significantly different ($p < 0.05$). Fisher's F value of casing (F(C)), time (F(t)), combined casing and time (F(C × t)), and time nested with casing (F(t(C))) factors calculated for each analytical determination. ANOVA significant differences were indicated by F values. ** $p < 0.01$. *** $p < 0.005$. n.d.—not detectable.

The major differences in FAA were observed during ripening, in which hydrophobic amino acids were accumulated. In addition, significant differences ($p < 0.05$) were observed for the greater amounts of Arg and Ala in MCB samples up to 30 days. This concentration appeared dramatically reduced at day 45, particularly for Arg in MCH samples and for Ala in MCB ones. In this respect, two hypotheses can be proposed: (1) the different environmental conditions present in MCB after 30 days could have selected microorganisms with a highly efficient arginine-converting machinery, with the aim of obtaining energy from arginine in the absence of glucose, as reported for some *Lactobacillus*, CNS and *Pseudomonas* species [38–40], and this might be reflected by the presence of *Pseudomonadaceae* at values of 5.11 ± 0.2 Log CFU/g in MCB samples at day 45; or (2) a possible oxidation of this amino acid could have happened by means of free radicals generated by lipolysis, leading to the formation of carbonyl groups [41]. In fact, amino acids such as lysine, threonine, arginine, and proline are easily attacked by these radicals.

In the case of MCH, the major FAA at the end of ripening was Ala with amounts of 123.20 mg/100 g of dry-matter.

3.5. Volatile Compounds Derived from Amino Acids

FAA are very important in fermented sausages, both for their contribution to the specific taste and for their involvement in degradation reactions that generate volatile compounds, which provide the flavor in this type of product. It is documented that the pH rise during fermentation is due to the microbial degradation of FAA by decarboxylation and deamination [42]. The transamination and decarboxylation of valine, isoleucine, and leucine, which are branched amino acids, produce the respective branched aldehydes, alcohols, and/or acids. Additionally, amino acids such as Phe, Thr, Try, Tyr, etc., are transformed into their respective aldehydes, such as phenylacetaldehyde from phenylalanine, and indole compounds from tryptophan, while the degradation of the sulfur amino acids cysteine and methionine produces sulfur volatile compounds [43]. In particular, we analyzed the accumulation dynamics of compounds derived from branched amino acids (branched aldehydes, alcohols, and carboxylic acids), such as 2-methylpropanal derived from valine (Val), 2-methylbutanal from isoleucine (Ile), 3-methylbutanal from leucine (Leu), and phenylacetaldehyde, benzaldehyde, phenylethyl alcohol, and ethyl benzoate ester that derived from phenylalanine (Phe) and the results are shown in Table 3.

In general, a greater relative abundance of branched chain aldehydes, alcohols, and acids from the catabolism of branched chain amino acids was detected in MCB samples. In particular, 3-Methyl-1-butanal was the most abundant compound in both types of samples, being more present during fermentation (up to 11 days) in MCH and during ripening in MCB samples. In this respect, other authors [44] suggested that 3-Methyl-butanoic acid and 3-Methyl-1-butanal are markers of the CNS activity in fermented meats.

On the other hand, the decrease in 3-Methyl butanol in MCB samples could be ascribed to its conversion into the corresponding 3-Methyl-butanoic acid (Table 3). MCB samples were characterized also by a major presence of 2-Methylpropanal and 2-Methylpropanoic acid, which increased over time and were not detected in MCH samples during the entire production period. On the contrary, phenyl ethyl alcohol concentration increased only in MCH batches.

Table 3. Relative abundance of branched chain compounds derived from branched chain amino acids in "*Mortadella di Campotosto*"-like sausages produced with beef (MCB) and hog (MCH) casings over time. Results are expressed as relative abundance × 10⁶.

	Time (Days)	2-MPA (%)	3-MBA (%)	3-MB (%)	PEA (%)	3-M1-B (%)	2-MP (%)
			Complete Design (CD)				
MCB	0	0.26 ± 0.01 de	1.18 ± 0.02 de	1.29 ± 0.07 c	1.63 ± 0.50 bc	7.93 ± 1.23 bc	0.49 ± 0.01 d
MCH	0	0.24 ± 0.01 de	1.18 ± 0.02 de	1.09 ± 0.09 c	1.49 ± 0.62 bc	7.93 ± 1.25 bc	0.52 ± 0.01 d
MCB	6	0.43 ± 0.03 cd	2.90 ± 0.16 abcd	7.37 ± 1.14 a	0.15 ± 0.01 c	2.64 ± 0.37 e	0.2 ± 0.03 d
MCH	6	n.d.	1.20 ± 0.20 cde	2.81 ± 0.48 bc	1.29 ± 0.26 bc	7.89 ± 0.77 bcd	n.d.
MCB	11	0.71 ± 0.07 bc	3.6 ± 0.49 ab	5.50 ± 1.17 ab	0.19 ± 0.04 c	5.42 ± 0.49 cde	0.7 ± 0.05 d
MCH	11	n.d.	1.50 ± 0.34 bcde	2.40 ± 0.62 bc	1.30 ± 0.29 bc	9.2 ± 0.68 abc	n.d.
MCB	18	0.88 ± 0.06 ab	4.75 ± 0.95 a	5.23 ± 1.76 ab	0.23 ± 0.04 c	12.7 ± 0.85 a	1.7 ± 0.34 c
MCH	18	0.26 ± 0.02 de	0.60 ± 0.10 e	0.2 ± 0.06 c	1.28 ± 0.23 bc	5.43 ± 1.09 cde	n.d.
MCB	30	n.d.	3.88 ± 0.10 a	n.d.	0.26 ± 0.03 c	10.94 ± 0.84 ab	2.8 ± 0.17 b
MCH	30	1.23 ± 0.13 a	0.65 ± 0.35 e	n.d.	1.32 ± 0.43 bc	7.63 ± 0.88 bcd	n.d.
MCB	45	n.d.	3.83 ± 0.12 a	n.d.	0.29 ± 0.05 c	7.32 ± 1.02 bcd	4.2 ± 0.53 a
MCH	45	1.01 ± 0.16 ab	1.07 ± 0.80 de	n.d.	4.33 ± 0.83 a	6.6 ± 0.31 bcde	n.d.d
F (C)		4.28 *	88.7 ***	25.5 ***	48.7 ***	0.45	206 ***
F (t)		14.9 ***	9.08 ***	17.0 ***	7.11 ***	6.06 ***	32.2 ***
F (C × t)		97.6 ***	5.54 **	5.48 **	8.21 ***	14.5 ***	35.9 ***
			Incomplete Design (CD + MCH 120 d)				
MCH	120	n.d.	3.44 ± 0.11 abc	n.d.	2.15 ± 0.20 b	3.7 ± 0.34 de	n.d.
F (C)		0.05	67.7 ***	34.3 ***	58.3 ***	3.68	242 ***
F (t(C))		60.2 ***	9.45 ***	11.2 ***	7.39 ***	11.7 ***	33.5 ***

2-MPA-2-Methylpropanoic acid; 3-MBA-3-Methylbutanoic acid; 3-MB-3-Methylbutanol; PEA-phenyl ethyl alcohol; 3-M1-B-3-Methyl-1-butanol; 2-MP-2-Methylpropanal. Means with different letters in the same column are significantly different ($p < 0.05$). Fisher's F value of casing (F(C)), time (F(t)), combined casing and time (F(C × t)), and time nested with casing (F(t(C))) factors calculated for each analytical determination. ANOVA significant differences were indicated by F values. * $p < 0.05$, ** $p < 0.01$, *** $p < 0.005$; n.d.—not detectable.

3.6. Texture Analysis

The textural properties of "*Mortadella di Campotosto*"-like sausages were studied both by stress relaxation and TPA (Texture Profile) analysis. TPA parameters of the two types of samples at the end of ripening are shown in Table 4. At the end of ripening, corresponding to 45 days for MCB and 120 days for MCH, the two types of samples showed very similar textural profiles, except for small differences in springiness and chewiness.

Table 4. Results of texture profile analysis and compression–relaxation test of ripened "*Mortadella di Campotosto*"-like sausages produced with beef (MCB) and hog (MCH) casings.

Product	Hardness (N)	Springiness (mm)	Cohesiveness ($J \times J^{-1}$)	Chewiness (N mm)	Relaxation Load (%)
MCB (45 days)	16.0 ± 3.4 [a]	1.91 ± 0.19 [b]	0.50 ± 0.04 [a]	15.2 ± 2.9 [b]	63.68 ± 0.63 [a]
MCH (120 days)	16.5 ± 1.7 [a]	2.06 ± 0.12 [a]	0.52 ± 0.04 [a]	17.6 ± 1.4 [a]	62.70 ± 0.82 [a]

Data in the same column with different letters are significantly different at a $p < 0.05$ level.

No statistically significant differences were found in hardness, despite MCB showing lower a_w and moisture values and a slightly higher proteolysis index (12.92% vs. 12.13%) than MCH. In general, protein breakdown during fermented sausages ripening contributes to hardness decrease [45]. However, beside proteolysis, drying is a major factor affecting the binding and textural properties of fermented meat products. In most cases, the effect of dehydration, which increases hardness by promoting the elastic behavior, could counteract and even overcome the effect of proteolysis [28,46].

MCH samples showed a more elastic physical behavior and a consequently higher chewiness. Chewiness resulted positively affected by proteolysis in many studies, independently from positive or negative hardness changes [28,47,48]. Since in TPA analysis, chewiness is the product of hardness × cohesiveness × springiness, the higher chewiness of the MCH product observed in this study is due to its higher springiness, since no differences were found in hardness and cohesiveness. Springiness, which is a measure of elasticity [18], is depleted by moisture content, since water acts as a plasticizer and promotes viscous behavior. Despite differences in springiness, observed by measuring the recovery of the deformation after uniaxial compression, no significant differences in elastic behavior were observed when a stress–relaxation test was applied, as the force dissipated by viscous flow was identical in the two samples (Table 4).

In this section, the effect of proteolysis and dehydration were discussed since they are the main factors affecting sausage texture, but it should be considered that also lipolysis may contribute to the final texture.

3.7. Biogenic Amines (BA) Content

High quantities of proteins, associated with the proteolytic activity of endogenous enzymes and decarboxylase activity of wild microbiota, can support the accumulation of biogenic amines in fermented sausages [49,50], although the final balance depends on the equilibrium between BAs formation and degradation [51]. Figure 3 depicts the BAs content in "*Mortadella di Campotosto*"-like samples up to the end of ripening (45 days for MCB, panel a; 120 days for MCH, panel b).

In general, tryptamine, phenylethylamine, and spermine were not detected, while tyramine (TYR) and polyamines such as cadaverine (CAD), putrescine (PUT), and spermidine (SPD) were found during the entire production process, although with differences between the two products. Histamine was not detected in MCH, while it was found in MCB at low concentration (up to 17 mg/Kg, after the drying step). In addition, during fermentation (up to 11 days), TYR and SPD were the most abundant amines in MCB sausages and were detected in similar concentrations in MCB and MCH samples at up to 45 days of ripening. Tyramine production has been associated with the presence of LAB and enterococci that usually possess high amino acid decarboxylase activity [52]. This characteristic is strain-dependent and could be expressed during drying and ripening [53].

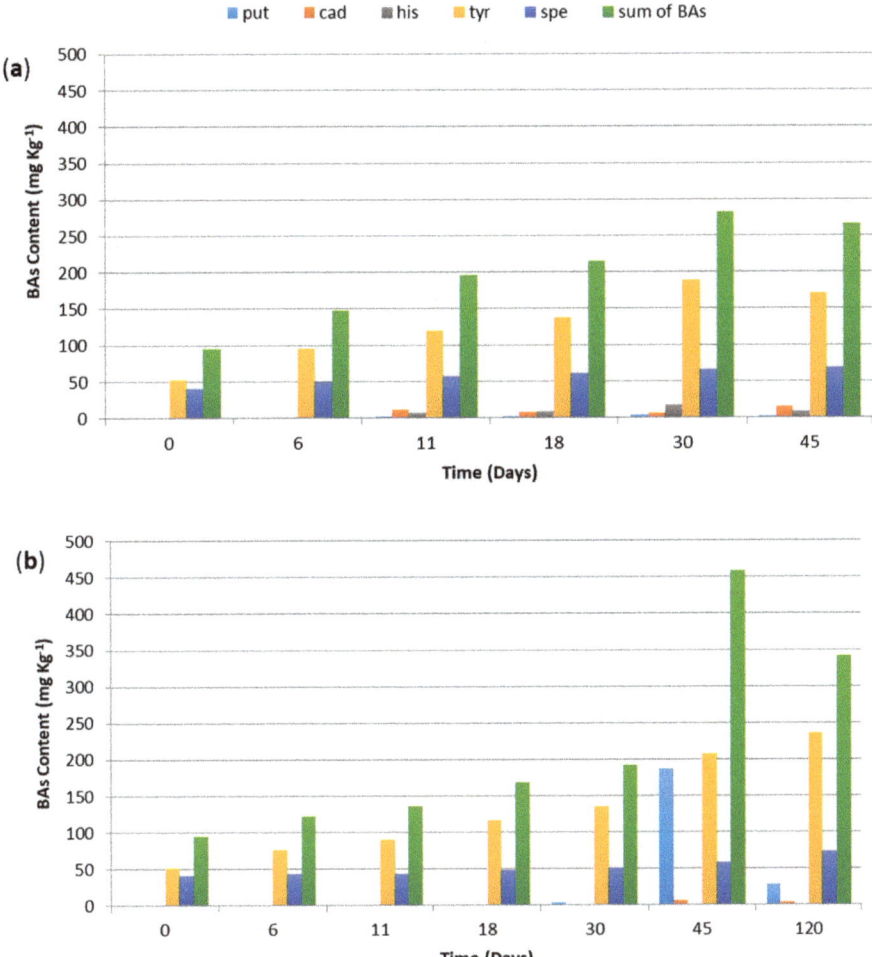

Figure 3. Putrescine (put), cadaverine (cad), histamine (his), tyramine (tyr), spermidine (spd), and sum of biogenic amines (as mg/Kg) content in "*Mortadella di Campotosto*"-like sausages produced with beef (panel (**a**), MCB) and hog (panel (**b**), MCH) casings, over time.

The sum of BAs content at the end of ripening resulted significantly different between the two types of products (265 ± 6 and 341 ± 23 mg/Kg, respectively, for MCB and MCH). These BAs levels are commonly found in other types of dry sausages produced by natural fermentation. Again, the differences in BAs content could be attributed to the higher water activity in MCH, as well as to the lower NaCl concentration due to scarce water loss, optimal for microbial development and BAs accumulation, in particular of tyramine and putrescine [54]. The significant reduction in total BAs at the end of ripening was associated with PUT decrease (more than 80%) in MCH samples, and with the decline of TYR, close to 40%, in MBH samples. Biogenic amines degradation was probably due to microorganisms possessing amino-oxidase enzymes, such as particular strains of the genera

Lactobacillus, Pediococcus, Micrococcus, as well as *Staphylococcus carnosus* [55]. The activity of these enzymes is pH-dependent and particularly active at pH values close to neutrality [56].

In the absence of a legal limit for biogenic amines content in dry fermented sausages, European Food Safety Authority (EFSA) stated that up to 50 mg of histamine and 60 mg of tyramine can be considered safe for healthy individuals; however, these limits fall dramatically if an individual takes anti-MAO drugs or is particularly sensitive to these amines [57]. Suzzi and Gardini [53] identified a sum of 200 mg/Kg of vasoactive amines (tyramine, histamine, tryptamine, and 2-phenylethylamine), as an indicator of good manufacturing procedure for fermented sausages. Among the investigated samples, only in MCH this limit was reached 45 days after the start of the manufacturing process and was still exceeded (although reduced) at the end of ripening.

4. Conclusions

The effect of different casing on some characteristics of dry fermented sausages produced at very low temperatures was investigated. This study demonstrated that *"Mortadella di Campotosto"*-like sausages did not show an intense proteolysis during fermentation and ripening, probably because production is carried out at very low temperatures. Nevertheless, the type of casing had a strong effect on ripening time, proteolysis, and production of some volatile compounds. On the other hand, although the presence of biogenic amines is considered as unavoidable in fermented meat products, the results highlighted that in *"Mortadella di Campotosto"*-like sausages processed with the traditional beef casing, the risk associated with the presence of bioactive amines is low. Furthermore, in addition to the better texture performance, when beef casing is used for this type of sausage, the process is significantly shorter in comparison to hog casing, with important positive effects on production costs for ripening and storage. For all these considerations, and despite its lower availability on the market, beef casings, traditionally used for this kind of product, are determinant for the final characteristics of this type of product.

Author Contributions: Conceptualization, A.P. and C.C.-L.; methodology, C.C.-L., A.S.; software, C.C.-L., G.S.; validation, A.S., C.C.-L. and A.P.; formal analysis, J.L., F.M., F.D., C.R.; investigation, J.L., F.M., F.D., C.R., M.M.; data curation, A.S., C.C.-L., A.P., M.M., G.S.; writing—original draft preparation, C.C.-L., A.S.; writing—review and editing, C.C.-L., A.S., A.P., G.S.; supervision, A.P.; project administration, A.P.; funding acquisition, A.P. All authors have read and agreed to the published version of the manuscript.

Funding: This research received no external funding.

Acknowledgments: The authors gratefully thank Macelleria "L'Olmo", sited in Scanno (AQ), Italy for the helpfulness, and for having provided all the experimental samples.

Conflicts of Interest: The authors declare no conflict of interest.

References

1. Toldrá, F. Characterization of proteolysis. In *Dry-Cured Meat Products*; Nip, W.K., Ed.; Wiley-Blackwell: Middletown, CT, USA, 2002; pp. 113–134. [CrossRef]
2. Djordjevic, J.; Pecanac, B.; Todorovic, M.; Dokmanovic, M.; Glamoclija, N.; Tadic, V.; Baltic, M.Z. Fermented sausage casings. *Procedia Food Sci.* **2015**, *5*, 69–72. [CrossRef]
3. Wu, Y.-C.; Chi, S.-P.; Christieans, S. Casings. In *Handbook of Fermented Meat and Poultry*; Toldrà, F., Ed.; Wiley Blackwell Publishing: Ames, IA, USA, 2010; pp. 86–96. [CrossRef]
4. Pisacane, V.; Callegari, M.L.; Puglisi, E.; Dallolio, G.; Rebecchi, A. Microbial analyses of traditional Italian salami reveal microorganisms transfer from the natural casing to the meat matrix. *Int. J. Food Microbiol.* **2015**, *207*, 57–65. [CrossRef] [PubMed]
5. AOAC. *Official Methods of Analysis of AOAC International*, 16th ed.; Association of Official Analytical Chemists: Gaithersburg, MD, USA, 1999.
6. Park, Y.W. Moisture and water activity. In *Handbook of Processed Meats and Poultry Analysis*; Nollet, L.M.L., Toldrà, F., Eds.; CRC Press: Boca Raton, FL, USA, 2009; pp. 36–67.

7. ISO 1841-2:1996. *Meat and Meat Products–Determination of Chloride Content. Part 1 Volhard Method*; ISO: Geneva, Switzerland, 1996.
8. AOAC. *Official Method of Analysis of AOAC International*, 17th ed.; Association of Official Analytical Chemists: Gaithersburg, MD, USA, 2002.
9. Martuscelli, M.; Lupieri, L.; Chaves-Lopez, C.; Mastrocola, D.; Pittia, P. Technological approach to reduce NaCl content of traditional smoked dry-cured hams: Effect on quality properties and stability. *J. Food Sci. Technol.* **2015**, *52*, 7771–7782. [CrossRef] [PubMed]
10. Martín-Sánchez, A.M.; Chaves-López, C.; Sendra, E.; Sayas, E.; Fenández-López, J.; Pérez-Álvarez, J.Á. Lipolysis, proteolysis, and sensory characteristics of a Spanish fermented dry-cured meat product (salchichón) with oregano essential oil used as surface mold inhibitor. *Meat Sci.* **2011**, *89*, 35–44. [CrossRef] [PubMed]
11. Bradford, M.M. A rapid and sensitive method for the quantification of microgram quantities of protein utilizing the principle of protein-dye binding. *Anal. Biochem.* **1976**, *72*, 248–254. [CrossRef]
12. Laemmli, U.K. Cleavage of structural proteins during the assembly of the head of bacteriophage T4. *Nature* **1970**, *227*, 68–685. [CrossRef] [PubMed]
13. Folkertsma, B.; Fox, P.F. Use of the Cd-ninhydrin reagent to assess proteolysis in cheese during ripening. *J. Dairy Res.* **1992**, *59*, 217–224. [CrossRef]
14. Berardo, A.; Devreese, B.; De Maerè, H.; Stavropoulou, D.A.; Van Royen, G.; Leroy, F.; De Smet, S. Actin proteolysis during ripening of dry fermented sausages at different pH values. *Food Chem.* **2017**, *221*, 1322–1332. [CrossRef]
15. Chaves-López, C.; Paparella, A.; Tofalo, R.; Suzzi, G. Proteolytic activity of *Saccharomyces cerevisiae* strains associated with Italian dry-fermented sausages in a model system. *Int. J. Food Microbiol.* **2011**, *150*, 50–58. [CrossRef]
16. Chaves-López, C.; Serio, A.; Mazzarrino, G.; Martuscelli, M.; Scarpone, E.; Paparella, A. Control of household mycoflora in fermented sausages using phenolic fractions from olive mill wastewaters. *Int. J. Food Microbiol.* **2015**, *207*, 49–56. [CrossRef]
17. Martuscelli, M.; Pittia, P.; Casamassima, L.M.; Lupieri, L.; Neri, L. Effect of intensity of smoking treatment on the free amino acids and biogenic amines occurrence in dry cured ham. *Food Chem.* **2009**, *116*, 955–962. [CrossRef]
18. Bourne, M.C. Texture Profile Analysis. *Food Technol.* **1978**, *32*, 62–66.
19. Khan, M.I.; Arshad, M.S.; Anjum, F.M.; Sameen, A.; Aneeq ur, R.; Gill, W.T. Meat as a functional food with special reference to probiotic sausages. *Food Res. Int.* **2011**, *44*, 3125–3133. [CrossRef]
20. Soriano, A.; Cruz, B.; Gómez, L.; Mariscal, C.; García Ruiz, A. Proteolysis, physicochemical characteristics and free fatty acids composition of dry sausages made with deer (*Cervus elaphus*) or wild boar (*Sus scrofa*) meat: A preliminary study. *Food Chem.* **2006**, *96*, 173–184. [CrossRef]
21. Nakagawa, T.; Watabe, S.; Hashimoto, K. Identification of the three major components in fish sarcoplasmic proteins. *Nippon Suisan Gakk* **1988**, *54*, 999–1004. [CrossRef]
22. Dalmış, Ü.; Soyer, A. Effect of processing methods and starter culture (*Staphylococcus xylosus* and *Pediococcus pentosaceus*) on proteolytic changes in Turkish sausages (sucuk) during ripening and storage. *Meat Sci.* **2008**, *80*, 345–354. [CrossRef] [PubMed]
23. Toldrà, F. Proteolysis and lipolysis in flavour development of dry-cured meat products. *Meat Sci.* **1998**, *49*, S101–S110. [CrossRef]
24. Ladrat, C.; Verrez-Bagnis, V.; Noël, J.; Fleurence, J. In vitro proteolysis of myofibrillar and sarcoplasmic proteins of white muscle of sea bass (*Dicentrarchus labrax* L.): Effects of cathepsins B, D and L. *Food Chem.* **2003**, *81*, 517–525. [CrossRef]
25. Casaburi, A.; Blaiotta, G.; Mauriello, G.; Pepe, O.; Villani, F. Technological activities of *Staphylococcus carnosus* and *Staphylococcus simulans* strains isolated from fermented sausages. *Meat Sci.* **2005**, *71*, 643–650. [CrossRef]
26. Xiong, Y.L.; Blanchard, S.P. Dynamic gelling properties of myofibrillar protein from skeletal muscles of different chicken parts. *J. Agric. Food Chem.* **1994**, *42*, 670–674. [CrossRef]
27. Fadda, S.; López, C.; Vignolo, G. Role of lactic acid bacteria during meat conditioning and fermentation: Peptides generated as sensorial and hygienic biomarkers. *Meat Sci.* **2010**, *86*, 66–79. [CrossRef] [PubMed]
28. Saccani, G.; Fornelli, G.; Zanardi, E. Characterization of textural properties and changes of myofibrillar and sarcoplasmic proteins in salame Felino during ripening. *Int. J. Food Prop.* **2013**, *16*, 1460–1471. [CrossRef]

29. Toldrá, F. The role of muscle enzymes in dry-cured meat products with different drying conditions. *Trends Food Sci. Technol.* **2006**, *17*, 164–168. [CrossRef]
30. Claeys, E.; Uytterhaegen, L.; Buts, B.; Demeyer, D. Quantification of myofibrillar proteins by SDS-PAGE. *Meat Sci.* **1995**, *39*, 177–193. [CrossRef]
31. Demeyer, D.; Raemaekers, M.; Rizzo, A.; Holck, A.; De Smedt, A.; ten Brink, B.; Hagen, B.; Montel, C.; Zanardi, E.; Murbrekk, E.; et al. Control of bioflavour and safety in fermented sausages: First results of a European Project. *Food Res. Int.* **2000**, *33*, 171–180. [CrossRef]
32. Roseiro, L.C.; Gomes, A.; Gonçalves, H.; Sol, M.; Cercas, R.; Santos, C. Effect of processing on proteolysis and biogenic amines formation in a Portuguese traditional dry-fermented ripened sausage "Chouriço Grosso de Estremoz e Borba PGI". *Meat Sci.* **2010**, *84*, 172–179. [CrossRef]
33. Di Cagno, R.; Chaves López, C.; Tofalo, R.; Gallo, G.; De Angelis, M.; Paparella, A.; Hammes, W.P.; Gobbetti, M. Comparison of the compositional, microbiological, biochemical and volatile profile characteristics of three Italian PDO fermented sausages. *Meat Sci.* **2008**, *79*, 224–235. [CrossRef]
34. Magistà, D.; Susca, A.; Ferrara, M.; Logrieco, A.F.; Perrone, G. *Penicillium* species: Crossroad between quality and safety of cured meat production. *Curr. Opin. Food Sci.* **2017**, *17*, 36–40. [CrossRef]
35. Benito, M.J.; Córdoba, J.J.; Alonso, M.; Asensio, M.A.; Nuñez, F. Hydrolytic activity of *Penicillium chrysogenum* Pg222 on pork myofibrillar proteins. *Int. J. Food Microbiol.* **2003**, *89*, 155–161. [CrossRef]
36. Beck, H.C.; Hansen, A.M.; Lauritsen, F.R. Catabolism of leucine to branched-chain fatty acids in *Staphylococcus xylosus*. *J. Appl. Microbiol.* **2004**, *96*, 1185–1193. [CrossRef]
37. Flores, M.; Olivares, A. Flavor. In *Handbook of Fermented Meat and Poultry*, 2nd ed.; Toldrà, F., Hui, Y.H., Astiasarán, I., Sebranek, J.G., Talon, R., Eds.; Wiley Blackwell: Hoboken, NJ, USA, 2014; pp. 217–225. [CrossRef]
38. Janssens, M.; Van der Mijnsbrugge, A.; Sánchez Mainar, M.; Balzarini, T.; De Vuyst, L.; Leroy, F. The use of nucleosides and arginine as alternative energy sources by coagulase-negative staphylococci in view of meat fermentation. *Food Microbiol.* **2014**, *39*, 53–60. [CrossRef] [PubMed]
39. Rimaux, T.; Vrancken, G.; Pothakos, V.; Maes, D.; De Vuyst, L.; Leroy, F. The kinetics of the arginine deiminase pathway in the meat starter culture *Lactobacillus sakei* CTC 494 are pH-dependent. *Food Microbiol.* **2011**, *28*, 597–604. [CrossRef] [PubMed]
40. Stalon, V.; Mercenier, A. L-arginine utilization by *Pseudomonas* species. *J. Gen. Microbiol.* **1984**, *130*, 69–76. [CrossRef] [PubMed]
41. Chen, Q.; Kong, B.; Han, Q.; Liu, Q.; Xu, L. The role of bacterial fermentation in the hydrolysis and oxidation of sarcoplasmic and myofibrillar proteins in Harbin dry sausages. *Meat Sci.* **2016**, *121*, 196–206. [CrossRef]
42. Toldrà, F.; Sanz, Y.; Flores, M. Meat fermentation technology. In *Meat Science and Application*; Hui, Y.H., Nip, W.K., Rogers, R., Eds.; CRC Press: Boca Raton, FL, USA, 2001. [CrossRef]
43. Ardö, Y. Flavour formation by amino acid catabolism. *Biotechnol. Adv.* **2006**, *24*, 238–242. [CrossRef]
44. Janssens, M.; Myter, N.; De Vuyst, L.; Leroy, F. Community dynamics of coagulase-negative staphylococci during spontaneous artisan-type meat fermentations differ between smoking and moulding treatments. *Int. J. Food Microbiol.* **2013**, *166*, 168–175. [CrossRef]
45. Barbut, S. Texture. In *Handbook of Fermented Meat and Poultry*; Toldrá, F., Hui, Y.H., Astiasarán, I., Nip, W.K., Sebranek, J.G., Silveira, E.T.F., Stahnke, L.H., Talon, R., Eds.; Blackwell Publishing: Ames, IA, USA, 2007; pp. 217–226. [CrossRef]
46. Ikonić, P.; Jokanović, M.; Petrović, L.; Tasić, T.; Škaljac, S.; Šojić, B.; Džinić, N.; Tomović, V.; Tomić, J.; Danilović, B.; et al. Effect of starter culture addition and processing method on proteolysis and texture profile of traditional dry-fermented sausage Petrovská klobása. *Int. J. Food Prop.* **2016**, *19*, 1924–1937. [CrossRef]
47. Feng, L.; Qiao, Y.; Zou, Y.; Huang, M.; Kang, Z.; Zhou, G. Effect of Flavourzyme on proteolysis, antioxidant capacity and sensory attributes of Chinese sausage. *Meat Sci.* **2014**, *98*, 34–40. [CrossRef]
48. Benito, M.J.; Rodríguez, M.; Cordoba, M.G.; Andrade, M.J.; Córdoba, J.J. Effect of the fungal protease EPg222 on proteolysis and texture in the dry fermented sausage 'salchichón'. *J. Sci. Food Agric.* **2005**, *85*, 273–280. [CrossRef]
49. Loizzo, M.R.; Spizzirri, U.G.; Bonesi, M.; Tundis, R.; Picci, N.; Restuccia, D. Influence of packaging conditions on biogenic amines and fatty acids evolution during 15 months storage of a typical spreadable salami ('Nduja). *Food Chem.* **2016**, *213*, 115–122. [CrossRef]

50. Paparella, A.; Tofalo, R. Fermented sausages: A potential source of biogenic amines. In *Biogenic Amines in Food: Analysis, Occurrence and Toxicity*; Saal, B., Tofalo, R., Eds.; The Royal Society of Chemistry: London, UK, 2020; pp. 103–118. [CrossRef]
51. Gardini, F.; Martuscelli, M.; Crudele, M.A.; Paparella, A.; Suzzi, G. Use of *Staphylococcus xylosus* as a starter culture in dried sausages: Effect on the biogenic amine content. *Meat Sci.* **2002**, *61*, 275–283. [CrossRef]
52. Serio, A.; Paparella, A.; Chaves López, C.; Corsetti, A.; Suzzi, G. *Enterococcus* populations in Pecorino Abruzzese cheese: Biodiversity and safety aspects. *J. Food Prot.* **2007**, *70*, 1561–1568. [CrossRef] [PubMed]
53. Suzzi, G.; Gardini, F. Biogenic amines in dry fermented sausages: A review. *Int. J. Food Microbiol.* **2003**, *88*, 41–54. [CrossRef]
54. Anastasio, A.; Draisci, R.; Pepe, T.; Mercogliano, R.; Delli Quadri, F.; Luppi, G.; Cortesi, M.L. Development of biogenic amines during the ripening of Italian dry sausages. *J. Food Prot.* **2010**, *73*, 114–118. [CrossRef] [PubMed]
55. Lorenzo, J.M.; Sichetti Munekata, P.E.; Dominiguez, R. Role of autochthonous starter cultures in the reduction of biogenic amines in traditional meat products. *Curr. Opin. Food Sci.* **2017**, *14*, 61–65. [CrossRef]
56. Martuscelli, M.; Crudele, M.A.; Gardini, F.; Suzzi, G. Biogenic amine formation and oxidation by *Staphylococcus xylosus* strains from artisanal fermented sausages. *Lett. Appl. Microbiol.* **2002**, *31*, 228–232. [CrossRef]
57. EFSA. Scientific opinion on risk based control of biogenic amine formation in fermented foods. *EFSA J.* **2001**, *9*, 2393. [CrossRef]

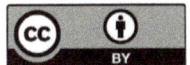

© 2020 by the authors. Licensee MDPI, Basel, Switzerland. This article is an open access article distributed under the terms and conditions of the Creative Commons Attribution (CC BY) license (http://creativecommons.org/licenses/by/4.0/).

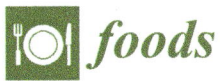

Article

Modeling Some Possible Handling Ways with Fish Raw Material in Home-Made Sushi Meal Preparation

Hana Buchtova [1,*], Dani Dordevic [2,3], Iwona Duda [4], Alena Honzlova [5] and Piotr Kulawik [4]

[1] Department of Meat Hygiene and Technology, Faculty of Veterinary Hygiene and Technology, University of Veterinary and Pharmaceutical Sciences Brno, 61242 Brno, Czech Republic
[2] Department of Plant Origin Foodstuffs Hygiene and Technology, Faculty of Veterinary Hygiene and Technology, University of Veterinary and Pharmaceutical Sciences Brno, 61242 Brno, Czech Republic; dordevicd@vfu.cz
[3] Department of Technology and Organization of Public Catering, South Ural State University, Lenin prospect 76, 454080 Chelyabinsk, Russia
[4] Department of Animal Product Technology, Faculty of Food Technology, University of Agriculture, 31-120 Krakow, Poland; iwona.duda@urk.edu.pl (I.D.); kulawik.piotr@gmail.com (P.K.)
[5] Department of Chemistry, State Veterinary Institute Jihlava, 58601, Jihlava, Czech Republic; honzlova@svujihlava.cz
* Correspondence: buchtovah@vfu.cz; Tel.: +42-0541-562-742

Received: 14 August 2019; Accepted: 4 October 2019; Published: 8 October 2019

Abstract: The aim of this work was to simulate selected ways of handling with raw fish after its purchase. The experiment was designed as three partial simulations: (a) trend in the biogenic amines formation in raw fish caused by breakage of cold chain during the transport after purchase, (b) the use of a handheld gastronomic unit as an alternative method of smoking fish with cold smoke in the household with regard to a possible increase in polycyclic aromatic hydrocarbon content, and (c) whether the cold smoked fish affects selected sensory parameters of nigiri sushi meal prepared by consumers. The material used in the research consisted of: yellowfin tuna (*Thunnus albacares*) sashimi fillets and the Atlantic salmon (*Salmo salar*) fillets with skin. The control (fresh/thawed tuna; without interrupting the cold chain) and experimental (fresh/thawed tuna; cold chain was interrupted by incubation at 35 °C/6 h) samples were stored at 2 ± 2 °C for 8 days and analyzed after 1st, 4th and 8th day of the cold storage. Histamine content was very low throughout the experiment, though one exception was found (thawed tuna without interrupting the cold chain: 272.05 ± 217.83 mg·kg^{-1}/8th day). Tuna samples contained more PAH (4.22 µg·kg^{-1}) than salmon samples (1.74 µg·kg^{-1}). Alarming increases of benzo(a)anthracene (1.84 µg·k^{-1}) and chrysene (1.10 µg·kg^{-1}) contents in smoked tuna were detected.

Keywords: nigiri sushi; polycyclic aromatic hydrocarbons; histamine; household smoker unit

1. Introduction

Currently, sushi meals are becoming popular worldwide [1]. Sushi meals have developed from a simple street food to sophisticated cuisine. Many studies have dealt with the health benefits and health hazards associated with the sushi cuisine [2]. In the past, high attention has been devoted to studies of microbiological [3], chemical [4,5] or parasitic [6] hazards in fishery products, like the toxicological risks of diseases after consumption of raw fish or foodstuffs that include raw fish flesh [1]. Recorded cases of acute gastric anisakiasis are a serious warning to consumers [7]. Sushi belongs to ready to eat foods and is predisposed to contamination with food pathogens, such as *Listeria monocytogenes* [8,9].

Consumer concerns about food safety might disrupt a healthy food choice [10]. Risks associated with the consumption of fish might impose barriers to consumption, though fish is considered an important component of the human diet [11].

A new look at research on sushi meal assessment, including simulation of model of real consumer behavior and culinary practices by chefs, should shift research to a higher level of knowledge. In recent years there has been an increase in collaboration between researchers and chefs in the field of gastronomy [12]. Modern trends of molecular gastronomy that works with human senses, is a fast food preparation method using portable, easy-to-use applications, developed specifically for chefs, to create new unusual flavors.

The biggest interruption in the cold chain occurs after product purchase and during its delivery to the household. Consumer behavior and the ambient temperature largely influence the shelf life and food safety [13].

In recent years, also in the Czech Republic, there has been a growing trend of self-preparation of sushi food by consumers. In our research, based on the buying habits of some consumers and their creativity approach to treat raw fish raw using a handheld smoker unit, we wanted to connect partial studies on fish handling and sushi preparation into one model experiment.

The experiment was designed in the form of three partial simulations: (a) trend in biogenic amines formation caused by severe breakage of cold chain during the transport of fish raw material after purchase to household, (b) the use of a handheld gastronomic unit as an alternative method of smoking fish with cold smoke in the household with regard to a possible increase in polycyclic aromatic hydrocarbons (PAH) content, and (c) whether the cold smoked fish affects selected sensory parameters of nigiri sushi meal prepared by consumers in their households.

2. Materials and Methods

Fresh sashimi fillets of the yellowfin tuna (*Thunnus albacares*, caught, FAO 71 area, category of fishing gear: seines) and fresh fillets with skin of the Atlantic salmon (*Salmo salar*, farmed, Norway) were bought from a retail shop (Ocean48, Brno, Czech Republic).

2.1. Trend in the Biogenic Amines Formation Caused by Severe Breakage of Cold Chain during the Transport of Fish Raw Material after Purchase Place to Household

Tuna sashimi fillet was used to a case study focused on simulating conditions sale of fresh and thawed fish and consumer behavior (compliance/interruption with/of the cold chain) and to determine how this behavior affects the formation of biogenic amines total content and its spectrum (tryptamine TRP, 2-phenylethylamine 2-PHE, putrescine PUT, cadaverine CAD, histamine HIS, tyramine TYR, spermidine SPD, spermine SPR). The experiment was carried out in four separate replicates. Tuna fillets purchased for the fifth repetition had to be excluded from the experiment because of the high histamine content at the start of the storage, which significantly exceeded the limit set out in Regulation (EC) No 2073/2005 [see in Appendix A1] at the start of storage (the possible reason for higher histamine content will be commented on in the Results and Discussion section).

The case study was based on the use of four different sashimi fillets (1, 2, 3, 4). Four types of samples A, B, C, D from each tuna fillet were prepared simultaneously. Characteristics of the samples were as follows: A: control sample, fresh tuna was cold stored at +2 ± 2 °C, without interrupting the cold chain after buying the fish in a store; B: experimental sample, fresh tuna, cold chain of fresh sample was interrupted before the cold storage in a laboratory by incubation of the sample (35 °C/6 h) to simulate the possible consumer behavior in the summer after buying the fish in a store, subsequently samples were cold stored at +2 ± 2 °C; C: experimental sample, thawed tuna, after buying the fish in a store the sample was experimentally frozen (−35 °C) and stored for two weeks in a frozen state (−18 °C), then the samples were thawed in the refrigerator (+2 ± 2 °C/12 h) and subsequently cold stored at +2 ± 2 °C; D: experimental sample, thawed tuna, after buying the fish in a store, the sample was experimentally frozen (−35 °C) and stored two weeks in a frozen state (−18 °C), the cold chain of thawed sample was interrupted by incubation the sample (35 °C/6 h) to simulate the possible consumer behavior in the summer after buying the fish in a store, the samples were subsequently cold stored at

+2 ± 2 °C. All samples (A, B, C, D) were stored at +2 ± 2 °C for 8 days, the samples were analyzed after 1st, 4th and 8th days of cold storage.

The biogenic amines analysis was performed according to the method described by [14]. The chromatographic separation was performed using a Dionex Ultimate 3000 HPLC apparatus (Thermo Scientific, Waltham, MA, USA) with a FLD 3400RS four channel fluorescent detector (Thermo Scientific) and a low pressure gradient pump with a four channel mixer. The detector settings were set to 340 nm for excitation and 540 nm for emission. The separation was performed on a Kromasil 100-5-C18 4.6 × 250 mm column (Akzo Nobel, Amsterdam, The Netherlands) and the column temperature of 30 °C. Flow rate was 0.8 mL/min with two mobile phases: (A) acetonitrile (Merck, Darmstadt, Germany) and (B) water (Merck). The detection limit for each biogenic amine was 0.005 mg·kg^{-1}. The samples were analyzed in duplicate and triplicate and injections into HPLC were carried out on each duplicate (N = 4 × 2 × 3).

2.2. The Part of the Research Consisting of Testing the Use of a Handheld Gastronomic Unit as an Alternative Method of Smoking Fish With Cold Smoke in the Household with Regard to a Possible Increase in Polycyclic Aromatic Hydrocarbons (PAH) Content and Whether the Cold Smoked Fish Affects Selected Sensory Parameters of Nigiri Sushi Meal Prepared by Consumers at Their Household

Tuna and salmon fillets were used for preparation of nigiri sushi with not-smoked (raw, control samples) and smoked (experimental samples) samples. Smoked muscle of both fish was prepared with application of a smoker unit (Super Aladin smoker, Manihi s.r.o., Praha, Czech Republic). Cold smoke (20 °C; Aladin oak chips) was applied on meat surface beneath the glass hatch for 5 min. The experiment was carried out in five separate replicates. Sensory attributes (saltiness, bitterness, juiciness, consistency) of sushi meal and a question focused on examining the fact whether the conscious consumption of smoked fish in sushi can affect the consumer's confidence in the health safety of this food were monitored by a group of trained evaluators and evaluated on the basis of questionnaires.

Nigiri sushi samples with tuna and salmon meat (smoked and not smoked) were prepared in the Sensory Laboratory at the Department of Meat Hygiene and Technology (Faculty of Veterinary Hygiene and Ecology, University of Veterinary and Pharmaceutical Sciences, Brno, Czech Republic). Fillets were frozen according to the Commission regulation (EC) No 853/2004 (Annex III, Section VIII, Chapter III, Part D, Point 2a [see in Appendix A2]) at −40 °C using quick freezing unit F.R.C. BF 031AF (Friulinox, Taiedo di Chions, Italy) to muscle core temperature of −20 °C and were stored in a frozen chamber with regulated temperature (−20 ± 2 °C) for 2 weeks. Then the samples were thawed in refrigerator (+2 ± 2 °C/12 h) and subsequently divided into two parts, the one was used as control (raw not smoked) samples for sushi preparation and the second one was used for cold smoking by Super Aladin smoker and for sushi preparation. The rice was cooked in rice cooker (42507 Design Reiskocher, Gastroback, Hollenstedt, Germany). Information about sushi ingredients are following: sushi rice (short grain variety, Yutaka, Italy), 8% vinegar (apple vinegar, Bzenecky Ocet, Bzenec, Czech Republic), 6% sugar (sugar crystal, producer: Korunni, Hrušovany nad Jevišovkou, Czech Republic) and 2% cooking salt with iodine (NaCl 98%, J 20-34 mg·kg^{-1}, K+S Czech Republic a.s., Olomouc, Czech Republic), wasabi paste (Yutaka, China). The experimental design is shown in Figure 1.

Sushi samples were sensory evaluated in the laboratory equipped according to ISO 8589:2008 [see in Appendix A3]. The protocol consisted of unstructured graphical scales of 100 mm length, with one edge of the scale representing the strongest expressed attribute and the second one the weakest expressed attribute. Saltiness (2% salt addition) was evaluated by respondents' comparison with sushi samples prepared without salt (0 point) and with 3% salt content (100 points) added to rice.

Twenty panelists took part in the sensory evaluation, where they assessed selected parameters: (saltiness, bitterness, juiciness, consistency) and consumer confidence in the food safety (expressed in their own words). Ingredients' weights (g) of nigiri sushi are given in Table 1.

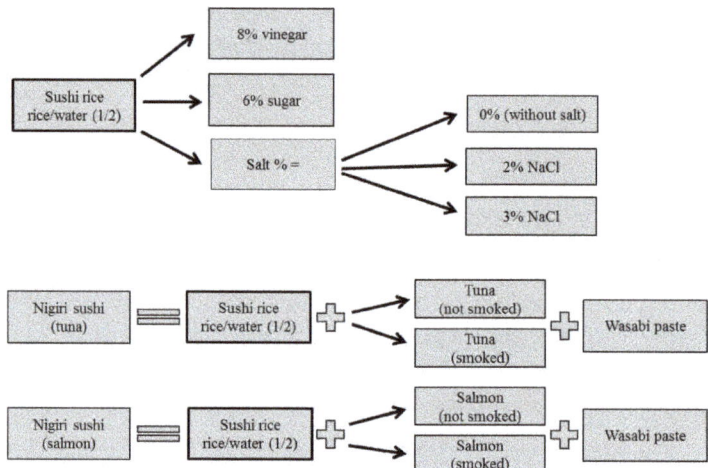

Figure 1. Experimental design of sushi production samples used in the research.

Table 1. Ingredients' portions (%) of nigiri sushi prepared with salmon and tuna.

Fish	Treatment	Rice	Seafood	Wasabi
Tuna	Not smoked	66.84 ± 0.53	37.24 ± 0.94	0.80 ± 0.06
	Smoked	63.02 ± 2.01	36.95 ± 1.04	0.75 ± 0.08
Salmon	Not smoked	66.76 ± 0.36	32.38 ± 0.34	0.86 ± 0.09
	Smoked	65.54 ± 0.25	33.31 ± 0.39	0.84 ± 0.07

The thawed raw tuna and salmon samples were used for chemical analysis (total protein, total fat and dry matter content). The same thawed not smoked and smoked tuna and salmon samples were used for determination of polycyclic aromatic hydrocarbons (PAH).

The total protein content (ISO 937:1978 [see in Appendix A4]) was determined as the amount of organically bound nitrogen (recalculating coefficient $f = 6.25$) using the analyzer Kjeltec 2300 (FOSS Tecator, Höganäs, Sweden). The total lipid content was determined quantitatively (ISO 1443:1973 [see in Appendix A5]) by extraction in solvents using Soxtec 2055 (FOSS Tecator). The dry matter was determined gravimetrically according to the Czech National Standard (ISO 1442:1997 [see in Appendix A6]) by drying the sample to a constant weight at +103 ± 2 °C (Binder FD 53, Tuttlingen, Germany).

PAH were determined by accredited method (no. 19 Standard operating procedure 8.15A) using HPLC/FLD in the laboratory of State Veterinary Institute Jihlava (Jihlava, Czech Republic). Each sample was analyzed in parallel. A thoroughly homogenized samples, after trituration with anhydrous sodium sulphate p.a. (Lach-Ner, sro, Tovarni 157, 27711, Neratovice, Czech Republic) and after addition of internal standard 2-methylchrysene (Dr. Ehrenstorfer GmbH, Augsburg, Germany) were extracted with diethyl ether. Extracts were filtered through glass fiber filter paper (Cat. No. 516-0867, VWR International bvba, Leuven, Belgien, the solvent was evaporated on a Büchi R-134 rotary evaporator (BÜCHI Labortechnik) AG, Flawil, Switzerland) at a maximum temperature of 30 °C. The residue was carefully blown off with a stream of nitrogen. The extracted fat was dissolved in chloroform (Cat. No. 20034-UT2-M2500-7 (Macron 6754), Lach-Ner, Ltd., Neratovice, Czech Republic). An aliquot of the solution was purified by gel permeation chromatography on a Gilson Aspec XL system (Gilson, Middleton, WI, USA) using a PAH prep column (500 × 8 mm) packed with gel (styrene divinylbenzene copolymer) (Watrex Praha, sro, Carolina Center, Prague, Czech Republic). Purified samples were evaporated to near dryness on a Büchi R-134 rotary evaporator at a maximum temperature of 30 °C or the remaining solvent was blown off with a stream of nitrogen. The residue was dissolved in acetonitrile and used for fluorescence detection by liquid chromatography.

Chromatographic analysis was performed on Waters Alliance e2695 liquid chromatograph with 2475 fluorescence detector (Waters Corporation, Milford, MA, USA) on Waters PAH column (250 mm × 4.6 mm × 5 µm) using gradient elution with mobile phase. Gradient mobile phase consisted out of acetonitrile/redistilled water (75/25 100/0), flow rate 0.7 mL/min, injection 10 µL, column temperature 30 °C. Detection was performed by fluorescence detector with programmable wavelength change (excitation wavelength—265 nm for benzo(a)anthracene and chrysene, 290 nm for benzo(b)fluoranthene and benzo(a)pyrene; wavelength 380 nm for benzo(a)anthracene and chrysene and 430 nm for benzo(b)fluoaranthene and benzo(a)pyrene). PAH Calibration Mix, CRM47940 (Supelco Analytical, Bellefonte, PA, USA) was used for the calibration. The limit of quantification was 0.25–0.29 µg/kg, the repeatability of the method was 10% and yield 65–95%.

2.3. Statistical Analysis

The results of chemical composition were evaluated (mean ± s. d.) in the program Microsoft Office Excel 2007 (Microsoft Corp., Redmond, WA, USA). Statistically significant differences of biogenic amines (BA) spectrum were performed at levels of $\alpha = 0.05$ ($p < 0.05$) using the UNISTAT 6.0 (Unistat® Ltd, London, UK) statistical package (multiple comparison, Tukey's HSD test).

3. Results and Discussion

Fresh fishery products are among the most perishable food commodities Their quality is influenced by a number of factors (the origin-wild/farmed, water temperature and level of environmental pollution, compliance with veterinary and hygienic standards during hunting and after capture, species and health and nutritional status/age/sex/phase of sexual cycle/size/weight of fish, way of treatment-gutting/cutting, initial microbiological contamination, keeping the cold chain) which can vary in time and therefore consequently the quality can vary significantly from batch to batch [15]. Freezing is an excellent way to extend shelf life of fish meat during long-term transport or frozen storage [16]. Offering thawed fishery products is a common way of selling fish in landlocked countries [17]. On the other hand, cold chain breakage can cause potentially serious alimentary intoxication, such as histamine content increment. Therefore, growth and activity of histamine-producing bacteria can become dangerous especially in fish which muscle tissue contain a high concentration (about 10,000 mg·kg^{-1}) of free histidine in muscle tissue as tuna fillets. Though, salmon has a low concentration (about 100 to 200 mg·kg^{-1}) of free histidine [18]. Especially, *Photobacterium phosphoreum* and psychrotolerant bacteria similar to *Morganella morganii* are known to be present in fresh fish tissue and form histamine at low temperatures (under 5 °C) [19]. Appearance freshness is often unlawfully restored by an injection or immersion of fillets in the nitrites solution to change the dark red or brown colour (visually less fresh meat) to red pigmentation. Meat after this application looks fresh but histamine levels can be high. Also, inappropriate practices of freezing with subsequent illegal treatment are often used (tuna fish originally of canning grade can be illegally sold as sushi grade of tuna). According to the regulation (EC) no 853/2004 [see in Appendix A2], fishery products shall be frozen below −18 °C, for canning industry; unprocessed fish initially is tolerated to be frozen in brine at −9 °C. Subsequent illegal treatment of tuna fillets and application of nitrites/nitrates (e.g., salt, additives or vegetable extracts containing high level of nitrites) or using of gas carbon monooxide (CO) is not authorized according to the regulation (EC) no 1333/2008 [see in Appendix A7]. Approximately 25,000 tons of tuna per year undergo this treatment [20].

Besides the fact that consumers may be deceived by the quality of fillets, their health can also be compromised. The high level of histamine can cause allergic syndrome [21], nitrites may lead to formation of nitrosamines that have carcinogenic effects [22]. As we wrote in the Materials and Methods section, fresh tuna fillets purchased for the fifth replicate of the experiment, could be hypothetically treated by any of the above illegal practices. Fresh/thawed samples were stored at +2 ± 2 °C; the samples contained in the 1st day of 781/195, 4th day of 1851/1542 and 8th day of 1717/2914 mg·kg^{-1} of histamine in meat. This fifth fillet was therefore excluded from the further experimentation. However, we have shown that even frozen tuna fillet can become a serious threat to human health due to the increment of BA.

3.1. Trends in Biogenic Amines Formation Caused by Severe Breakage of the Cold Chain during the Transport to Households of Fish Raw Material after Purchase

Significant qualitative and quantitative variability in the observed BA was found between sample groups (A, B, C, D) depending on the sampling day (Table 2) as well as between the individual sampling days within one particular group (Table 3).

Regarding the criteria for foodstuffs (Regulation (EC) No 2073/2005, Chap. I, Point 1.26 [see in Appendix A1]), histamine content was very low throughout the experiment, with one exception (C/8 day) which will be further commented (Table 2). The fresh sample of tuna (A) contained the highest ($p < 0.05$) histamine content in the samples measured after 4 days (Table 3).

The fresh samples (group B) that were exposed to 35 °C/6 h and subsequently cold-stored at +2 ± 2 °C during 8 days had almost the same histamine contents during the storage period (Table 3). Distinctly higher histamine contents were found in C samples (thawed/subsequently cold-stored at +2 ± 2 °C), after 8th day of storage (the mean of four different batches: 272.05 ± 217.83 mg·kg^{-1}). The noticeably high value of the standard deviation (s. d.) draws attention to possible differences in quality among purchased lots of fillets; due to these differences the results of thawed fillets (C) obtained for the 8th day of sampling are presented in Table 4. Based on the partial results for each of the four lots, it can be concluded that the three lots were probably more contaminated with microorganisms capable to decarboxylation activity. Due to their activities, histamine content of three tuna lots (8 days of storage) increased to 354.74 ± 185.67 mg·kg^{-1}; PUT, CAD and TYR contents were significantly ($p < 0.05$) higher and caused five times higher total biogenic amine content (563.32 ± 252.61 mg·kg^{-1}) for these three tuna lots compared to the fourth one (Table 4).

In the fourth lot, the HIS content (23.98 ± 0.93 mg·kg^{-1}) was very low, but compared to the other three lots, the fillet contained significantly more SPD, though the BA total was low overall (108.67 ± 1.67 mg·kg^{-1}) (Table 4). In the thawed samples of group D tuna, that were experimentally exposed to temperatures of 35 °C/6 h and subsequently cold-stored at +2 ± 2 °C during 8 days, the HIS content remained virtually unchanged between 1 and 4 days, and we found only a significant reduction in the HIS content on day 8 (Table 3). Based on higher standard deviation (s. d.) for PUT, CAD, TYR, SPD (Table 2), differences in quality were observed for group D tuna batches (similar to the batches of group C tuna). Three batches were found to have significantly ($p < 0.05$) higher amounts of CAD. Consequently, the total BA content in three batches of fillets was approximately two times higher ($p < 0.05$) in comparison to the fourth fillet (Table 4).

The total BA contents of all sample groups were less than 100 mg·kg^{-1}, except for samples from group C and D/8 days (Table 2, BA sum). Each of studied sample groups (A, B, C, D) showed a different trend depending on the storage time (Table 3). BA contents in fresh (A) and thawed samples (C) without cold chain break taken on the day 1 were very low ($p > 0.05$) (Table 2).

Table 2. Qualitative and quantitative biogenic amine spectrum (in mg·kg^{-1}) for groups (A, B, C, D) depending on the sampling day.

Day	Sample	Tryptamine	2-Phenyl-Ethylamine	Putrescine	Cadaverine	Histamine	Tyramine	Spermidine	Spermine	Sum of BAs
1st	A	0.03 ± 0.05 [a]	1.05 ± 0.68 [a]	3.21 ± 1.77 [ab]	2.99 ± 1.35 [ab]	2.00 ± 1.40 [a]	10.21 ± 5.31 [a]	11.08 ± 8.08 [a]	0.75 ± 0.44 [a]	31.31 ± 13.74 [a]
	B	0.32 ± 0.57 [a]	2.15 ± 0.99 [bc]	5.06 ± 6.27 [b]	4.25 ± 2.24 [ab]	3.31 ± 3.04 [ab]	19.31 ± 20.84 [a]	16.82 ± 3.82 [ab]	32.45 ± 20.54 [b]	83.66 ± 38.47 [b]
	C	0.27 ± 0.23 [a]	1.27 ± 1.23 [ab]	0.99 ± 0.41 [a]	1.48 ± 0.31 [a]	3.53 ± 1.15 [ab]	6.71 ± 6.87 [a]	19.49 ± 6.15 [bc]	3.16 ± 1.66 [a]	36.90 ± 11.68 [a]
	D	0.07 ± 0.05 [a]	2.61 ± 0.64 [c]	2.74 ± 1.29 [ab]	7.23 ± 7.40 [b]	6.06 ± 3.62 [b]	10.77 ± 7.34 [a]	24.10 ± 1.62 [c]	2.20 ± 0.38 [a]	55.78 ± 14.66 [a]
Statistical significance						$p < 0.05$				
4th	A	1.67 ± 1.27 [b]	3.03 ± 1.45 [b]	4.29 ± 3.81 [ab]	6.56 ± 4.87 [a]	18.55 ± 16.46 [b]	23.31 ± 10.57 [b]	22.58 ± 5.69 [bc]	1.06 ± 1.92 [a]	81.05 ± 30.95 [bc]
	B	0.97 ± 1.55 [ab]	0.98 ± 1.12 [a]	1.39 ± 0.89 [a]	5.85 ± 4.71 [a]	3.73 ± 2.57 [a]	7.87 ± 4.46 [a]	23.67 ± 10.86 [c]	4.65 ± 4.58 [b]	49.12 ± 23.46 [ab]
	C	0.09 ± 0.05 [a]	0.58 ± 0.38 [a]	3.79 ± 0.62 [ab]	4.28 ± 3.19 [a]	3.45 ± 0.67 [a]	11.77 ± 4.58 [a]	7.32 ± 3.07 [a]	1.30 ± 0.22 [a]	32.59 ± 5.33 [a]
	D	0.34 ± 0.44 [a]	2.38 ± 1.26 [b]	8.10 ± 7.37 [b]	28.11 ± 28.35 [b]	13.59 ± 12.59 [ab]	28.36 ± 15.46 [a]	15.55 ± 3.85 [b]	3.39 ± 0.99 [ab]	99.82 ± 61.65 [c]
Statistical significance						$p < 0.05$				
8th	A	2.31 ± 1.68 [b]	1.35 ± 0.46 [b]	2.87 ± 1.29 [a]	4.60 ± 2.95 [a]	6.11 ± 3.95 [a]	4.95 ± 1.62 [a]	7.84 ± 2.35 [a]	21.34 ± 3.31 [b]	51.37 ± 9.29 [a]
	B	0.40 ± 0.06 [a]	0.31 ± 0.09 [a]	5.23 ± 4.10 [a]	5.05 ± 3.58 [a]	3.84 ± 0.38 [a]	6.66 ± 3.60 [a]	15.39 ± 11.04 [a]	4.29 ± 5.44 [a]	41.16 ± 20.47 [a]
	C	2.77 ± 2.87 [b]	0.74 ± 0.46 [ab]	22.93 ± 15.04 [b]	75.91 ± 52.06 [b]	272.05 ± 217.83 [b]	61.69 ± 20.53 [b]	12.08 ± 6.69 [a]	1.50 ± 0.57 [a]	449.66 ± 297.81 [b]
	D	0.14 ± 0.16 [a]	1.41 ± 1.61 [b]	17.66 ± 12.51 [b]	45.96 ± 32.37 [b]	3.11 ± 0.94 [a]	46.12 ± 19.72 [a]	16.56 ± 11.60 [a]	1.79 ± 0.79 [a]	132.74 ± 56.44 [a]
Statistical significance						$p < 0.05$				

Statistically significant differences ($p < 0.05$) between values for each day of storage (lower cases "a", "b", "c" in indexes in columns).

Table 3. Statistically significant differences ($p < 0.05$) for a particular biogenic amine (lower case "a", "b" in columns) depending on the sampling day and between biogenic amines (capital letters "A" to "D" in italic in rows) for the sampling day are given.

Day	Sample	Tryptamine	2-Phenylethylamine	Putrescine	Cadaverine	Histamine	Tyramine	Spermidine	Spermine	Sum of BAs
1st	A	a *A*	a *AB*	a *BCD*	a *BCD*	a *BC*	a *D*	a *CD*	a *AB*	a
4th		b *A*	b *AB*	a *AB*	b *ABC*	b *BC*	b *C*	b *C*	a *A*	b
8th		b *AB*	a *A*	a *AB*	ab *ABC*	a *BCD*	a *BC*	a *CD*	b *D*	a
1st	B	a *A*	b *AB*	a *ABC*	a *BCD*	a *ABC*	b *CD*	a *D*	b *D*	b
4th		a *A*	a *A*	a *AB*	a *BCD*	a *ABC*	ab *CD*	a *D*	a *ABC*	a
8th		a *AB*	a *A*	a *CD*	a *CD*	a *CD*	a *CD*	a *D*	a *BC*	a
1st	C	a *A*	a *AB*	a *ABC*	a *ABC*	a *CD*	a *BCD*	b *D*	b *BCD*	a
4th		a *A*	a *A*	a *BC*	a *BC*	a *BC*	a *C*	a *C*	a *AB*	a
8th		b *A*	a *A*	b *BCD*	b *CD*	b *D*	b *CD*	a *ABC*	a *AB*	b
1st	D	a *A*	a *B*	a *AB*	a *B*	ab *BC*	a *BC*	b *C*	a *AB*	a
4th		a *A*	a *AB*	a *BC*	ab *CD*	b *BCD*	b *D*	a *CD*	b *ABC*	ab
8th		a *A*	a *A*	b *A*	b *CD*	a *ABC*	c *D*	a *BCD*	a *AB*	b

Table 4. Qualitative and quantitative BA spectrum (in mg·kg^{-1}) for three batches and for one batch for groups C and D/8th day of sampling in a detailed view.

Day/Sample		Tryptamine	2-Phenyl-Ethylamine	Putrescine	Cadaverine	Histamine	Tyramine	Spermidine	Spermine	Sum of BAs
8th	3/C	3.67 ± 2.77 ^{aA}	0.83 ± 0.51 ^{aA}	27.96 ± 14.04 ^{bA}	97.22 ± 41.03 ^{bA}	354.74 ± 185.67 ^{bB}	68.68 ± 18.96 ^{bA}	8.64 ± 2.91 ^{aA}	1.58 ± 0.64 ^{aA}	563.32 ± 252.61 ^{b}
	1/C	0.05 ± 0.00 ^{aA}	0.46 ± 0.01 ^{aAB}	7.83 ± 0.15 ^{aC}	11.97 ± 0.03 ^{aD}	23.98 ± 0.93 ^{aF}	40.71 ± 0.34 ^{aG}	22.39 ± 0.10 ^{bE}	1.28 ± 0.15 ^{aB}	108.67 ± 1.67 ^{a}
	S. s.	*	*	$p < 0.05$	$p < 0.05$	$p < 0.05$	$p < 0.05$	$p < 0.05$	*	$p < 0.05$
	3/D	0.16 ± 0.18 ^{aA}	1.67 ± 1.80 ^{aAB}	20.30 ± 13.56 ^{aB}	58.93 ± 26.15 ^{bC}	3.36 ± 0.97 ^{aAB}	52.99 ± 17.96 ^{aC}	12.89 ± 11.15 ^{aAB}	1.73 ± 0.91 ^{aAB}	152.04 ± 52.01 ^{b}
	1/D	0.06 ± 0.01 ^{aA}	0.62 ± 0.02 ^{aA}	9.75 ± 0.35 ^{aD}	7.04 ± 0.19 ^{aC}	2.36 ± 0.10 ^{aB}	25.51 ± 0.59 ^{aE}	27.59 ± 0.25 ^{aF}	1.94 ± 0.05 ^{aB}	74.87 ± 1.12 ^{a}
	S. s.	*	*	*	$p < 0.05$	*	$p < 0.05$	*	*	$p < 0.05$

Statistically significant differences ($p < 0.05$) for a particular biogenic amine (lower case "a", "b" in columns) and between biogenic amines (capital letters "A" to "G" in italic in rows) depending of number of batches are given. * values are without statistically significant differences (S. s.).

The BA content in fresh samples (A) from day 4 was significantly higher compared to day 1, followed by a significant ($p < 0.05$) decrease in BA content on the day 8 (Table 3). Thawed samples (C) contained very low levels of BA on day 1 and day 4, while BA samples were significantly ($p < 0.05$) 13 times higher on day 8. In the group of fresh (B) and thawed samples (D), where the cold chain was experimentally broken, the BA formation dynamics was more uniform, but the trend was the opposite. Overall, the BA content of Group B samples gradually decreased (significant differences were observed between days 1 and 4, 8); in contrast, in samples of group D, BA content increased gradually (significant differences were found between days 1 and 8) (Table 3).

The spectrum of BA was formed in larger quantities (above 10 mg·kg^{-1}) mainly TYR and SPD and in isolated cases PUT (C and D/8th day), CAD (D/4th and 8th day). HIS contents were already discussed (A and D/4th day, C/8th day), same as SPR (B and D/1st day, D/4th and 8th day). TRP and 2-PHE levels were very low and oscillated between 0 and 3.0 mg·kg^{-1} in individual samples. Statistically significant ($p < 0.05$) differences between the biogenic amine values are given for each group and each day of the storage in Table 3 (capital letters "A" to "D" in rows).

3.2. Testing of Use of a Handheld Gastronomic Unit as an Alternative Method of Smoking Fish with Cold Smoke in the Household with Regard to a Possible Increase in Polycyclic Aromatic Hydrocarbons (PAH) Content and Whether the Cold Smoked Fish Affects Selected Sensory Parameters of Nigiri Sushi Meal Prepared by Consumers at Their Household

The factors affecting food or meal acceptance among consumers have changed rapidly. Sushi is admired by many consumers worldwide due to its appearance and taste [23–25].

A new non-traditional or unusual treatment of meal can increase consumer interest in its taste and, maybe, in its safety. We have found no previous reports of sushi meal containing tuna or salmon smoked with cold smoke for a very short period. It is possible to predict that Super Aladin smoker will be used more frequently in the practice of molecular gastronomy or home-made sushi preparation to imitate its sensory qualities and bring it closer to that of Philadelphia rolls, which is sometimes prepared with salmon smoked with cold or hot smoke.

Appearance, touch, odor, texture and taste represent the sensory properties of foods/meals. Sensory properties are one of the main factors influencing consumers' acceptance and purchase of meals. Health consciousness (including lowering sodium content, the presence of biogenic amines or smoked products) is another factor that can have significant influence on meal acceptance. Certain sushi ingredients (such as vinegar, wasabi and sugar) provide specific sensory properties to this meal.

The sensory properties of prepared sushi samples, smoked and not smoked, are shown in Table 5. Higher values estimated by panelists for juiciness and consistency indicate worse evaluation of these sensory properties. Bigger values for bitterness are emphasizing savoury intensity. Juiciness of sushi prepared without salt was evaluated with higher values then the rest of sushi samples, though statistical significance was not observed ($p > 0.05$).

Health aspects of certain meal are getting priority over shelf life and nutritional profile [26]. Dealing with issues concerning salt consumption is also important due to the fact that salty foods belong to the group of foods toward which consumers can develop addictive tendencies [27].

Sodium intake according to World Health Organization (WHO) should not exceed 2 g per day or 5 g of natural salt (NaCl) [28]. Worldwide salt intake exceeds this limit and ranges from 9 g/day to 12 g/day, which is equivalent to 3.6 g/day to 4.8 g/day [29].

Published information about cold-smoked tuna is sparse, though cold-smoked tuna processing is similar to that of cold-smoked salmon, in which both processing and product characteristics have been extensively studied [4,18].

Warm or hot smoked seafood is accepted and consumed by consumers due to its unique taste, texture and color. Additionally, due to dehydrating, bactericidal and antioxidant properties, smoking processes increase food shelf life. The problem with smoking of foods is that during the process of smoking considerable amount of polycyclic aromatic hydrocarbons (PAH) can be formed due to incomplete wood combustion. Phenols present in wood smoke belong to desirable molecules, since they positively affect food sensory properties and shelf life, but PAH compounds are undesirable molecules [30].

Table 5. Sensory attributes evaluation for nigiri sushi meal with not smoked and smoked samples of tuna and salmon fillets.

Sushi	Treatment	Salt %	Saltiness	Bitterness	Juiciness	Consistency
tuna	not smoked	0		16.25 ± 23.13	32.8 ± 36.15	34.15 ± 36.88
		2	55.55 ± 20.45	29.6 ± 38.57	16.7 ± 21.72	9.6 ± 8.45
		3		20.00 ± 30.60	27.45 ± 25.43	9.1 ± 10.93
	smoked	0		20.09 ± 30.71	26.18 ± 29.02	21.95 ± 26.67
		2	59.68 ± 17.84	23.45 ± 30.08	18.36 ± 20.27	9.64 ± 6.47
		3		17.91 ± 24.48	25.00 ± 23.34	14.45 ± 15.05
salmon	not smoked	0		14.6 ± 10.87	18.25 ± 6.88	18.1 ± 26.23
		2	53.9 ± 23.68	11.25 ± 9.58	13.55 ± 7.12	9.2 ± 5.71
		3		18.1 ± 14.59	20.25 ± 7.38	11.4 ± 5.21
	smoked	0		20.80 ± 17.32	21.25 ± 18.92	19.10 ± 18.58
		2	48.22 ± 20.33	18.35 ± 19.50	12.10 ± 6.48	7.85 ± 4.54
		3		17.60 ± 12.32	22.00 ± 13.19	16.60 ± 13.51

Saltiness (2% salt addition) was evaluated by respondents' comparison with sushi samples prepared without salt (0 point) and with 3% salt content (100 points) added to rice.

Table 6 shows contents of polycyclic aromatic hydrocarbons (PAH) in the samples of smoked and not smoked tuna and salmon. Tuna samples contained more PAH (4.22 µg·kg^{-1}) than salmon samples (1.74 µg·kg^{-1}).

Table 6. The content of polycyclic aromatic hydrocarbons (PAH) in µg·kg^{-1}.

Fish	Treatment	B(a)a	Chr	B(b)f	B(a)p	Sum of Pah
tuna	not smoked	<0.24	<0.28	<0.28	<0.27	*
	smoked	1.84	1.10	0.52	0.76	4.22
salmon	not smoked	<0.24	<0.28	<0.28	<0.27	*
	smoked	<0.24	0.77	0.37	0.60	1.74

B(a)A—benzo[a]anthracene; CHr—chrysene; B(b)F—benzo[b]fluoranthene; B(a)P—benzo[a]pyrene; * values under limit of detection (LOD).

Despite alarming content findings of B(a)A (1.84 µg·kg^{-1}) and CHr (1.10 µg·kg^{-1}) in smoked tuna, the content of B(a)P and sum of PAH in our samples were lower than the maximum levels written in the regulation (EC) no. 1881/2006, Annex, Section 6 (B(a)P [see in Appendix A8]: 2 µg·kg^{-1}, sum of PAH: 12 µg·kg^{-1}).

The existence of several factors affecting PAH content in smoked fish has been scientifically confirmed. PAHs are produced during combustion processes and smoke formation. The type of used matrix (wood), combustion temperature, smoke generation technique, filtration, temperature and smoke composition. Following factors are also influencing PAH formation: size, treatment and chemical composition of smoked fish. Regarding the effect on food (fish), the diffusion intensity of PAH below its surface into the muscle is relatively low. This fact that PAHs are mainly concentrated in the surface layers means that their content in the food is determined by food surface, same as total weight of the food. Surface/weight ratio is also probably responsible for higher levels of PAH in smoked tuna. Certainly, shape of smoked food (thickness and weight) are influencing PAH levels too. The content of PAHs is also associated with the fat content of food. Reference [31] also found that B(a)A content can differ significantly in dependence of seafood species.

Higher fat content in salmon samples influences higher PAH contents than in tuna samples [4,32,33]. The findings of these authors are not in agreement with the results of our chemical composition analysis

(Table 7). However, the fat content, which we determined in our samples, did correspond to published values [34]. Fluctuations in filtering capacity of the smoker could also influence PAH amounts, though the processes of sample smoking took place in the laboratory under the same conditions (time of smoke/cover of samples with glass lid).

Table 7. Chemical composition of sashimi tuna fillets and salmon fillets with skin (in %).

Samples	Protein	Fat	Dry Matter
tuna	29.02 ± 0.06	0.83 ± 0.01	30.09 ± 0.70
salmon	20.46 ± 0.98	23.46 ± 0.96	43.63 ± 0.00

Beside the antibacterial and antioxidant properties of smoking that are connected with phenolic compounds present in wood smoke, from our results a negative impact of seafood smoking represented as an increase of PAH compounds can be also seen. The importance of PAH level control in food is important, since these compounds are carcinogenic, mutagenic and endocrine disrupting. PAH compounds (there are more than 660 identified PAH compounds) are produced in wood smoke during pyrolysis (depolymerisation) of lignin and then condensation of the lignin components in lignocelluloses at temperature above 350 °C [35,36]. Aside from PAH increment, smoking changes color of food due to Maillard reaction (change coloration occurs due to the reaction of carbonyl groups in smoke with amino groups present on the surface of smoked food [36]. Phenols from wood smoke enter seafood by diffusion and capillary action, changing its flavor, color and prolonging shelf life [30]. PAH compounds in canned smoked tuna were 17.67 $\mu g \cdot kg^{-1}$ [37].

4. Conclusions

The main finding of the research is highlighting a food safety issue that was found by the experiments with a gastronomic smoking unit due to increased amounts of polycyclic aromatic hydrocarbons. The Super Aladin smoker unit is a patented product, but the manufacturer does not comment on the PAH hazards associated with food safety in the user documentation. The producers of this smoker units should at least include in the manuals the maximum smoking time depending on the type of food and its fatness. In this way they would alert users to the possible danger, which is the adhesion of harmful PAH on smoked food. The minimum or maximum exposure time of food to smoke is not specified or restricted for specific food types. For prolonged smoking (up to 24 h!), the manufacturer recommends intermittent repeated batches of smoke under the hatch at multiple time intervals as required (optical smoke density control under the hatch). In addition to commercial hardwood chips (oak, beech, Jack Daniels), users can use other alternative matrices including aromatic oils for the development of smoke. Due to the lipophilic nature of PAH, these substances could hypothetically be added to the smoke and subsequently increase PAH level to even more harmful concentrations. Certainly, that further experiments with household gastronomic smokers, such as, Super Aladin smoker, will probably give broader and more precise picture about all possibilities and issues concerning these types of devices.

In the case of the experiment aimed at monitoring the content of biogenic amines in tuna samples, we found much more favorable results than expected. Serious interruption of thawed tuna samples cold chain after purchase did not result in an increase of biogenic amines to levels that could represent a health risk for consumers. Manufacturers inform consumers that they should store purchased fish at 0–2 °C and consume it within 2 days. According to the results obtained in our experiment, tuna samples could be considered suitable for consumption after 4 days in terms of BA content and even up to 8 days (except for thawed samples without cold chain interruption) after purchase. However, we cannot recommend this practice due to the possibility that purchased tuna could have higher histamine content developed before purchase. The risk of intoxication with histamine becomes more realistic with each new day of storage. Laboratory examinations of fish species associated with high histamine content in muscle should therefore be a normal part of quality controls by sellers so that they do not have to passively rely on written statements from fish suppliers regarding histamine content in commercial or veterinary evidences of their origin.

Author Contributions: H.B. conceived and designed the experiments. H.B. and D.D. performed the basic chemical and sensory analyses and processed all laboratory data including statistical analysis, A.H. carried out the determination of the polycyclic aromatic hydrocarbons include software service and validation of this methodology. I.D. and P.K. carried out the determination of the biogenic amine spectrum include software service and validation of this methodology. The first draft of the manuscript was prepared by H.B. and D.D. and it was revised and substantially improved by D.D. and H.B.

Funding: This research received no external funding.

Conflicts of Interest: The authors declare no conflict of interest.

Appendix A

Appendix A.1 Legislation and Procedures

1. Commission Regulation (EC) No 2073/2005 of 15 November 2005 on microbiological criteria for foodstuffs. Available online. https://eur-lex.europa.eu/legal-content/EN/TXT/?qid=1565694175620&uri=CELEX:02005R2073-20190228 (accessed on 28 February 2019).
2. Regulation (EC) No 853/2004 of the European Parliament and of the Council of 29 April 2004 laying down specific hygiene rules for food of animal origin. Available online: https://eur-lex.europa.eu/legal-content/EN/TXT/?qid=1565693935604&uri=CELEX:02004R0853-20190101 (accessed on 1 January 2019).
3. International Organization for Standardization ISO 8589:2008 Sensory analysis—General guidance for the design of test rooms
4. International Organization for Standardization ISO 937:1978 Meat and meat products—Determination of nitrogen content (Reference method)
5. International Organization for Standardization ISO 1443:1973 Meat and meat products—Determination of total fat content. (Reference method)
6. International Organization for Standardization ISO 1442:1997 Meat and meat products—Determination of moisture content (Reference method)
7. Regulation (EC) No 1333/2008 of the European Parliament and of the Council of 16 December 2008 on food additives. Available online: https://eur-lex.europa.eu/legal-content/EN/TXT/?qid=1565693786967&uri=CELEX:02008R1333-20190618 (accessed on 18 July 2019).
8. Commission Regulation (EC) No 1881/2006 of 19 December 2006 setting maximum levels for certain contaminants in foodstuffs. https://eur-lex.europa.eu/legal-content/EN/TXT/?qid=1565694263939&uri=CELEX:02006R1881-20180319 (accessed on 19 March 2018).

References

1. Fusco, V.; den Besten, H.M.W.; Logrieco, A.F.; Rodriguez, F.; Skandamis, P.N.; Stessl, B.; Teixeira, P. Food safety aspects on ethnic foods: Toxicological and microbial risks. *Curr. Opin. Food Sci.* **2015**, *6*, 24–32. [CrossRef]
2. Feng, C.H. Tale of sushi: History and regulations. *Compr. Rev. Food Sci. Food Saf.* **2012**, *11*, 205–220. [CrossRef]
3. Puah, S.M.; Tan, J.A.M.A.; Chew, C.H.; Chua, K.H. Diverse Profiles of Biofilm and Adhesion Genes in Staphylococcus Aureus Food Strains Isolated from Sushi and Sashimi. *J. Food Sci.* **2018**, *83*, 2337–2342. [CrossRef] [PubMed]
4. Storelli, M.M.; Stuffler, R.G.; Marcotrigiano, G.O. Polycyclic aromatic hydrocarbons, polychlorinated biphenyls, chlorinated pesticides (DDTs), hexachlorocyclohexane, and hexachlorobenzene residues in smoked seafood. *J. Food Prot.* **2003**, *66*, 1095–1099. [CrossRef] [PubMed]
5. Rahmani, J.; Miri, A.; Mohseni-Bandpei, A.; Fakhri, Y.; Bjørklund, G.; Keramati, H.; Moradi, B.; Amanidaz, N.; Shariatifar, N.; Khaneghah, A.M. Contamination and Prevalence of Histamine in Canned Tuna from Iran: A Systematic Review, Meta-Analysis, and Health Risk Assessment. *J. Food Prot.* **2018**, *81*, 2019–2027. [CrossRef]

6. EFSA (European Food Safety Authority) Panel on Biological Hazards (BIOHAZ). Scientific Opinion on risk assessment of parasites in fishery products. *EFSA J.* **2010**, *8*, 1543. [CrossRef]
7. Fukita, Y.; Asaki, T.; Katakura, Y. Some like It Raw: An Unwanted Result of a Sushi Meal. *Gastroenterology* **2014**, *146*, E8–E9. [CrossRef] [PubMed]
8. Škaljac, S.; Jokanović, M.; Tomović, V.; Ivić, M.; Tasić, T.; Ikonić, P.; Sojic, B.; Dzinic, N.; Petrović, L. Influence of smoking in traditional and industrial conditions on colour and content of polycyclic aromatic hydrocarbons in dry fermented sausage "Petrovská klobása". *LWT-Food Sci. Technol.* **2018**, *87*, 158–162. [CrossRef]
9. Josewin, S.W.; Ghate, V.; Kim, M.J.; Yuk, H.G. Antibacterial effect of 460 nm light-emitting diode in combination with riboflavin against *Listeria monocytogenes* on smoked salmon. *Food Control.* **2018**, *84*, 354–361. [CrossRef]
10. De Jonge, J.; van Trijp, H.; Renes, R.J.; Frewer, L. Understanding consumer confidence in the safety of food: Its two-dimensional structure and determinants. *Risk Anal.* **2007**, *27*, 729–740. [CrossRef] [PubMed]
11. Verbeke, W.; Sioen, I.; Pieniak, Z.; Van Camp, J.; De Henauw, S. Consumer perception versus scientific evidence about health benefits and safety risks from fish consumption. *Public Health Nutr.* **2005**, *8*, 422–429. [CrossRef] [PubMed]
12. Fooladi, E.; Hopia, A.; Lasa, D.; Arboleya, J.C. Chefs and researchers: Culinary practitioners' views on interaction between gastronomy and sciences. *Int. J. Gastron. Food Sci.* **2019**, *15*, 6–14. [CrossRef]
13. Geczi, G.; Korzenszky, P.; Szakmar, K. Cold chain interruption by consumers significantly reduces shelf life of vacuum-packed pork ham slices. *Acta Aliment. Hung.* **2017**, *46*, 508–516. [CrossRef]
14. Kulawik, P.; Dordevic, D.; Gambuś, F.; Szczurowska, K.; Zając, M. Heavy metal contamination, microbiological spoilage and biogenic amine content in sushi available on the Polish market. *J. Sci. Food Agric.* **2018**, *98*, 2809–2815. [CrossRef] [PubMed]
15. Sharifian, S.; Alizadeh, E.; Mortazavi, M.S.; Moghadam, M.S. Effects of refrigerated storage on the microstructure and quality of Grouper (*Epinephelus coioides*) fillets. *J. Food Sci. Technol. Mys.* **2014**, *51*, 929–935. [CrossRef] [PubMed]
16. Duflos, G.; Le Fur, B.; Mulak, V.; Becel, P.; Malle, P. Comparison of methods of differentiating between fresh and frozen-thawed fish or fillets. *J. Sci. Food Agric.* **2002**, *82*, 1341–1345. [CrossRef]
17. Reis, M.M.; Martinez, E.; Saitua, E.; Rodriguez, R.; Perez, I.; Olabarrieta, I. Non-invasive differentiation between fresh and frozen/thawed tuna fillets using near infrared spectroscopy (Vis-NIRS). *LWT-Food Sci. Technol.* **2017**, *78*, 129–137. [CrossRef]
18. Emborg, J.; Laursen, B.G.; Dalgaard, P. Significant histamine formation in tuna (*Thunnus albacares*) at 2 degrees C - effect of vacuum- and modified atmosphere-packaging on psychrotolerant bacteria. *Int. J. Food Microbiol.* **2005**, *101*, 263–279. [CrossRef]
19. Holland, J. Brussels warns against the illegal treatment of tuna with vegetable extracts. Sea Food Source News 9. 2016. Available online: https://www.seafoodsource.com/news/food-safety-health/brussels-warns-against-the-illegal-treatment-of-tuna-with-vegetable-extracts (accessed on 7 February 2019).
20. European Commission. Food fraud network EU-ccoordinated case: Illegal treatment of Tuna: From canning grade to Sushi grade. 2017. Available online: https://ec.europa.eu/food/sites/food/files/safety/docs/food-fraud_succ-coop_tuna.pdf (accessed on 7 February 2019).
21. Bhangare, R.C.; Sahu, S.K.; Pandit, G.G. Nitrosamines in seafood and study on the effects of storage in refrigerator. *J. Food Sci. Tech. Mys.* **2015**, *52*, 507–513. [CrossRef]
22. De Gennaro, L.; Brunetti, N.D.; Locuratolo, N.; Ruggiero, M.; Resta, M.; Diaferia, G.; Rana, M.; Caldarola, P. Kounis syndrome following canned tuna fish ingestion. *Acta Clin. Belg.* **2017**, *72*, 142–145. [CrossRef]
23. Drewnowski, A.; Moskowitz, H.R. Sensory characteristics of foods: New evaluation techniques. *Am. J. Clin. Nutr.* **1985**, *42*, 924–931. [CrossRef] [PubMed]
24. Desmet, P.M.A.; Schifferstein, H.N.J. Sources of positive and negative emotions in food experience. *Appetite* **2008**, *50*, 290–301. [CrossRef] [PubMed]
25. Dordevic, D.; Buchtova, H. Factors influencing sushi meal as representative of non-traditional meal: Consumption among Czech consumers. *Acta Alim. Hung.* **2017**, *46*, 76–83. [CrossRef]
26. Fellendorf, S.; O'Sullivan, M.G.; Kerry, J.P. Effect of different salt and fat levels on the physicochemical properties and sensory quality of black pudding. *Food Sci. Nutr.* **2017**, *5*, 273–284. [CrossRef] [PubMed]

27. Mies, G.W.; Treur, J.L.; Larsen, J.K.; Halberstadt, J.; Pasman, J.A.; Vink, J.M. Prevalence of food addiction in a large sample of adolescents and its association with addictive substances. *Appetite* **2017**, *118*, 97–105. [CrossRef] [PubMed]
28. World Health Organisation (WHO). *Guideline: Sodium Intake for Adults and Children*; WHO: Geneva, Switzerland, 2012. Available online: https://www.ncbi.nlm.nih.gov/books/NBK133309/ (accessed on 22 June 2018).
29. Rust, P.; Ekmekcioglu, C. Impact of salt intake on the pathogenesis and treatment of hypertension. In *Advances in Experimental Medicine and Biology*, 1st ed.; Islam, M.S., Ed.; Springer: Cham, Switzerland, 2017; Volume 956, pp. 61–84.
30. Remy, C.C.; Fleury, M.; Beauchêne, J.; Rivier, M.; Goli, T. Analysis of PAH residues and amounts of phenols in fish smoked with woods traditionally used in French Guiana. *J. Ethnobiol.* **2016**, *36*, 312–325. [CrossRef]
31. Swastawati, F.; Surti, T.; Agustini, T.W.; Riyadi, P.H. Benzo(α)pyrene potential analysis on smoked fish (Case study: Traditional method and smoking kiln). *KnE Life Sci.* **2015**, *1*, 156–161. [CrossRef]
32. Afolabi, O.A.; Adesula, E.A.; Oke, O.L. Polynuclear aromatic hydrocarbons in some Nigerian preserved freshwater fish species. *J. Agric. Food Chem.* **1983**, *31*, 1083–1090. [CrossRef]
33. Lawrence, J.F.; Weber, D.F. Determination of polycyclic aromatic hydrocarbons in some Canadian commercial fish, shellfish and meat products by liquid chromatography with confirmation by capillary gas chromatography-mass spectrometry. *J. Agric. Food Chem.* **1984**, *32*, 789–794. [CrossRef]
34. Anonymous Salmon vs Tuna. Diffen.com. Diffen LLC, n.d. 2019. Available online: https://www.diffen.com/difference/Salmon_vs_Tuna (accessed on 19 February 2019).
35. Essumang, D.K.; Dodoo, D.K.; Adjei, J.K. Effect of smoke generation sources and smoke curing duration on the levels of polycyclic aromatic hydrocarbon (PAH) in different suites of fish. *Food Chem. Toxicol.* **2013**, *58*, 86–94. [CrossRef]
36. Nithin, C.T.; Ananthanarayanan, T.R.; Yathavamoorthi, R.; Bindu, J.; Joshy, C.G.; Gopal, T.S. Physico-chemical Changes in Liquid Smoke Flavoured Yellowfin Tuna (*Thunnus albacares*) Sausage during Chilled Storage. *Agric. Res.* **2015**, *4*, 420–427. [CrossRef]
37. Novakov, N.J.; Mihaljev, Ž.A.; Kartalović, B.D.; Blagojević, B.J.; Petrović, J.M.; Ćirković, M.A.; Rogan, D.R. Heavy metals and PAHs in canned fish supplies on the Serbian market. *Food Addit. Contam. Part B Surveill.* **2017**, *10*, 208–215. [CrossRef] [PubMed]

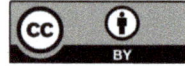

© 2019 by the authors. Licensee MDPI, Basel, Switzerland. This article is an open access article distributed under the terms and conditions of the Creative Commons Attribution (CC BY) license (http://creativecommons.org/licenses/by/4.0/).

MDPI
St. Alban-Anlage 66
4052 Basel
Switzerland
Tel. +41 61 683 77 34
Fax +41 61 302 89 18
www.mdpi.com

Foods Editorial Office
E-mail: foods@mdpi.com
www.mdpi.com/journal/foods

www.ingramcontent.com/pod-product-compliance
Lightning Source LLC
LaVergne TN
LVHW070736100526
838202LV00013B/1251